LWW PHARMACY TECHNICIAN E

STANDARDS OF PRACTICE *for the* PHARMACY TECHNICIAN

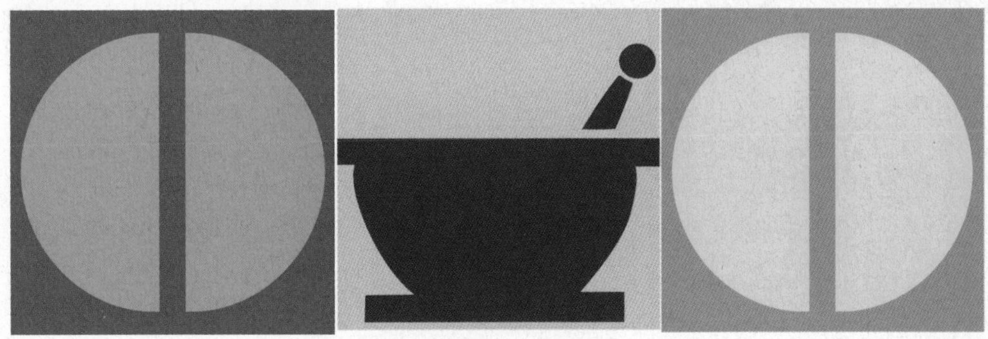

LWW PHARMACY TECHNICIAN EDUCATION SERIES

STANDARDS OF PRACTICE *for the* PHARMACY TECHNICIAN

MARY E. MOHR, RPH, MS

Pharmacy Technician Program Director
Clarian Health Partners, Inc.
Methodist Campus
Indianapolis, Indiana

President
Pharmacy Technician Educator Council, 2007–2009

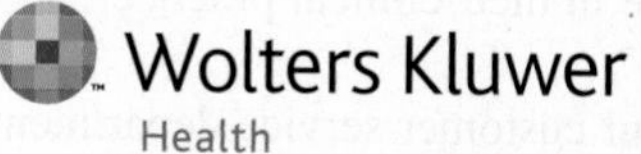

Lippincott Williams & Wilkins

Philadelphia • Baltimore • New York • London
Buenos Aires • Hong Kong • Sydney • Tokyo

Acquisitions Editor: David B. Troy
Managing Editor: Meredith Brittain
Marketing Manager: Zhan Caplan
Production Editor: Julie Montalbano
Designer: Doug Smock
Compositor: Maryland Composition, Inc.

351 West Camden Street
Baltimore, MD 21201

530 Walnut Street
Philadelphia, PA 19106

Printed in China.

9 8 7 6 5 4 3

Library of Congress Cataloging-in-Publication Data
Mohr, Mary E.
Standards of practice for the pharmacy technician / Mary E. Mohr.
p. ; cm.
Includes bibliographical references and index.
ISBN 978-0-7817-6617-3
1. Pharmacy technicians—Standards. I. Title.
[DNLM: 1. Clinical Competence—standards. 2. Pharmacists' Aides—standards. 3. Pharmaceutical Preparations—administration & dosage. 4. Pharmacy—methods. QV 21.5 M699s 2009]
RS122.95.M643 2009
615′.1—dc22

2008026602

DISCLAIMER

Care has been taken to confirm the accuracy of the information present and to describe generally accepted practices. However, the authors, editors, and publisher are not responsible for errors or omissions or for any consequences from application of the information in this book and make no warranty, expressed or implied, with respect to the currency, completeness, or accuracy of the contents of the publication. Application of this information in a particular situation remains the professional responsibility of the practitioner; the clinical treatments described and recommended may not be considered absolute and universal recommendations.

The authors, editors, and publisher have exerted every effort to ensure that drug selection and dosage set forth in this text are in accordance with the current recommendations and practice at the time of publication. However, in view of ongoing research, changes in government regulations, and the constant flow of information relating to drug therapy and drug reactions, the reader is urged to check the package insert for each drug for any change in indications and dosage and for added warnings and precautions. This is particularly important when the recommended agent is a new or infrequently employed drug.

Some drugs and medical devices presented in this publication have Food and Drug Administration (FDA) clearance for limited use in restricted research settings. It is the responsibility of the health care provider to ascertain the FDA status of each drug or device planned for use in their clinical practice.

To purchase additional copies of this book, call our customer service department at **(800) 638-3030** or fax orders to **(301) 223-2320**. International customers should call **(301) 223-2300**.

Visit Lippincott Williams & Wilkins on the Internet: http://www.lww.com. Lippincott Williams & Wilkins customer service representatives are available from 8:30 am to 6:00 pm, EST.

CCS0713

Dedication

This book is dedicated to my mother, Mary Steinberger, RN, and my father, George Steinberger, RPh, who taught me the value of excellent patient care and instilled a love of health care in our family. These values have been passed on to our sons, Mike and Tom, and our daughters, Marcia and Susie, and will continue to guide our grandchildren, Makayla, Amelia, and Mitchell.

This Book and the LWW Pharmacy Technician Education Series

Standards of Practice for the Pharmacy Technician is part of a series of texts that embodies a shift between eras. Previously, on-the-job training of technicians was considered acceptable, but the recent realization of those in the field is that pharmacy technicians must be educated professionals. The changing role of the pharmacist and the emergence of a new definition of pharmaceutical care dictate that competent, well-trained technicians be prepared to assume most of the dispensing functions previously performed by pharmacists. The conceptual organizational approach of the LWW Pharmacy Technician Education Series is to educate the technician as an invaluable member of the pharmacy team and to assist in the development of the decision-making ability required for the technician's practice.

Current texts emphasize the mechanics of performing functions under the direct supervision of a pharmacist. This concept of direct supervision is beginning to change and will continue to evolve as pharmacists assume responsibility for greater numbers of technicians. Technicians need the tools to make important decisions and the confidence to trust their decisions, while retaining the ability to discern when pharmacist consultation is needed. The LWW Pharmacy Technician Education Series is written by premier educators in the field of pharmacy technician education to provide technician students with the confidence-based knowledge required for their practice today and in the future. Each title is accompanied by a strong ancillary package of instructor and student resources.

The following titles appear in the series:

Standards of Practice for the Pharmacy Technician by Mary Mohr

Practical Pharmacology for the Pharmacy Technician by Joy Sakai

Pharmaceutical Calculations for the Pharmacy Technician by Barbara Lacher

Lab Experiences for the Pharmacy Technician by Mary Mohr

In *Standards of Practice for the Pharmacy Technician,* Mary Mohr, a respected educator with years of experience in retail, hospital, home care, and mail order pharmacy practice settings and pharmacy technician education, has presented a complex subject in a format that can be readily understood by the pharmacy technician student. Her experience as a pharmacist and an educator brings an authenticity to the text, which provides guidance for instructors and facilitates comprehension by the student. This book is an up-to-date, comprehensive pharmacy practice text that will prepare technician students for their expanded role in pharmacy practice.

Preface

Standards of Practice for the Pharmacy Technician provides a roadmap for the exciting journey that will enable a beginning technician student to become an accomplished pharmacy technician professional. The text discusses standards of practice, scope of practice, and projections for the future practice of an emerging professional in the modern world of pharmacy. The reader will follow the developmental stages of the pharmacist from an unregulated dispenser of herbal remedies to an educated licensed professional, and the development of the technician from a pill counter to an educated technician with the ability to assist the pharmacist in providing pharmaceutical care to patients.

Throughout the text, various patients and realistic pharmacy technicians interact and deal with everyday critical thinking decisions pertinent to the practice of pharmacy. The ultimate goal is to instill in the student a feeling of competence, an ability to utilize critical thinking skills for problem solving, and an innate comprehension of the concepts of *professionalism* and *professional judgment.* This knowledge will enable the pharmacy technician to function in the future model of pharmacy practice, which will require more independence on the part of the pharmacy technician and a complete understanding of the difference between the professional judgment of a technician and the professional judgment of a pharmacist.

The text is intended for use in a formal, instructor-guided education program. The student will be best served by a curriculum that includes medical terminology, pharmacy calculations, anatomy and physiology, communication and pharmacology, studied either prior to or concurrently with the general pharmacy practice course outlined in this text.

The student should have access to a reasonable complex of pharmacy reference books, including *Facts and Comparisons, Remington's Science and Practice of Pharmacy, Trissel's Handbook of Injectable Drugs, PDR for Nonprescription Drugs,* and the *Pediatric Dosage Handbook.* Laboratory facilities with basic equipment and chemicals will allow for hands-on experiences to reinforce learning.

Organizational Philosophy

Standards of Practice for the Pharmacy Technician is divided into seven units: Unit I: Evolution of the Pharmacy; Unit II: Pharmacy Law, Ethics, and Confidentiality; Unit III: Technician's Role in Assuring Patient Rights; Unit IV: Mechanics of Medication Dispensing and Inventory Control; Unit V: Extemporaneous Compounding; Unit VI, Compounded Sterile Products, and Unit VII: Professionalism and Career Exploration. Within each unit are chapters that discuss various topics related to the unit.

The chapters lead the student from a broad general understanding of the humble beginnings of pharmacy through its development into a scientific study of medications and their potential to treat disease and positively impact the lives of patients. Likewise, the emergence of the pharmacist from a peddler of herbs to an educated, respected professional providing excellent pharmaceutical care to patients will be used as a model for the development of the pharmacy technician as a professional.

Unit 1 provides an overview of past and present pharmacy models and some possible directions for the future. From this beginning, the remaining units present the specifics of the scope and standards of practice for the pharmacy technician.

Chapter Structure

The chapter format consists of the following:

- **Objectives:** A list of educational competencies that should be achieved during the study of the chapter.
- **Key Terms:** Terminology pertinent to the chapter that is bolded in the text and defined in the margins and the glossary for quick reference.
- **Chapter introduction:** An introductory paragraph that explains the purpose of the subject matter.
- **Sample prescriptions and medication orders:** Documents written by physicians that will help students develop the ability to interpret and evaluate written orders.
- **Preparation Method boxes:** Lists of step-by-step techniques for compounding procedures. When a video reel icon appears next to the Preparation Method title, it indicates that a video of the procedure can be found on the book's companion CD-ROM and website.

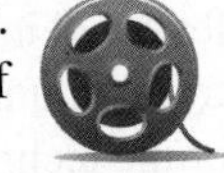

- **Professional Judgment Scenario boxes:** Realistic professional and ethical scenarios requiring the technician to use professional judgment to formulate a response.
- **Tips:** Reminders of important points.
- **Cautions:** Alerts of potential hazards.
- **Tables:** Demonstrations and consolidations of key points.
- **Figures:** Illustrations or photos used to bring clarity to the text.
- **Case Studies:** Real-life scenarios involving technicians and patients to provide for student discussion.
- **Chapter Summary:** Important points from the chapter text formatted for a quick review.
- **Review Questions:** Designed to stimulate critical thinking skills and reinforce chapter content.
- **Learning Activities:** Hands-on activities that present opportunities for research and discussion to further student learning.
- **Suggested Readings:** Suggestions for additional information to enhance students' learning.

Instructor and Student Ancillaries

Additional Resources

Standards of Practice for the Pharmacy Technician includes additional resources for both instructors and students that are available on the book's companion website at thePoint.lww.com/mohrpractice. Resources are also available via an Instructor's Resource CD-ROM and the Student Resource CD-ROM packaged with this text.

Instructors

Approved adopting instructors will be given access to the following additional resources:

- Brownstone test generator
- PowerPoint presentations
- Image bank with figures and tables
- Lesson plans
- Game show interactivities
- Answers to questions from the text
- Discussion of Case Studies and Professional Judgment Scenario boxes from the text
- Blank forms for classroom use
- Blank prescriptions and labels
- WebCT and Blackboard-ready cartridges

Students

Students who have purchased *Standards of Practice for the Pharmacy Technician* have access to the following additional resources:

- Video clips
- Quiz bank of Pharmacy Technician Certification Board Review Questions
- Flash cards
- Math exercises
- Learning activities
- English-to-Spanish phrases

In addition, purchasers of the text can access the searchable Full Text Online by going to the *Standards of Practice for the Pharmacy* website at http://thePoint.lww.com. See the inside front cover of this text for more details, including the passcode you will need to gain access to the website.

Reviewers

Dodi Craft
Program Director
Pharmacy Technician Department
Vatterott College
Omaha, NE

George Fakhoury, MD, DORCP, CMA, RMA
Curriculum Manager
Heald College, LLC
San Francisco, CA

Stephanie Garthrite, CPhT
Lead Pharmacy Technician Instructor
Remington College
Cleveland, OH

Tina Hansen, CPhT, MS, BS
Instructor
Respiratory Therapy Department
Maric College
Salida, CA

Scott Higgins, MA
Department Chair
Pharmacy
Technology Education College
Columbus, OH

Cristina Kaiser, CPhT, MA
Curriculum Technician, Health Studies
Academic Affairs Department
San Joaquin Valley College
Visalia, CA

Stacie Ling
Instructor
Vatterott College
Springfield, MO

Marisa Maron
Pharmacy Technician
Pharmacy Technician Instructor/Medical Programs Externship Coordinator
Education Department
Institute of Technology, Inc.
Clovis, CA

Ivan Martinez, BS, CPhT
Program Coordinator
Pharmacy Technology
Keiser Career College
Miami Lakes, FL

John J. Smith, EdD, MS, BS
Senior Director, Health Sciences
Academic Affairs Department
Corinthian Colleges, Inc.
Santa Ana, CA

Acknowledgments

The assistance of the very professional staff at Lippincott Williams and Wilkins has been invaluable in the preparation of this text. Meredith Brittain has provided outstanding guidance and support. My thanks to Dr. Robert Beardsley and the students from the University of Maryland School of Pharmacy—Vicky Hsu, Hanpin Lim, Ravi Kona, Harris Howland, and Antonia Tolson—for their assistance in preparing for and participating in the photo/video shoot. Thanks also to Carol Dunham for preparing the glossary and to the reviewers, named previously, for their insights and advice as this text was being prepared. Lastly, thanks to my husband, John, for his continued support during this process.

Contents

UNIT I

Evolution of the Pharmacy

- **Chapter 1**
  Pharmacy History
- **Chapter 2**
  Pharmacy of Today and Tomorrow
- **Chapter 3**
  Professional Roles in the Pharmacy

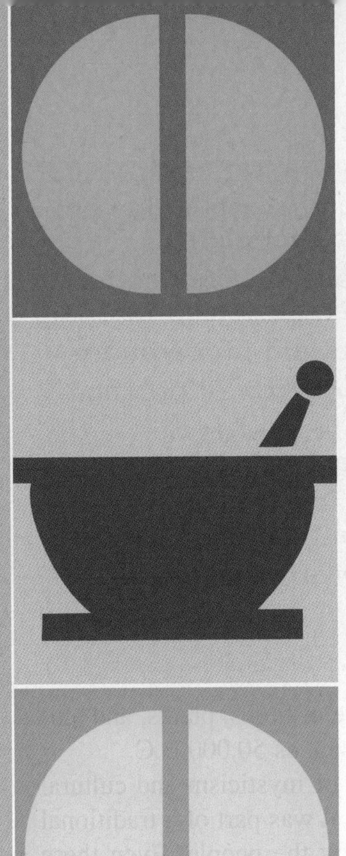

Chapter 1

Pharmacy History

OBJECTIVES

After reading this chapter, the student will be able to:

- Explain the historical relationships of culture, religion, and medicine.
- Define pharmacopoeia and discuss its origins.
- Discuss the efforts of early Greek philosophers to create a scientific approach to medicine.
- List some of the contributions of Hippocrates to the medical field.
- Define the humoral system of medicine introduced by Galen.
- Explain the importance of Britain's Apothecaries Act of 1815 in the transition to modern pharmacy.
- List the organizations established in the United States to provide standards for the practice of pharmacy.
- Compare and contrast the practice of pharmacy before and after the emergence of large chain pharmacies.
- Discuss the impact of prescription insurance on the practice of pharmacy.
- Create a time line for the establishment of pharmacy laws.
- Correlate the evolution of pharmacists as professionals with the emergence of technicians as professionals.
- Discuss the importance of mandatory education and certification in being respected as a professional pharmacy technician.

KEY TERMS

- American Pharmaceutical Association (APhA)
- American Society of Health-System Pharmacists (ASHP)
- apothecaries
- Apothecaries Act of 1815
- bowl of Hygeia
- counter-prescribing
- Drug Abuse Control Amendments
- Durham-Humphrey Amendment
- Ebers papyrus

- Federal Food, Drug and Cosmetic Act
- Food and Drug Administration (FDA)
- Food and Drugs Act
- Galen
- germ theory
- Hippocrates
- Hippocratic oath
- humoral system
- humors of the body
- IV admixture
- Kefauver-Harris Amendment
- Louis Pasteur
- medication error
- model curriculum for pharmacy technician training
- paradigm shift
- patent medicines
- pharmacopeia
- Pharmacy Practice Act
- pharmacy technicians
- professional judgment of a technician
- scope of practice for pharmacy technicians
- shotgun preparations
- standards of practice
- state boards of pharmacy (BOPs)
- United States Pharmacopeia (USP)
- William Proctor, Jr.

Historians and anthropologists have uncovered evidence of herbs, plants, and animal parts being utilized for medicinal purposes as far back as 50,000 B.C.

Certainly, in the early days there was a great deal of mysticism and cultural lore associated with the healing process. In many cases it was part of a traditional ceremony conducted by a religious leader appointed by the people. Even these early civilizations sought an understanding of the cycle of life and death, and searched for ways to alleviate suffering and preserve good health. Although medicine, religion, and pharmacy were originally intertwined, they became separated for many years, and are now often seen as coming together again. There are lessons we can learn from exploring the beginnings of medicinal treatments and examining the emergence of pharmacy as a trusted profession.

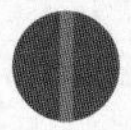

Egyptian History

Ebers papyrus Document discovered in ancient Egypt that demonstrated the use of a list of herbs and drugs used to improve health. It is considered the precursor to the pharmacopeia of today.

pharmacopeia Term used to denote an official listing of drugs.

As historical documentation became more reliable, a series of Egyptian documents from the 16th century B.C. were discovered. The most famous of these is the Ebers papyrus, which was composed in 1552 B.C. and discovered between the knees of a mummy. This scroll is similar to a "mini" pharmacopeia and consists of compounding formulas for drug preparations that involve many drugs still in use today. Included in the list are aloes, opium, peppermint, and castor oil. A fibrous seed used by the early Egyptians for its laxative properties was the psyllium seed, which is found on pharmacy shelves today as Metamucil. In addition to plant and animal parts, the early Egyptians had begun to utilize mineral compounds such as iron, lead, and copper, as well as powdered precious stones such as emeralds and sapphires. The ancient Egyptian writings describe many of the same types of preparations used today, such as infusions, inhalations, and gargles. Some historians believe that the Rx sign (see Fig. 1.1), which is so prominent on every prescription, was derived from an ancient Egyptian eye symbol. Others believe it is an abbreviation for the Latin verb *recipere*, meaning "to receive."

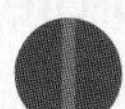

Greek Influence

The writings of ancient Greek philosophers such as Socrates, Plato, and Aristotle encouraged people to embrace a thought process that would lead to a more scientific approach to health and healing and away from the primarily supernatural

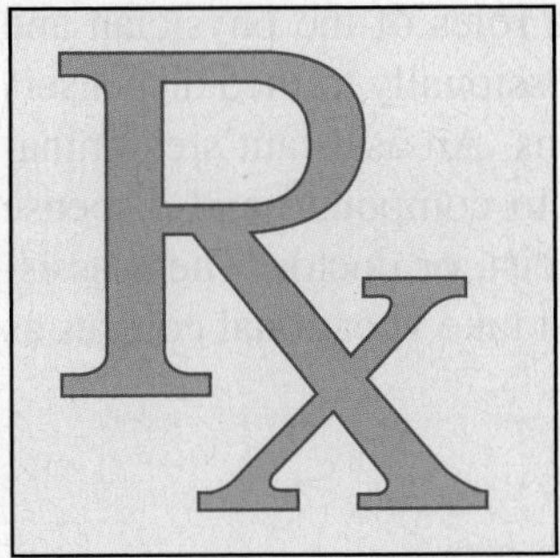

Figure 1.1 The Rx symbol is thought to stand for the Latin word *recipere*, meaning "to receive."

approach. Still, even in the seventh century B.C., sanctuaries devoted to healing the sick were scattered across the country. The bowl of Hygeia (see Fig. 1.2), which is the symbol of pharmacy, was named after the daughter of a mythical god and used in religious ceremonies for offerings to the goddess of health.

Later Greek history yielded the physician Hippocrates, who is considered to be the father of medicine and was the namesake of the Hippocratic oath, which is still used to guide physicians today. Although he was a physician, Hippocrates' writings contained many references to drugs and compounding processes. He attempted to explain illness by balancing four environmental elements—earth, air, fire, and water—with the four humors of the body (black bile, blood, yellow bile, and phlegm). Physicians who followed this thinking would recommend dietary and lifestyle modifications first, and if those failed, they would compound their own prescriptions.

Another Greek physician who was influential in the science of medicine was Galen. Although he lived in the second century A.D., his influence stayed with us until the 16th century, as he had created a system of pathology and therapy that laid the foundation for future scientific research. Galen adapted the humoral system introduced by Hippocrates, which balanced the humors of an ill individual with a drug that would act in an opposing manner to the problem being treated. An example of this would be to apply a cool cloth to an area that is inflamed. He also utilized "shotgun preparations," which are still being employed today by some physicians.

British Apothecaries

During the 17th century in Britain, the apothecaries began to be differentiated from the grocers as professionals who practiced a professional skill. When Britain passed the Apothecaries Act of 1815, it included a requirement that an apothecary

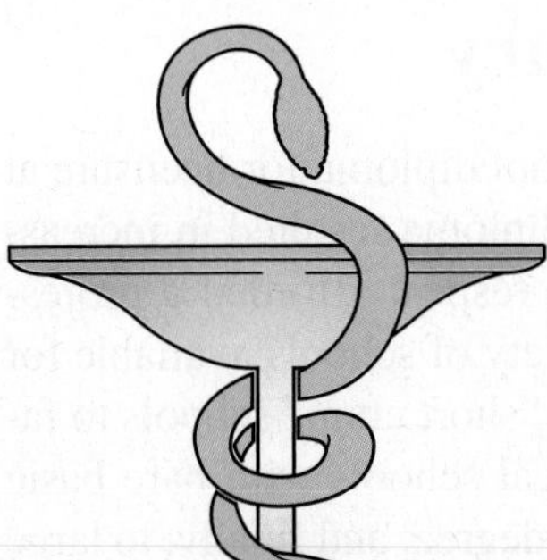

Figure 1.2 The goddess Hygeia, daughter of the god of healing and medicine, was pictured holding a cup with a snake coiled around her. The symbol of a cup with a snake coiled around it has become a modern emblem for pharmacy.

bowl of Hygeia Bowl with a snake coiled around it, often depicted as a symbol of pharmacy. Hygeia was the Greek goddess of health.

Hippocrates Ancient Greek physician considered to be the father of medicine.

Hippocratic oath Code of ethics still recited by physicians today, attributed to the teachings of Hippocrates outlining the responsibilities of the physician to the patient.

humors of the body Blood, black bile, yellow bile, and phlegm.

Galen Early Greek physician who practiced in Rome and created a system of therapy, based on humors of the body, that influenced the practice of medicine for decades.

humoral system A system set forth by Galen to establish a treatment plan based on the assumption that disease is caused by an imbalance of one or more of the four humors of the body (blood, black bile, yellow bile, and phlegm).

shotgun preparations Involves using a combination of drugs in the hope that one or more of them will be effective in treating a condition of unknown cause.

apothecaries Name given to early dispensers of medicines and their shops in Great Britain.

Apothecaries Act of 1815 Separated the apothecaries from the grocers and established the apothecaries as professionals who were required to be licensed.

pharmacy technicians Well trained, educated professionals who have complied with the requirements of the Pharmacy Practice Act of the state in which they practice and are qualified to assist the pharmacist in providing pharmaceutical care to patients.

United States Pharmacopeia (USP) The official listing of drugs and the quality standards they must meet to be considered official. The USP also establishes guidelines for the proper preparation of drugs used in the pharmacy.

American Pharmaceutical Association (APhA) Founded in 1852 to provide for more uniform standards of education.

William Proctor, Jr. Considered the father of American pharmacy for his lifelong dedication to service in the profession as a retail pharmacist, professor of pharmacy, member of the USP Revision Committee, editor of the *American Journal of Pharmacy*, and leader in founding the American Pharmaceutical Association.

state boards of pharmacy (BOPs) Groups of pharmacists, usually appointed by the governor of each state, who convene on a regular basis to govern and direct the practice of pharmacy in that state.

patent medicines Medicines for which a patent has been applied and received, allowing marketing to the general public and restricting duplication by another person or company.

be licensed, and it also differentiated more clearly the roles of the physician and the pharmacist. Pharmacists began to employ non-professionally trained dispensers to assist with compounding and dispensing medications. An assistant's examination was offered to qualified candidates who wished to compound and dispense drugs under the supervision of an apothecary, pharmacist, or doctor. These assistants are now known as pharmacy technicians and most take vocational courses as part of their training.

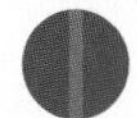

American Pharmacy Pre-1900

As the pharmacy profession evolved in the United States, the need for a system of standards, quality control, and an approved formulary became apparent. The United States Pharmacopeia (USP) was founded in 1820 and became the official compendium in 1848. In an effort to establish better communication among pharmacists and to provide for more uniform standards of education, the American Pharmaceutical Association (APhA) was founded in 1852. William Proctor, Jr., was the first secretary of the APhA and later served as president. His many years of service to the profession in different capacities earned him the title "Father of American Pharmacy." In the late 1800s, states began establishing state boards of pharmacy (BOPs) to regulate the practice of pharmacy in their respective states. Apothecary shops began to take on a more uniform appearance and became the main distributors of patent medicines. Physicians fostered the education and training of professional pharmacists as a vital link to medical care. However, the relationship between physicians and pharmacists began to sour as pharmacists began to treat customers by counter-prescribing, and physicians began to dispense medications. At first, pharmacists rejected the idea that formal education and licensing would enhance their professionalism, and believed it would interfere with their freedom to practice. Near the end of the 19th century, pharmacists began to establish themselves as professionals through university degrees, state licensing, and other certifications. In this way they put an educational gap between their profession and public understanding of their work.

In 1878 Louis Pasteur presented a scientific paper to the French Academy of Sciences that would change the practice of medicine and pharmacy. In the paper he introduced the germ theory, describing experiments in the laboratory in which he had grown anthrax bacilli in a sterile culture and produced the disease by inoculating an animal with it. This revolutionized scientific theory about the causes and cures of disease, and opened the door to research and the eventual discovery of antibiotics.

Pharmacy in the 20th Century

Although state laws did not yet mandate a pharmacy school diploma for licensure at the beginning of the century, the prestige attached to a diploma resulted in increasing expectations from the public and an increase in the respect afforded a professional who had attained this milestone. There were a variety of schools available for the students' educational experiences. They ranged from "short cram" schools to facilitate passing the state board examination, to small local schools with bare basic education, to local pharmacy schools offering a two-year degree, and finally, to large universities offering a four-year degree. During this transitional time, the pharmacy profession solidified as a dispenser of medicines, although the dispensing of patient counseling was forbidden until much later. During the 20th century, the minimum requirement for a pharmacist to practice was increased to a four-year degree and some apprenticeship time in a pharmacy. In the sixties, the educational requirement was raised to a five-year degree, and by the end of the 20th century the entry-level degree became a six-year PharmD degree, which includes a year of clinical rotations and in some cases is followed by a residency. This expansion of education transformed the pharmacist into the most knowledgeable professional in medications and their uses and interactions.

At the beginning of the 20th century, family-owned (or "mom and pop") pharmacies began to appear in large cities and small towns across the country. Most were owned and operated by a pharmacist with the help of his (there were very few female pharmacists at this time) spouse and children or perhaps a non-related employee or two. The pharmacist kept the drugs and tools of the trade in the "back room" and the other workers took care of the front of the store, which almost always included a soda fountain. The soda fountain became a community gathering place where many lively discussions took place. Customers would bring in a prescription from a doctor or, in some cases, would bring a family member who needed advice and ask to speak to the pharmacist. Although some proprietary medicines were available, up to 70% of medications had to be compounded by the pharmacist. Each pharmacist had a recipe book of compounds he could mix up to treat various symptoms for customers who were unable or unwilling to see a physician. Proprietary or patent medicines could still be marketed with false or misleading therapeutic claims, and there was no law requiring a prescription for the sale of drugs that required medical supervision. Although Louis Pasteur had already established the germ theory of disease, and the search for more vaccines and therapeutic drugs was continuing, the public still clung to the outdated theories held by Galen and was often misled by the advertising claims of patent medicine salesmen about their so-called "wonder drugs." In the hospital setting, IV admixture was often performed by nurses on the patient floor without the benefit of laminar flow hoods and with little training in aseptic technique. During this time, American physicians began to view the services provided by the pharmacist as a valuable link to the provision of healthcare to their patients. Professional pharmacy organizations became more influential but often did not agree on their focus. Although they could establish best practices, these organizations could not legislate. The Food and Drugs Act was passed by Congress in 1906, but it only prohibited interstate commerce in misbranded and adulterated foods, drinks, and drugs. The Food and Drug Administration (FDA) was officially named in 1930 to regulate standards of quality for foods and drugs.

During World War I, sulfanilamide was used very successfully to prevent infections from gunshot and other types of wounds. Researchers believed it would also be effective for throat infections, but the taste made it unsuitable for oral use. In 1937, in an attempt to make sulfanilamide more palatable, it was combined with diethylene glycol. Diethylene glycol is a very sweet liquid and masked the taste of the drug. One hundred and seven people, many of them children, died after ingesting the compound. Diethylene glycol is used as antifreeze in automobiles today. This tragic incident emphasized the need to establish firm standards for drug safety. The Federal Food, Drug and Cosmetic Act was passed by Congress in 1938. This act required drugs to be proven safe prior to marketing, provided for safe tolerances to be set for poisonous substances, and authorized factory inspections. In the early 1940s, the need for a national organization of hospital pharmacists was

counter-prescribing Common practice involving patients describing their symptoms and the pharmacist prescribing an over-the-counter drug without consulting a physician.

Louis Pasteur French scientist who developed the germ theory to explain infectious diseases.

germ theory Major breakthrough in modern medicine originated by Pasteur after he grew anthrax bacilli in the laboratory and theorized that some diseases are caused by bacteria.

IV admixture Process of preparing intravenous fluids using aseptic technique.

Food and Drugs Act Original act passed by Congress in 1906 to prohibit misbranded or adulterated foods and drugs to be sold across state lines.

Food and Drug Administration (FDA) The regulating body established by Congress to enforce rules regarding the sale of food and drugs.

Federal Food, Drug and Cosmetic Act Act passed by Congress in 1938 that required new drugs to be proven safe before marketing. It also extended controls to cosmetics and therapeutic devices.

recognized. A constitution and by-laws were compiled and approved, and in 1942 the American Society of Health-System Pharmacists (ASHP) was formed, establishing minimum standards for pharmaceutical services in hospitals. Pharmacy was becoming a more structured and regulated profession.

By the middle of the 20th century the FDA was well established as the watchdog for violations of pharmacy regulations. Pharmacists had established themselves as professional dispensers of drugs. Although they were highly respected by customers, they were still subservient to physicians and functioned mostly with a "count and pour" mentality despite all their education. In 1951 the Durham-Humphrey Amendment classified drugs as those that could be safely used by consumers without medical supervision and those that would require a prescription. The pharmacy profession had progressed tremendously up to that point, but more change was on the horizon. The Kefauver-Harris Amendment, passed in 1962, required manufacturers to prove to the FDA that a drug was effective for the indication it was being marketed to treat. Then, in 1965, the Drug Abuse Control Amendments were enacted to regulate depressants, stimulants, and hallucinogens that could be addicting.

American Society of Health-System Pharmacists (ASHP) Founded in 1942 to establish minimum standards for pharmaceutical services in hospitals.

Durham-Humphrey Amendment Law mandating that certain drugs require a prescription written by a licensed practitioner.

Kefauver-Harris Amendment Amendment passed in 1962 that requires manufacturers to prove the effectiveness of products before marketing them.

Drug Abuse Control Amendments Amendments enacted in 1965 to deal with abuse of stimulants, depressants, and hallucinogens.

Several things happened in the next two decades to completely change the world of pharmacy. The first was the arrival on the scene of large chain drugstores with mass merchandising and discount prices. The pharmacist became the manager of a store with a large inventory, many employees, great managerial responsibilities, and a growing prescription volume. The small corner drugstore began to disappear, choked by the competition. The chain stores grew in size and numbers. During this same time period, the major pharmaceutical manufacturers realized the economic feast that could result from the research, manufacture, and marketing of new drug entities to a world very ready for a "magic pill." The other factor that entered the picture at this time was third-party payers. The fact that many prescriptions were now being paid for by insurance companies, coupled with the emerging mentality that a pill could solve any problem, and the ever-increasing population, caused the volume of prescriptions to skyrocket. The pharmacist could no longer handle all the responsibilities alone. In desperation, pharmacists began asking a "trusted" clerk to help out in the pharmacy during busy hours. This could mean anything from taking in the prescriptions, filling out insurance forms, or accepting payment, to counting pills and labeling bottles. Training was strictly "on the job," but many clerks became very capable assistants and the position of pharmacy technician emerged as a vital link to the healthcare field.

Development of the Pharmacy Technician's Role

People who assist pharmacists have been called many names over the years, including pharmacy helpers, aides, and clerks. Only in the last several decades have they been called pharmacy technicians. These dedicated people assist pharmacists in many ways and often perform many of the same duties as pharmacists, but they always work under the supervision of a pharmacist. A pharmacist is required to check their work, and the ultimate responsibility for any medication errors rests with the supervising pharmacist. Responsibilities are limited to the duties that each individual pharmacist feels comfortable in relinquishing to a nonpharmacist. Pharmacy assistants soon learn that each pharmacist has a very

medication error Any variation from the correct patient, medication, dosage form, route of administration, or time of administration.

specific way of doing things and very specific ideas about what are acceptable duties for a nonlicensed person to perform. The pharmacist on one shift might ask a technician to type labels, count tablets, and pour liquids, whereas the pharmacist on another shift might only allow them to fill out insurance forms and collect money. This was and continues to be a source of great frustration for many experienced technicians.

Hospitals were the first pharmacy practice settings to establish positions and training for pharmacy technicians. The roles played by hospital pharmacy technicians began to change during the last few decades of the 20th century as many technicians gained experience and competence, especially in IV admixture. Pharmacists began to rely more heavily on them and expect more professionalism from them as the demands on the pharmacists' time increased. This paradigm shift in their roles prompted the hospitals to establish more formal training programs, which may have involved some classroom experience but were often in the form of a self-study manual. This manual would have self-study modules to be completed according to a time schedule established by the department. On completion of each module, a written exam would evaluate learning. In addition to this, there would be on-the-job training and a check list to be completed when each competency was attained adequately by the technician. The technician would often be awarded a certificate of completion by the hospital and allowed to assume certain responsibilities as a result of this certification. This certificate was not very portable if the technician moved to another location or accepted another position, because there was no standardization of the training. Most states did not include any mention of pharmacy technicians in their Pharmacy Practice Act.

By the late 1900s, the technicians' responsibilities were increasing and the need for more formalized education and training became evident. At this time the ASHP developed an accreditation process for pharmacy technician training programs so that a standardization process could begin to evaluate educational criteria on a national basis. In 1994 the Model Curriculum for Pharmacy Technician Training Programs was developed by a group of educators convened by the ASHP. This document, which includes goals and objectives for a comprehensive technician education and training program, serves as a guidepost for the development of training programs nationwide. Over 90 pharmacy technician training programs have been accredited by the ASHP. In 1995 the Pharmacy Technician Certification Board developed a national certification exam to verify and document the knowledge of technicians. Since then, over 200,000 technicians have passed the exam to demonstrate their competency. The scope of practice for pharmacy technicians began to change, and the Model Curriculum was updated in the year 2000 to reflect the new responsibilities of technicians.

Although technician education is mandatory in a few states, many states still have no requirements for the practice of pharmacy by technicians. The scope of practice for technicians continues to mushroom as they are asked to assume greater responsibilities in pharmaceutical care. Their knowledge base reaches far beyond the role of a dispenser of drugs. As the population ages and healthcare becomes more available to a larger population, the expertise of the pharmacist must be directed to the clinical provision of pharmaceutical care in hospitals and an expanded role in counseling patients in outpatient settings. This will necessitate an expanded role for the many technicians practicing in pharmacies around the world. The standards of practice for technicians must be realigned to facilitate this new model of the pharmacy world. Pharmacy technicians must be taught to develop the professional judgment of a technician.

paradigm shift A change in the format or basic design of a model. (The model of a pharmacy technician is undergoing a paradigm shift from a clerk or assistant to a pharmacy professional.)

Pharmacy Practice Act Legal document passed by the legislature of each state to outline laws governing the practice of pharmacy in that state.

model curriculum for pharmacy technician training Comprehensive set of guidelines for effective pharmacy technician education in a formal program.

scope of practice for pharmacy technicians List of functions that pharmacy technicians can perform as part of their duties in the pharmacy.

standards of practice Quality-assurance guidelines that define the competence required for the performance of pharmacy technician duties.

professional judgment of a technician Requires knowledge of the scope and standards of practice for technicians, the state and federal laws governing their practice, and the job description of the practice site to facilitate a competent decision-making process.

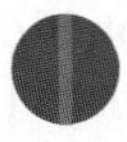 Scope of Practice for Pharmacy Technicians

The scope of practice for pharmacy technicians is being driven by a mandate for pharmacists to fully utilize their professional expertise to provide pharmaceutical care to all patients through increased patient counseling, increased clinical consultations with other health professionals, and participation in administrative and legislative decisions at the state and national levels that will affect the health of patients. For this to take place, there must be an expanded scope of practice for technicians. The scope of practice is a list of responsibilities that a technician is legally qualified and approved to perform in the work place. From the broad list of acceptable competencies included in the State Pharmacy Practice Act, each practice setting will specify those that are considered a technician's responsibilities. These responsibilities will be outlined in the departmental policy and procedure handbook and/or the technician's job description. It is the professional responsibility of each technician to know the scope of practice for his/her practice setting and abide by it in the performance of daily technician duties. Each technician must consistently perform all responsibilities with the utmost professionalism and concern for the care of the patient.

TIP **Continue to demonstrate professionalism by creating new responsibilities within the scope of practice.**

 Standards of Practice

The term "standards of practice" is a measure of quality of performance rather than a list of competencies. For each responsibility included in the scope of practice for technicians, there is a corresponding level of competency that is expected from a qualified technician. Failure to meet this standard may result in performance-improvement counseling, loss of the pharmacist's trust, patient medication errors, and possibly legal action. When a legal action is brought against a technician, the judgment will be based on the opinions of other technicians and pharmacists as to whether the technician involved followed accepted standards of practice or was negligent.

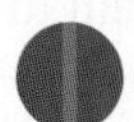 Professional Judgment

It has often been stated that pharmacy technicians perform duties that do not require professional judgment. This may have been true in the past, but certainly it is no longer the case. There is definitely a difference between the professional judgment of a pharmacist and that of a technician. The pharmacist has the knowledge and expertise to evaluate the medication regimen of a patient and assist in clinical decision-making to improve the health of the patient. The technician has or must attain the knowledge to evaluate the information on a written prescription, be alert for drug interactions and drug-disease contraindications with other prescriptions or over-the-counter medicines, accurately fill the prescription, and communicate effectively with the patient to ascertain when he or she may need pharmacist counseling even if he or she refuses it. In a busy pharmacy the technician often must be the eyes and ears of the pharmacist, and use professional judgment to alert the pharmacist about situations that may require pharmacist intervention.

Technician Development

Technician education must become mandatory in all states, and the education provided must be visionary in its scope. Students must be prepared today for future roles as competent professionals. The provision of excellent pharmaceutical care by pharmacists depends on the education and training of competent technicians who are capable of using the professional judgment of a technician to assist the pharmacist. Later chapters will delineate current standards and scope of practice, and possible future standards for educated professional technicians.

The various pharmacy organizations will be discussed in more detail in later chapters, but it is vitally important that technician students and all practicing technicians become involved in organizations where they can have an impact on the future direction of their profession. This means membership in state and local pharmacy organizations, as well as national pharmacy technician organizations. Technicians should also become acquainted with their BOPs and state legislators. The Pharmacy Practice Act of each state legislates the regulations for the practice of pharmacists and technicians in that state. This is a legal document and any changes require legislation. Let your voice be heard so that these important people understand your abilities and professionalism. Re-read the section earlier in the chapter about the progression of pharmacists from herbalists to respected professionals, and the part that mandatory education played in that process. This chapter has planted the roots of the profession of pharmacy technicians. There is a strong foundation for future growth nourished by quality education and dedication to assisting the pharmacist in providing excellent pharmaceutical care to the patient.

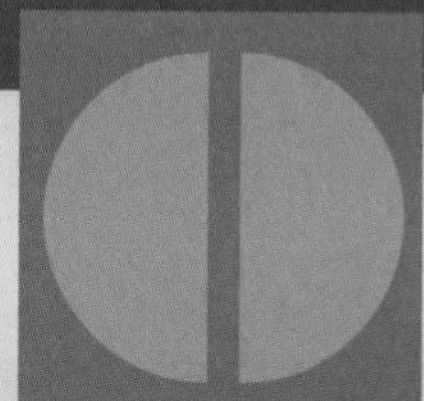

Case Study 1.1

Jill is a pharmacy technician at Nickelson's Super Pharmacy, which is a major chain pharmacy in a large Midwestern city. Initially her responsibilities consisted of greeting the patients and receiving their prescriptions, answering the telephone, and operating the cash register. After receiving on-the-job training, she began to assume other roles in inventory control and data entry. At this time, she begins to realize the seriousness of the pharmacy profession and the opportunities that might exist for a pharmacy technician with more knowledge about drugs and their uses and interactions. She has begun a dialogue with her pharmacist, Marie, who is a wonderful mentor, and together they decide that Jill should pursue a formal pharmacy technician education program to supplement her on-the-job training.

Together, Marie and Jill search the Internet for local programs and compare the educational offerings. They decide on a nearby career school with a curriculum that offers background courses in communication skills, calculations, law and ethics, medical terminology, anatomy, and physiology, along with a beginning course in pharmacy practice for technicians.

Jill continues to work part-time as she matriculates through these courses, and discovers an immediate sense of self-satisfaction as she incorporates her learning into her daily duties as a technician. In a communications class she learns to address patients with empathy and communicate with each patient in an appropriate manner. Learning medical terminology has helped her to understand more fully the directions on the prescriptions, and law and ethics classes guide her in making better legal and ethical decisions in her daily practice. The pharmacy practice course reinforces her current duties and brings a new understanding of procedures for processing prescriptions. We will follow Jill's learning progress throughout this book as she interacts with patients and develops new competencies in her profession.

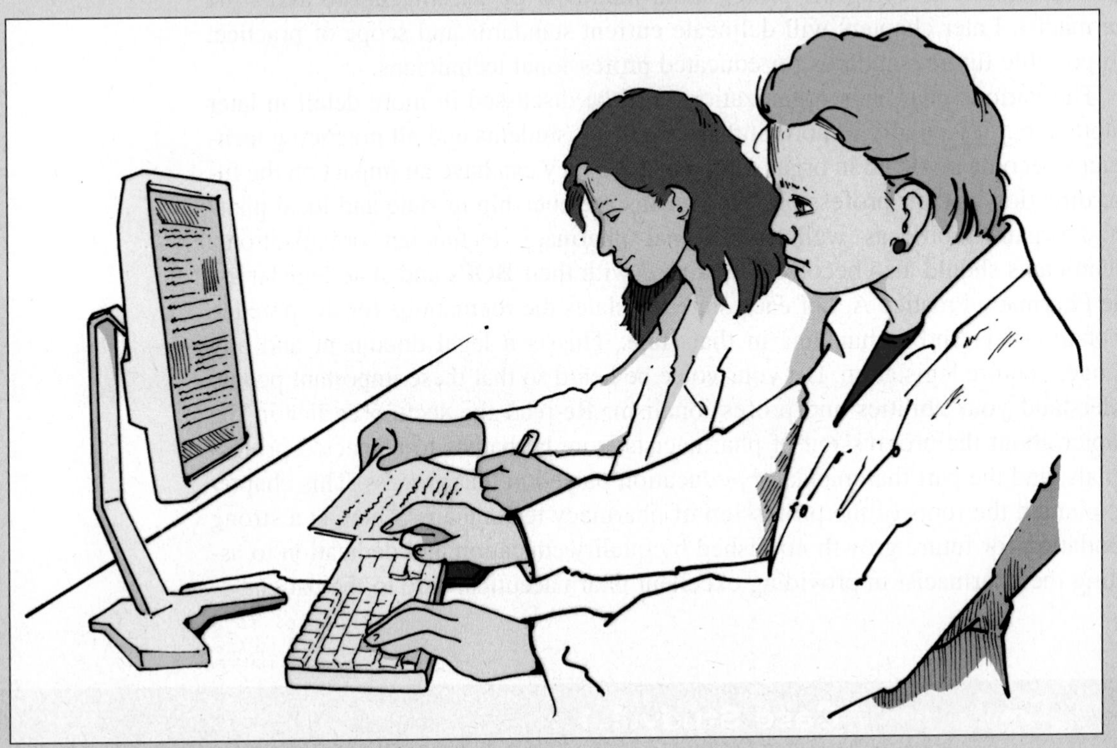

Case Study 1.2

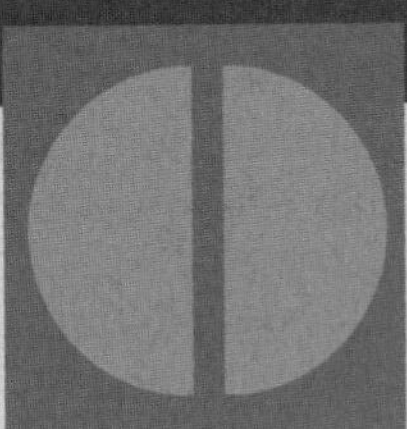

The Johnson family has just moved into the area and decides to shop at Nickelson's for their pharmacy needs. Mr. Johnson is an attorney with a local law firm and suffers from hypertension and arthritis. He is 43 years old and a heavy smoker. Mrs. Johnson is a stay-at-home mother of three children: 14-year-old Scott, 10-year-old Sara, and 3-year-old Jenna. Mrs. Johnson has recently been diagnosed with diabetes and suffers from occasional migraines. Jenna is being treated for asthma.

As Jill is checking the inventory, Mrs. Johnson arrives at the pharmacy counter. "Hello, Mrs. Johnson, how may I help you?" asks Jill in her most pleasant voice.

Mrs. Johnson smiles and replies, "My three-year-old daughter, Jenna, has a cold and a runny nose. Could you recommend a cold medicine that would be appropriate for a 3-year-old?"

Jill starts to call Marie to make the recommendation, but realizes that Marie is on the phone consulting with a physician. Jill does not want to interrupt their conversation, and Mrs. Johnson seems to be in a hurry to return to her ill daughter. Jill remembers that Marie had recommended a cold medicine earlier in the day for a 3-year-old, so she believes it would be all right to offer the same medicine to Mrs. Johnson. She takes the package from the shelf and helps Mrs. Johnson find the appropriate dose for her child. Jill feels proud that she was able to help Mrs. Johnson without disturbing Marie. An hour later there is a call from Mrs. Johnson, who is very upset. She asks to speak with the pharmacist. Marie speaks with her in a calm voice and apologizes for the error. When Marie hangs up the phone, she explains to Jill that the medication she recommended for Jenna had a warning that it was not to be used in a patient with asthma, and the medicine precipitated an asthma attack in the child.

1. Discuss this scenario and how it relates to the scope of practice and professional judgment.
2. What mistakes did Jill make in this incident? Describe how she could have handled the situation better.

Case Study 1.3

Mr. Laker is an 80-year-old man who suffers from congestive heart failure and has frequent angina attacks. He takes warfarin to thin his blood, furosemide to control excess fluid, and digoxin for his heart. Mr. Laker is very forgetful and not always compliant with his medication.

Mr. Laker enters the store and shuffles his way back to the pharmacy counter. He is out of breath and looks very pale. Jill takes the refill bottles from him and asks him to be seated. When she enters the refill numbers in the computer, she sees that his refills are several weeks overdue. She asks Mr. Laker if he has been taking his medication correctly every day. He responds that sometimes he forgets. He doesn't see very well and often gets his medicines mixed up. Marie is busy counseling a patient and Jill wants to get Mr. Laker on his way as quickly as possible, so she fills the prescription and asks Marie to check it because Mr. Laker isn't feeling well. Marie carefully checks the drugs' strengths and directions, but doesn't notice that the refills are overdue and does not see Mr. Laker. Because these are refills, he refuses counseling so he can return home. A short time later, Jill hears a siren and sees an ambulance turn into the pharmacy parking lot. On investigating, she discovers that Mr. Laker suffered a heart attack before he reached his car.

1. Discuss how Jill might have acted differently to provide better pharmaceutical care to Mr. Laker. Relate this incident to scope of practice and standards of practice for technicians.
2. Compare and contrast the terms "scope of practice" and "standards of practice" as they apply to pharmacy technicians.
3. It has been said in the past that technicians perform functions that do not require professional judgment. Discuss the importance of the professional judgment of a technician and how it differs from the professional judgment of a pharmacist.

Chapter Summary

- Early civilizations often used cultural lore, mysticism, and religion combined with herbs and plants to treat illness.
- The Ebers papyrus, which was a type of pharmacopoeia or compounding list, was composed as early as the 16th century B.C. in Egypt.
- Ancient Greek philosophers searched for a scientific approach to health.
- The humoral approach to illness referred to the four humors of the body: black bile, blood, yellow bile, and phlegm.
- Britain's Apothecaries Act of 1815 laid the groundwork for a more modern practice of pharmacy.
- The USP was established as the official list of drugs in 1820.
- National pharmacy organizations, such as the APhA and ASHP, were established in the mid 1800s to provide guidance and support for pharmacists.
- State BOPs were formed in the late 1800s to regulate the pharmacies in each state.
- In 1878 Louis Pasteur introduced the germ theory after successfully cultivating the anthrax bacillus in a sterile medium in the laboratory.
- In the early 20th century, various types of pharmacy schools began to appear as pharmacists realized that education would bring them the knowledge and respect they sought.
- Pharmacists compounded medications in small apothecary shops or neighborhood "drugstores" for customers who came to them with their illnesses.
- In 1965 the Drug Abuse Control Amendments were passed to regulate depressants, stimulants, and hallucinogens.
- Large chain pharmacies and mass merchandising added a new dimension to retail pharmacy, while pharmaceutical manufacturers increased the number of patent medications for sale.
- Third-party insurance claims increased the work load of the pharmacist as prescription volume skyrocketed.
- Clerks began to help fill out insurance forms, count pills, and operate the cash register, and hospitals trained pharmacy assistants to perform IV admixture and fill patient medicine carts.
- The Model Curriculum for Pharmacy Technician Training Programs was developed in 1994.
- A national certification exam for pharmacy technicians was developed in 1995 by the Pharmacy Technician Certification Board.

Review Questions

Multiple Choice

Choose the best answer for the questions below:

1. The Greek physician considered to be the "father of medicine" is
   a. Socrates
   b. Galen
   c. Hippocrates
   d. Aristotle

2. A pharmacopoeia
   a. lists standards of practice for pharmacies
   b. provides rules for state boards of pharmacy
   c. lists quality standards for an approved list of drugs
   d. requires pharmacists to be licensed
3. The germ theory about the cause and cure of disease was introduced by
   a. Galen
   b. Pasteur
   c. Hippocrates
   d. Socrates
4. The act passed by Congress in 1938 that required drugs to be proven safe before marketing was the
   a. Durham-Humphrey Amendment
   b. Kefauver-Harris Amendment
   c. Federal Food, Drug and Cosmetic Act
   d. Food and Drugs Act
5. Pharmacies in the United States are regulated by
   a. the Apothecaries Act of 1815
   b. the National Association of Boards of Pharmacy
   c. state boards of pharmacy
   d. the American Pharmaceutical Association

Fill in the Blanks

Fill in the blanks with the correct term:

6. The Model Curriculum for Pharmacy Technician Training Programs was developed in 1994 by educators convened by ___________________________.
7. The legal document used by state boards of pharmacy to set standards for pharmacies in each state is called ___________________________.
8. The ______________________Amendments were passed in 1965 to regulate the sale of drugs that may be addicting.
9. A list of competencies that a technician is allowed to perform is called a ___________________________.
10. Education, training, and good judgment will enhance the ________________ of technicians and result in greater respect and higher pay.

True/False

Mark the following statements True or False. If the statement is false, change it to make it true.

11. ________ The humoral system of treating illness was based on the theory that illness is caused by an invading organism.
12. ________ The American Pharmaceutical Association was established primarily to organize and set guidelines for hospital pharmacists.

13. ________ Technician education is mandatory in all states in the United States.

14. ________ The bowl of Hygeia was named after the daughter of a mythical god and used in religious ceremonies for offerings to the goddess of health.

15. ________ William Proctor, Jr., is considered the father of American pharmacy.

Matching

Match the following terms:

16. _____ Durham-Humphrey Amendment
17. _____ Food and Drug Administration
18. _____ Federal Food, Drug and Cosmetic Act
19. _____ Drug Abuse Control Amendment
20. _____ Kefauver-Harris Amendment

A. regulated depressants, stimulants and hallucinogens
B. classified drugs according to those requiring a prescription and those which could be safely used by consumers without supervision
C. Organization responsible for regulating standards of quality for food and drugs.
D. required manufacturers to prove the drug was effective for the indication it was marketed to treat
E. required drugs to be proven safe prior to marketing

LEARNING ACTIVITY

Using the material in this chapter, the suggested readings, and any other references, compare and contrast the development of pharmacy as a trusted profession and the development of the profession of pharmacy technician as a trusted professional. Discuss the roles of scientists, manufacturers, educators, and pharmacists in both developments. Project the continued development of the pharmacy technician as an educated, well-paid, respected, professional, and discuss important factors involved in this process. Prepare a presentation either as a group project or individually for class discussion. Be creative in your projections about the future roles of technicians. Include a job description for your ideal job as a technician. List steps you can take to make this a reality.

Suggested Readings

A History of Pharmacy in Pictures. Taken from Bender GA. Great Moments in Pharmacy. Copyright © Parke, Davis & Company 1965. Available online at http://www.pharmacy.wsu.edu/History. Accessed July 7, 2008.

Gennaro AR, ed. Remington: The Science and Practice of Pharmacy. Baltimore: Lippincott Williams & Wilkins, 2006.

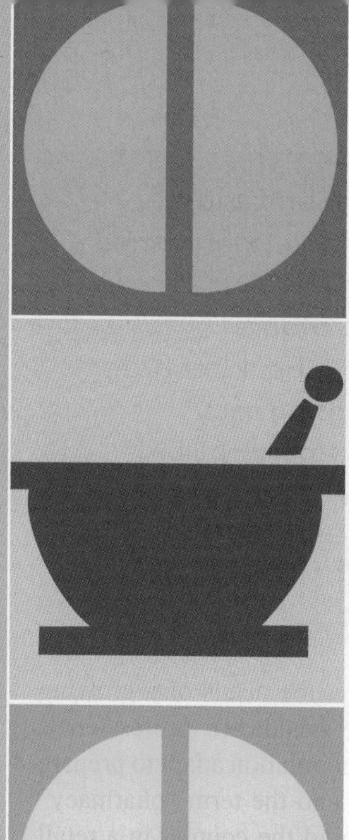

Chapter 2

Pharmacy of Today and Tomorrow

OBJECTIVES

After completing this chapter, the student will be able to:

- List some pharmacy practice settings that are available for technician employment in an outpatient community pharmacy.
- Describe some responsibilities that are performed by technicians in outpatient practice settings.
- Describe technological advances and tell how they are changing the role of technicians in outpatient pharmacies.
- Discuss the education and skills that are needed to prepare for outpatient responsibilities.
- List some inpatient hospital responsibilities that are being performed by technicians today.
- Describe how technological advances are changing the technician's role in an inpatient setting. Discuss the education and training required to adequately prepare technicians for these tasks.
- Discuss opportunities for technicians in home infusion pharmacies.
- Explore other practice settings, such as nuclear medicine, compounding pharmacies, and pharmacies specializing in disease management.

KEY TERMS

- aseptic conditions
- biohazard spill
- broth test
- chemotherapeutic drugs
- convalescent supplies
- DEA number
- drug–disease interaction
- drug–drug interaction
- drug duplication
- durable medical equipment (DME)
- emergency drug kits (EDKs)
- enteral feedings

- extemporaneous compounds
- good manufacturing practices
- hospital protocols
- inhalers
- insurance information
- intravenous medication
- inventory control
- IV admixture
- license number
- Medication Administration Record (MAR)
- microbiology
- on-line adjudication
- parenteral dose form
- patient profiles
- peak flow meters
- prioritizing phone calls
- receiving and verifying prescriptions
- reconstituted
- satellite pharmacies
- spacers
- stat orders
- tech-check-tech
- telepharmacy
- third-party billing
- Total Parenteral Nutrition (TPN)
- USP Chapter 797

The practice of pharmacy is constantly evolving to meet the needs of a growing and aging population. It is vitally important that the healthcare professionals responsible for the pharmaceutical care of this dynamic population adapt to prepare for the future needs of the profession. Just a few years ago the term "pharmacy" described a profession in which a pharmacist stood behind the counter in a retail store and dispensed prescriptions or worked in a hospital pharmacy sending medications to patients on the various floors. Pharmacists were dispensers of drugs, and technicians counted tablets and answered phones. Pharmacists were discouraged, and in some cases forbidden, to use their knowledge for patient counseling, and technicians received only on-the-job training. Fortunately, this model for the practice of pharmacy has been replaced by a new paradigm that allows and even encourages pharmacists and technicians to reach their full potential as professionals dedicated to the pharmaceutical care of patients. This chapter will demonstrate ways in which pharmacists and technicians are working together to achieve optimal patient outcomes.

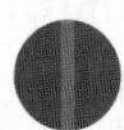

Community Pharmacy

Independently Owned Pharmaceutical Centers

The category of independently owned pharmaceutical centers includes pharmacy centers that stock only prescription and over-the-counter (OTC) drugs, specialty pharmacies dedicated to the management of certain diseases, and full-service pharmacies that stock a wide array of merchandise. The technician's responsibilities vary according to the type of pharmacy and the services offered. In a full-service pharmacy the technician may be required to function in all departments of the store depending on the size of the store, the number of employees, and the prescription volume of the pharmacy. Inventory control is an important duty that technicians routinely perform. It is vitally important that an adequate stock of medications be available in the pharmacy so that patients can receive their treatment in a timely manner. There are various ways to control inventory, but most pharmacies use a computerized method. Prioritizing phone calls helps the pharmacist concentrate on patient-care concerns by directing calls that do not truly require the pharmacist's attention to other employees or having the technician respond to questions when possible. Technicians may take refill phone orders from patients. A new prescription from a doctor must be transferred to the pharmacist. A refill

inventory control
Management of products that are bought and sold, and the resulting profit and loss.

prioritizing phone calls
Answering the phone and transferring the call to the correct person at a time consistent with the workflow.

order from the doctor may be accepted by the technician if there is no change in the medication strength or directions.

Receiving and verifying prescriptions require the expertise of a competent technician. The process begins with the technician greeting the patient and accepting the written prescription(s). The patient's name, address, and phone number should be verified with the patient and double-checked with the data in the patient's computer profile. Insurance information should also be verified and updated if necessary. A prescription for a controlled drug will require a picture ID in some states.

receiving and verifying prescriptions The technician must check the prescription for completeness of information, legibility, and accuracy.

The patient should be asked about drug allergies each time a new prescription is presented.

TIP

insurance information A series of plan numbers, group numbers, and member ID numbers that when entered into the computer database will identify patients and their benefits.

The technician will then check the body of the prescription for drug name, strength, amount, directions, physician information, and refills. If the technician has any concerns (e.g., regarding legibility, drug strength, or directions), they should be brought to the attention of the pharmacist before the prescription is entered into the computer.

Guessing the meaning of illegible handwriting may result in medication errors.

CAUTION

Missing prescriber information, such as the DEA number or license number, can be verified by the technician with a call to the prescriber's office. The technician should then document the information on the prescription, including the name of the verifying office personnel and the date and initials of the technician. When the prescription information is complete, the technician may enter the prescription into the computer and retrieve the correct medication from the shelf.

DEA number Number issued by the Drug Enforcement Administration to authorize the prescribing and dispensing of controlled drugs.

Be sure to check the drug and label three times.

CAUTION

The medication may then be counted or poured and placed into an appropriate container. The prescription label should be neatly placed on the container along with any auxiliary labels needed. The completed prescription and paper work should be placed in an organized manner in the designated area for the pharmacist to check. After the pharmacist has checked and initialed the prescription, the patient may be called to the counter. Each patient should be offered counseling by the pharmacist as mandated by OBRA '90. The prescription sale may then be completed.

license number The identifying number from the license of the prescriber. Most insurance plans require this number for insurance coverage.

Tips when filling a medication order:

1. **The size and type of the container should match the amount and type of the medication and be secured with a child-safety cap.**
2. **Keep each patient's prescriptions together.**
3. **Watch for OTC purchases of products that may interact with the prescription dispensed and alert the pharmacist.**

TIP

There are numerous ways in which community pharmacy technicians can assist the pharmacist with record-keeping. One very important responsibility is entering new patient information into the computer and updating the patient profiles of existing customers. Accuracy is vitally important because this information will verify that you have the correct patient and will trigger the drug duplication and drug interaction alerts that assist the pharmacist in patient counseling. One of the most

patient profiles Computer files that list a patient's medication history, including allergies, diagnoses, age, weight, and all medications ordered.

drug duplication Computer alert to signal the data entry of a drug that is already in the patient's profile.

third-party billing Billing process utilized when the patient's prescriptions are paid for by an insurance company.

on-line adjudication Process of submitting an insurance claim for a prescription through a computer modem and receiving a response indicating the amount of coverage.

peak flow meters Devices used in the management of asthma to determine a patient's optimum expiration volume and establish a danger zone to indicate when the patient needs to seek help.

inhalers Aerosolized medications containing medications to treat asthma.

spacers Devices that can be attached to an oral inhaler to serve as a holding area for the medication until the patient is ready to inhale.

convalescent supplies Medical needs such as catheters, braces, Band-Aids, slings, etc.

durable medical equipment (DME) Reusable medical equipment, such as crutches or wheelchairs.

time-consuming aspects of retail pharmacy is third-party billing. On-line adjudication eliminates much of the paper work involved with third-party billing, but may cause conflicts with patients who are not familiar with the restrictions of their insurance plan. Communication skills are vital in assuring the patient that their needs are being met, and helping to resolve conflicts with insurance companies. Many technicians become experts in this constantly changing task, and this allows the pharmacist to concentrate on patient care.

Many independently owned community pharmacies have developed a specialty that distinguishes them from other pharmacies and provides a service to their patients that they may not find elsewhere. Technicians are a vital link in these specialty pharmacies. Some pharmacies have begun to offer immunizations as a service to patients. Technicians in these pharmacies may take extra training to be qualified to administer immunizations under the supervision of a pharmacist, or they may serve in documenting records, monitoring inventory, and setting up supplies for the person administering the immunizations. There are also pharmacies that specialize in managing one or more diseases, such as diabetes or asthma. The technician may be specially trained to assist patients with the purchase of diabetes supplies and the use of testing equipment while the pharmacist offers counseling and supervision of blood glucose levels. An asthma clinic would afford the technician an opportunity to become familiar with the sale and use of peak flow meters, inhalers, and spacers while the pharmacist counsels the patient on their disease state and how to monitor peak flow levels. Providing convalescent supplies and durable medical equipment (DME) is another specialty where a competent technician can assist patients in fitting braces and supplying other medical equipment. These special competencies will be discussed further in subsequent chapters, but this is an overview of some possibilities for a fulfilling career as a community pharmacy professional.

Retail Chain Pharmacies

A retail chain pharmacy could be a group of three or more pharmacies owned by one or more individuals, or it could be a local chain with many pharmacies in the state or region. The term could also refer to a large national chain owned by a corporation. Chain pharmacies generally have standard operating procedures that apply to all pharmacies in the system. On-the-job training, technician responsibilities, and general employee regulations are usually described during an orientation period and are often documented in a policy and procedure book and/or employee handbook. Many of the retail technician's responsibilities will be the same as, or similar to, those expected of a technician in an independently owned retail pharmacy. Large chain pharmacies will often have a higher prescription volume and may have many more employees. There may be several pharmacists and many technicians depending on the location and size of the pharmacy. Some of these pharmacies may be open 24 hours and technicians may always work the same shift or take turns rotating through the morning, evening, and overnight shifts. Technician responsibilities, such as serving as a third-party specialist or performing inventory control or telephone triage, may be assigned to certain technicians on each shift or everyone may perform these duties as needed. Communication among the technicians and the pharmacists is vitally important to ensure the smooth operation of the pharmacy department. There may be one or more lead technicians to assist in training and scheduling, but everyone must work together in a professional manner to ensure excellent pharmaceutical care for the patients.

Workflow is an important factor in a pharmacy with multiple employees. Technicians can often make suggestions to improve workflow and minimize errors. In one workflow model, one or two technicians may work with each pharmacist and complete the prescription process from start to finish for one patient before going on to the next patient. After verifying the prescription information, one technician enters the prescription into the computer while the other technician retrieves the correct medication from the shelf and counts or measures the correct amount of medication. In this model, both technicians are responsible for accuracy and must double-check each other's work. The pharmacist may then perform the final check on the prescription(s) and offer counseling to the patient. Many pharmacists allow the offer of counsel to be extended by the technician. Communication skills may determine whether the patient accepts or refuses counseling. A common way to offer counseling is to ask patients if they have any questions for the pharmacist. Most patients are in a hurry and don't have enough knowledge about the medication to know what questions to ask. Consequently they refuse the offer of counseling. A more acceptable way would be to let them know that the pharmacist would like to speak with them about their medications. At this point they may still refuse the offer, but at least a sincere offer has been made to the patient. While the pharmacist is counseling the patient, the technicians can begin serving the next patient. This will ensure a smooth workflow.

Another workflow model involves an assembly-line type of operation where each technician is responsible for one part of the prescription processing. This would involve one technician greeting the patient and verifying the information. The prescription(s) would then be transferred to the next station for data entry into the patient profile in the computer. During this step, there is the possibility of a drug–drug interaction or drug–disease interaction alert, or an allergy alert being displayed on the computer screen. It is vitally important that the pharmacist be called to check the interaction and make the decision to override the interaction or to call the prescriber and consult with him or her about the interaction.

drug–drug interaction
An adverse event that may occur as the result of two incompatible drugs being used together.

drug–disease interaction
An interaction created by the addition of a drug that will cause a problem with a disease or condition of the patient.

CAUTION

It is not legal for a technician to override an interaction.

This is an area that involves the professional judgment of a pharmacist, and the professional judgment of the technician will afford the pharmacist the opportunity to demonstrate that professionalism. After data entry has been completed and any interaction issues have been resolved by the pharmacist, the prescription is ready to fill. The filling technician retrieves the medication from the shelf and measures or pours the correct amount of medication into an appropriate container. The label is applied and the finished prescription is placed in the assigned area to be checked by the pharmacist. The pharmacist or technician then offers counseling to the patient, and the technician or pharmacy clerk completes the sale.

Clinic Pharmacies

Many outpatient clinics have an on-site pharmacy to ensure that patients are able to begin their prescribed treatment immediately. Clinic pharmacies generally serve only patients who see physicians located in the clinic building. This provides some unique advantages for the prescriber, the patient, and the pharmacy. There is a great opportunity for the pharmacists and technicians to develop a wonderful working relationship with the prescribers and other healthcare professionals employed in the various areas of the clinic. The prescribers will feel more at ease in calling or visiting the pharmacy with questions about formulary items, drug information, and requests for special orders. The pharmacist will be able to participate in clinical decisions affecting the health of the patients. The technicians will enjoy participating in dialogue with other healthcare professionals and developing increasing knowledge about diseases and their treatments. The patients will benefit from having a team of professionals dedicated to improving their health by providing excellent pharmaceutical care.

Technology in Outpatient Pharmacies

The size and prescription volume of an outpatient pharmacy determine the amount of technology that is routinely utilized. In a relatively small operation, tablets and capsules may be manually counted using a counting tray and a pharmacy spatula. Individual stand-alone counting machines, such as the one shown in Figure 2.1, are available that can count tablets and capsules as they are slowly poured into a feed tube at the top of the machine and released into a funnel at the bottom of the machine, where they can be collected in a vial. Larger operations with a higher prescription volume may utilize a more complex counting system consisting of many individual counting cells, each programmed for a particular tablet or capsule, that will count the desired number of doses while the labels are being prepared (see Fig. 2.2). More sophisticated automation (for example, see Fig. 2.3) will complete the labeling and filling process from data entered into the computer system. Technicians are generally responsible for cleaning and maintaining these automated machines. It is imperative that the automated cells be accurately filled with the correct drug to prevent medication errors.

TIP **When transferring medication from automated machines to dispensing vials, visually check to verify that all tablets or capsules are the same size and color.**

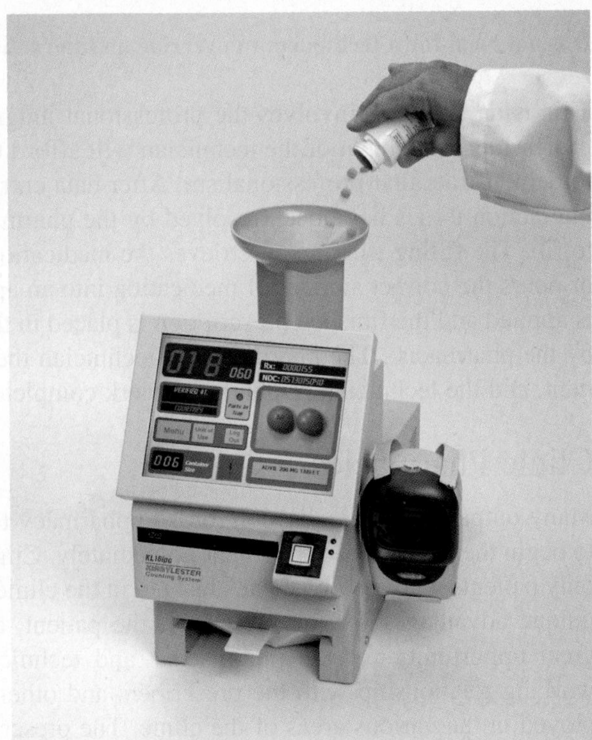

Figure 2.1 Kirby Lester tablet and counting machine. The tablets are poured through the opening at the top and fed into a vial at the bottom after being counted. (Courtesy of Kirby Lester, LLC.)

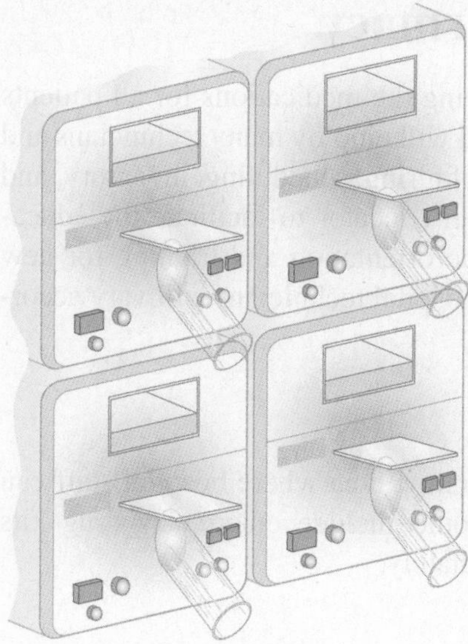

Figure 2.2 Baker cells. A modular system of counting cells specific to each tablet or capsule. It can count up to 600 tablets per minute.

Technician Education for Retail Pharmacy Practice

Technician education for practice in a retail community pharmacy should include basic background subjects such as anatomy, physiology, and medical terminology to develop an understanding of the language of medicine and the structure and functions of the body. Communication skills must be developed to ensure professional dialogue with patients and their caregivers, and other health professionals. Classes in law and ethics will assist the health professional in forming a basis for understanding general healthcare laws and provide guidance for making moral and ethical decisions. This will also lay the groundwork for the study of specific federal and state laws governing the practice of pharmacy. Computer and keyboarding skills must be adequate to perform accurate data entry in a timely manner. Pharmacy math will facilitate the calculation of accurate doses, amounts of medication to dispense, days' supply, and inventory management. The heart of technician education is a pharmacy practice course that will outline all aspects of pharmacy practice for technicians with a special emphasis on dosage forms, routes of administration, confidentiality, pharmacy laws, and professionalism, and include a laboratory for hands-on practice in dispensing procedures and basic compounding techniques. A pharmacology course for technicians should also be included to learn the brand and generic names of drugs, drug classes, common side effects, and drug interactions. These should be the minimum requirements for a professional technician who will be preparing medications that will profoundly affect the health of patients.

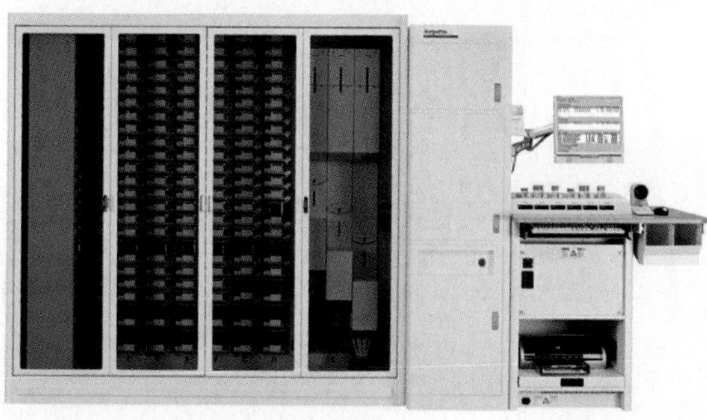

Figure 2.3 ScriptPro SP 200. A robotic dispensing system that counts the tablets or capsules, dispenses them into a vial, and labels the vial. (Courtesy of ScriptPro.)

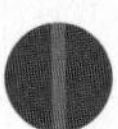

Inpatient Hospital Pharmacy

Hospital pharmacies are responsible for supplying the medications for all patients during their stay in the hospital. A large hospital will employ many technicians and often have a technician supervisor to take care of hiring, scheduling, inventory, and documentation. There may also be a technician educator to facilitate the educational needs of the technician staff and provide orientation and training for new employees. The responsibilities performed by hospital technicians will vary according to the size and type of hospital involved.

Front Area

Most hospitals will have a front counter or window area where hospital staff can pick up items needed on the floors. This would include emergency drug kits (EDKs) and other items that are needed immediately.

emergency drug kits (EDKs) Kits that are kept stocked with drugs that may be needed in an emergency situation; they are kept readily available in strategic locations.

Emergency Drug Kits

EDKs contain a standard list of drugs that may be needed in an area for a possible emergency. It is the technician's responsibility to check the returned EDKs for items that have been removed and enter the patient billing information into the computer (see Fig. 2.4 for an EDK). The kit is then refilled with all items on the list, expiration dates are checked, and the earliest expiration date is listed on the outside of the box.

Pneumatic Tube System

There may also be a pneumatic tube system at or near the front window for sending items to other stations accessed by the tube (see Fig. 2.5 for a pneumatic tube). Often items that need to be "tubed" will be brought to the technician at the front window for periodic transfer to designated units.

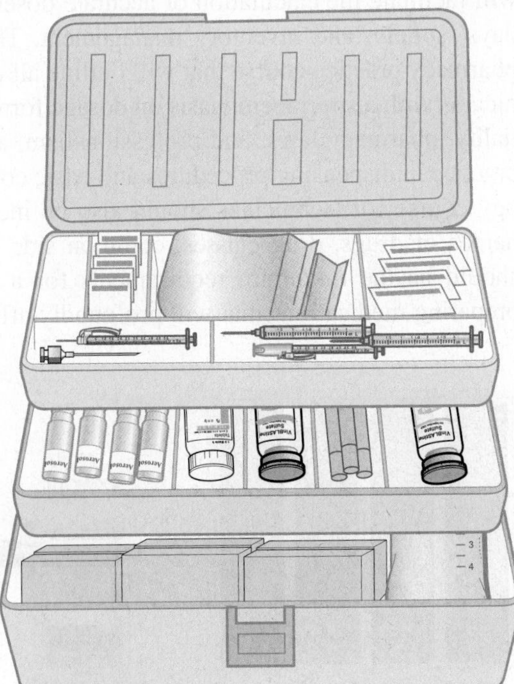

Figure 2.4 EDK. A kit containing drugs needed for an emergency situation in a hospital. The technician checks the kit, bills for items used, refills the kit, and puts a proper expiration date on the kit.

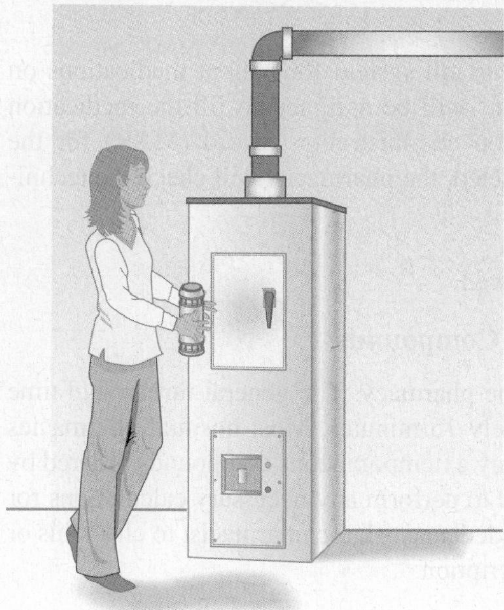

Figure 2.5 A pneumatic tube system is an efficient way to transfer medications and supplies to other parts of the hospital.

Depending on the security of the tubing system, there will be a list of medications that cannot be placed in the tube system, and the technician must be cognizant of this list. Here are some examples of medications that should not be sent through the pneumatic tube:

- Abciximab
- Alprostadil
- Beractant
- Caspofungin
- Chlorambucil
- Cyclosporin
- Darbepoetin alfa
- Digoxin Immune Fab
- Eptifatide
- Etanercept
- Filgrastim
- Infliximab
- Interleukin
- Nesiritide
- Sargramostim
- Somatropin
- Tirofiban

This list will vary according to institutional policy. Generally, any liquid hazardous substances should be hand delivered. Any glass ampules, vials, or oral liquids that may come open in the tube should be carefully sealed in plastic. Controlled substances should not be "tubed" unless there is assurance that they will be retrieved by an authorized person and cannot be intercepted by another person.

medication administration record (MAR) A form used by the nursing staff to document the administration of medication to the patient. The forms are often prepared by a pharmacy.

Cart Fill

A small hospital may have a manual cart fill system for patient medications on the floors. If this is the case, technicians will be assigned to fill the medication carts and possibly provide a medication administration record (MAR) for the nursing staff. After the cart fill is completed, the pharmacist will check the technician's work.

TIP In some states, tech-check-tech **is allowed.**

tech-check-tech Process in which two certified technicians are allowed to check each other's work without a final check by the pharmacist.

Stat Orders and Extemporaneous Compounds

Often a stat order will be received in the pharmacy. The general turnaround time expected for a stat order is approximately 15 minutes. Most hospital pharmacies will also have a compounding area for any extemporaneous compounds ordered by the physicians. The technician will need to perform any necessary calculations for the preparation, gather the materials needed, and ask the pharmacist to check his or her work before compounding the prescription.

TIP Some commonly used formulations will be recorded in a formula book kept in the compounding area.

stat orders Medication orders written in a hospital setting that should be delivered within 15 minutes.

extemporaneous compounds Medications compounded in the pharmacy pursuant to a prescriber's order for a given patient.

enteral feedings Measured liquid nutritional supplements that can be inserted into a stomach tube or consumed orally by patients who need additional nourishment because they are unable or unwilling to consume adequate amounts of food.

IV admixture Process of preparing intravenous fluids using aseptic technique.

parenteral dose form Injectable doses of medications to be delivered subcutaneously, intramuscularly, or intravenously.

aseptic conditions Conditions in which there is a complete absence of living pathogenic organisms.

After preparing and labeling the compound, the technician should leave the completed compound and paper work in the designated area. The compounding directions and each ingredient measurement should be documented with the dates, expiration dates, and lot numbers of ingredients on the compounding formula sheet and left for the final check by the pharmacist.

Some hospital pharmacies will prepare infant formulas and enteral feedings for patients with a stomach tube. There is usually a set schedule for technicians to make regular runs to deliver medications to the floors. This can be time-consuming in a large hospital, so it is important for the technician to learn the layout of the hospital and the abbreviations for each unit to facilitate this process.

IV Admixture

One of the major responsibilities of hospital pharmacy technicians is IV admixture. Many hospitalized patients are unable to take oral medications, and many of the medications utilized in the hospital setting are only available in a parenteral dose form. IV admixture involves the preparation of intravenous medications under aseptic conditions. See Figure 2.6 for a picture of a technician working in IV admixture. It is essential to follow hospital protocols because these preparations will be delivered directly into the bloodstream and cannot be retrieved. Often an intravenous medication must first be reconstituted before being added to the IV bag. Pharmacy calculations must be accurate during this procedure and proper aseptic technique is essential. Later chapters will elaborate on the microbiology governing possible infection, and the USP Chapter 797 regulations for IV admixture.

Satellite Pharmacies

Inpatient hospital pharmacies often have satellite pharmacies in addition to the central pharmacy. One example would be a satellite pharmacy in the surgery area stocked with medications generally used in surgery. Often there will be a list of medications that are usually required for certain types of surgeries or are requested

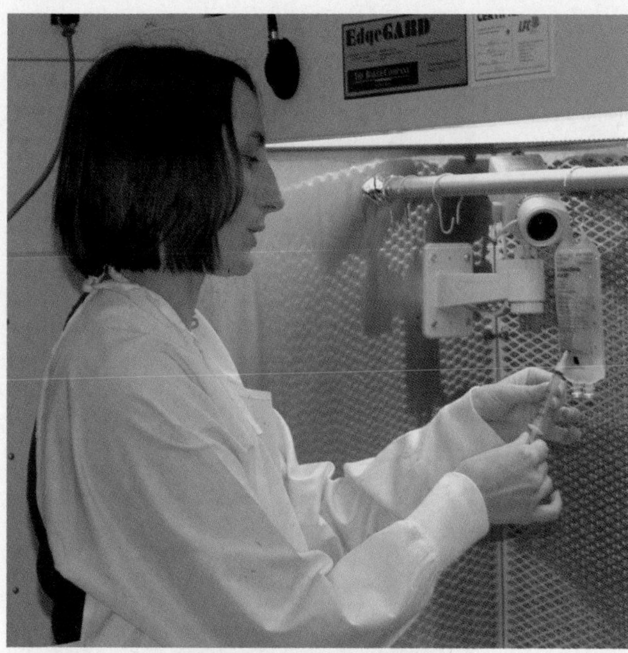

Figure 2.6 Technician working in IV admixture. An important aspect of a hospital technician's job is to perform IV admixture. (Reprinted with permission from Lacher BE. Pharmaceutical Calculations for the Pharmacy Technician. Baltimore, MD: Lippincott Williams & Wilkins, 2008.)

by certain surgeons. The technician can check the surgery schedule each day and prepare the medicine trays accordingly. There may be a satellite pharmacy on the pediatric floor or the intensive care unit (ICU) to serve the special needs of those patients. Assignment to a satellite pharmacy creates an opportunity for the technician to become somewhat of a specialist in the designated area through constant interaction with health professionals, and to continue to grow in knowledge about the drugs and procedures commonly used in that area.

Generally, there will be a pharmacist assigned to each satellite, but one pharmacist may rotate among several satellites. This is an opportunity for a technician to demonstrate the professional judgment of a competent technician, working independently while unsupervised, but knowing when to call the pharmacist for a final check or to respond to a question. Earning the trust and respect of the pharmacist and other health professionals, and attaining a sense of confidence will result in a great sense of self-satisfaction.

Inpatient Technology

The development of automated medication systems for inpatient pharmacies is a fast-growing industry. The amount of technology available in a hospital pharmacy is determined by the size and medication volume of the hospital, the available space, the need to improve workflow, a desire to decrease medication errors, and the finances available to the department. The utilization of dispensing cabinets, such as the Pyxis MedStation SN shown in Figure 2.7, has greatly impacted the job functions of the hospital technician. Cabinets are strategically placed in hospital units and loaded with medications according to the needs of the unit. The nurse can access the needed medication using a personal identification code, and can remove the medication and adjust the inventory count. When the medication needs to be replaced by the pharmacy, a pick list will be printed on a designated computer in the pharmacy. The technician will then collect the needed items and enter a personal ID code in each machine to replace the dispensed item and adjust the

hospital protocols Policies established by a hospital to standardize procedures in different departments.

intravenous medication A medication that is prepared under aseptic conditions and formulated to be injected or infused into the veins of a patient.

reconstituted Purified water or an appropriate liquid is added to a powder to produce a solution or suspension for oral administration.

microbiology The study of microscopic organisms.

USP Chapter 797 Guidelines established to provide standards for the areas, personnel, and techniques involved in IV admixture.

satellite pharmacies Small pharmacy locations away from the central pharmacy that provide services to a specific area, such as the surgery.

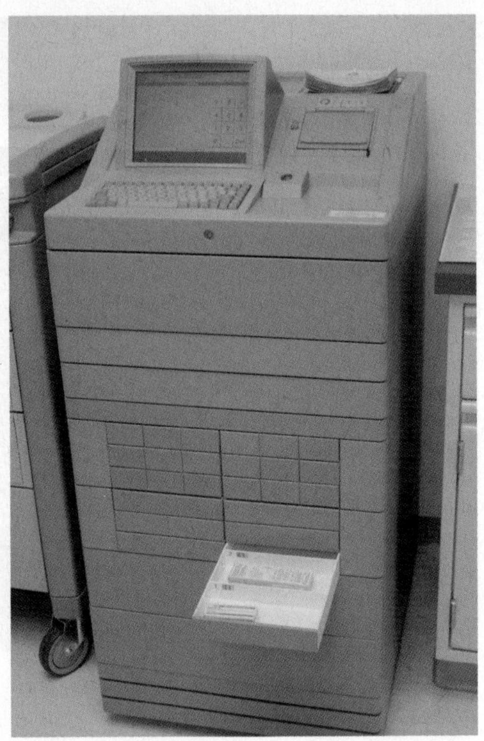

Figure 2.7 Pyxis MedStation SN. An automated dispensing cabinet for distributing and tracking medications on patient floors.

machine inventory. Robotic cart fill systems greatly shorten the time-consuming task of filling patient med carts for the hospital units. The technician may be responsible for keeping the robot stocked, or the robot may stock itself. The technician may still need to remove the patient drawer from the med cart and place it on the conveyor belt so the robot can read the bar code. Then as the robot fills the cart, the technician will check the computer for the list of drugs that are not stocked on the robot, and these items will be hand-filled by the technician. The hand-filled drugs will need to be checked by a pharmacist, but the robot does not need to be checked because it does not make errors. Preparing total parenteral nutrition (TPN) bags has become less time-consuming and more accurate since the invention of automixing machines. A TPN compounder (see Fig. 2.8) measures and adds the base fluids to the TPN bag, and can be programmed to add the correct amount of each electrolyte to the bag.

total parenteral nutrition (TPN) Intravenous therapy designed to provide nutrition for patients who cannot or will not take in adequate nourishment by mouth.

chemotherapeutic drugs Drugs used in the treatment of cancer that can destroy normal living cells. Extra precautions are needed to ensure the safety of the compounder.

biohazard spill The spill of a chemotherapeutic drug that is capable of causing damage to living cells through contact or inhalation.

broth test Another name for a media fill procedure used to assess the aseptic technique of a technician performing IV admixture. Fluid is withdrawn from one container and injected into another, then incubated for a period of time and checked for microbial growth.

Education and Training for the Hospital Technician Practice

The hospital technician will need to study all of the basic allied health courses in the curriculum of an outpatient technician. In addition, a classroom-based course outlining the principles of asepsis, as well as an understanding of microbiology and the causes of infection, will be needed. Such courses should be taken concurrently with a laboratory-based course in sterile products. Hours of supervised hands-on practice in gowning and gloving, drawing up fluids, reconstituting vials of powders, and injecting fluids into IV bags should precede any mixing for actual patients. Special gowning and gloving and safe handling requirements for chemotherapeutic drugs must be taught. Proper technique for cleanup and disposal of a biohazard spill should be practiced. Each technician should be graded with a check list of competencies and a written exam before mixing products for patients. A broth test should also precede mixing for patients.

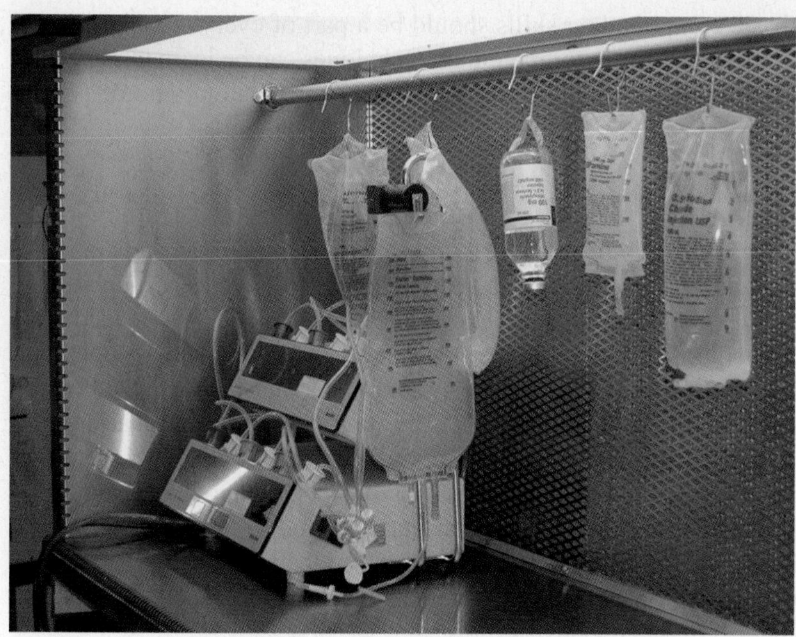

Figure 2.8 A TPN compounder. (Reprinted with permission from Lacher BE. Pharmaceutical Calculations for the Pharmacy Technician. Baltimore, MD: Lippincott Williams & Wilkins, 2008.)

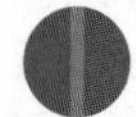

Home Infusion Pharmacies

Home infusion pharmacies are increasing in number with the spiraling cost of inpatient services and the limits on inpatient coverage by insurance companies. Terminally ill patients also often choose to remain in the home, given the availability of hospice services. A technician's responsibilities often include packing IV medications and medical supplies for shipping or transport to the patient's home. However, the primary responsibility will be accurate IV admixture using the strictest aseptic technique in a cleanroom. Broth tests should be performed periodically. IV bags sent into a patient home may be kept for several days to a week before use, so any break in aseptic technique that could allow the growth of organisms would be critical for an already compromised patient. Home infusion pharmacies offer many opportunities for advancement into administrative roles for qualified technicians desiring this type of position. Educational requirements for home infusion technicians would be the same as for inpatient hospital technicians, with a strong emphasis on sterile products.

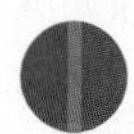

Compounding Pharmacies

Although extemporaneous compounding may be a part of a technician's duties in any of the practice settings, there are many pharmacies that specialize in compounding medications for a specific patient on the order of a physician. Responsibilities would include assisting the pharmacist in compounding lotions, solutions, ointments creams, lozenges, suppositories, and numerous other preparations to meet the special medication needs of individual patients when manufactured products on the market are not appropriate.

good manufacturing practices Regulations that set minimum standards to be followed by the manufacturing industry for human and veterinarian drugs. Standards should also be observed for extemporaneous compounds.

TIP

Knowledge of good manufacturing practices that outline accepted procedures established by the FDA for compounding medications is important.

Although basic compounding skills should be a part of every technician's education and training, additional compounding techniques can be learned by receiving on-the-job training or completing a compounding certificate program.

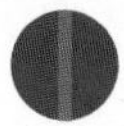

Nuclear Pharmacy

Nuclear pharmacy is a specialty area that focuses on the compounding and dispensing of radioactive materials for use in nuclear medicine procedures. Compounding of radioactive materials is done behind leaded glass shields and with leaded glass syringes. The material is contained in lead containers. A technician's responsibilities in a nuclear pharmacy may include generating computer labels for radiopharmaceuticals, performing calculations for specific unit doses of radiopharmaceuticals, managing inventory and documenting records for radioactive materials, repackaging and labeling unit doses from bulk containers, compounding and properly measuring and packaging radiopharmaceuticals, and performing and documenting quality control tests. All of these functions are performed under the direct supervision of a nuclear pharmacist after the technician completes intense education and training.

Education and training should be in addition to the course work required for hospital pharmacy technicians. A comprehensive nuclear pharmacy technician certificate should be completed. Education must include additional regulatory requirements for working with radioactive materials, radiopharmaceutical medical terminology, abbreviations, symbols, brand and generic names, and diagnostic and therapeutic uses of radioactive drugs. Extensive training in dose calculations for radiopharmaceuticals and closely supervised compounding techniques should be completed before compounding for patient use. A site-specific understanding of functions that require the professional judgment of a pharmacist, and any state or federal regulations affecting technicians' responsibilities should be clearly understood. There are a relatively small number of technicians practicing in this specialty, but the number of nuclear pharmacies is growing and opportunities are available in nearly every state.

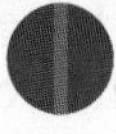

Telepharmacy

telepharmacy Use of audio and video links in addition to a computer system so that a pharmacist at a central location can perform the final check and patient counseling for a patient at a remote site whose medication has been prepared by a certified technician.

Many areas have no pharmacy services within a reasonable driving distance, which creates a hardship for patients. With a telepharmacy, certified technicians can prepare prescriptions for dispensing and have the prescription checked by a pharmacist at a central location through the use of audio and video computer links. A telepharmacy consists of a central pharmacy with one or more remote sites. The central pharmacy and the remote sites are connected by audio, video, and computer links. The patient receives counseling from the pharmacist using the telecommunication equipment. The technician is afforded the opportunity to have a fulfilling position managing the inventory and sales of the site, working independently to assist patients in receiving their medication without having to drive long distances, and functioning under the guidance and supervision of the pharmacist at the central site. The pharmacy technician must be a graduate of an approved pharmacy technician education program and have one year of experience as a technician. The pharmacist continues to be responsible for any activity at the remote site and is immediately available to the technician and the patient.

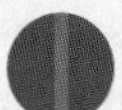

Long-Term Care Pharmacies

Long-term care pharmacies service nursing homes in a state or regional area. They employ drivers or delivery persons to distribute the medications daily to the homes that have contracted with them for services. Pharmacy technicians are a vital link in the timely provision of these services. Orders from the homes are usually faxed to the pharmacy in the morning. Generally they are in the form of inpatient medication orders. There may be a pool of data entry technicians who type the medication orders into the computer to produce labels for the medications. These technicians must be well versed in interpreting medication orders and accurately entering them in the computer.

Long-term care pharmacies also carry many nursing-home supplies, including IV tubing, catheters, colostomy supplies, and other convalescent needs. Technicians must familiarize themselves with all of the ancillary supplies so that the correct items will be sent. Periodically during the day, the data entry department will run all the labels entered in a given time period. At this point, one or more pharmacists will check the labels produced against the original medication orders received. The labels will be verified by the pharmacist or returned to data entry for any correction needed.

Once the labels are verified, they are passed on to the filling technicians, who begin to fill them in a manner appropriate for the facility being served. Many facilities utilize a system in which a 30-day supply of each medication is sealed in a blister pack (often called a "bingo card"; see Fig. 2.9). Each individual dose of medication can be punched out of its compartment and administered to the patient. The technician is responsible for placing the medication into the pockets in the card, heat-sealing the card, and placing the correct label on the card. This process may also be accomplished by automation if it is available. High-volume products

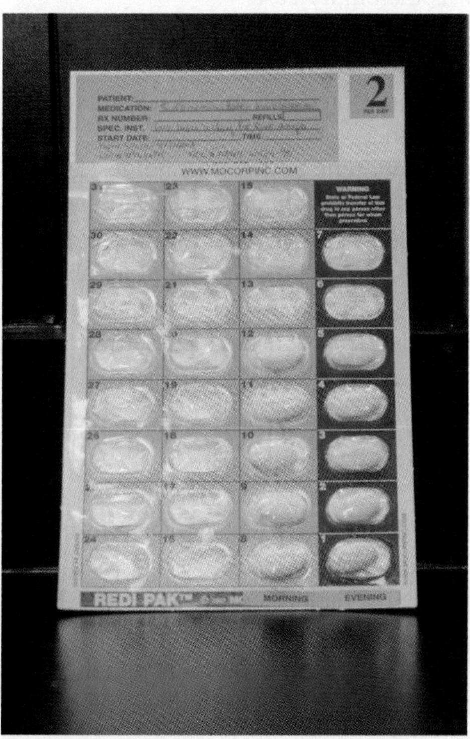

Figure 2.9 Thirty-day dose card, sometimes called a bingo card. Each bubble contains one dose of medication for easy dispensing in a nursing home or assisted-living facility.

are often sealed in cards ahead of time and placed in a storage area for easy retrieval when needed. These products are required to meet all the regulations for repackaging of drugs.

TIP **Repackaged products must have correct expiration dates, lot numbers, and brand or generic name, and be entered into a logbook and verified by a pharmacist.**

When the medication orders are filled, they are placed in a central checking area to be verified by the pharmacist. For any compounds ordered, the labels go to the compounding area, where a technician is assigned to process them. The compounding process is supervised by a pharmacist. IV medications will be processed by the IV technician and checked by the pharmacist. Homes with a pediatric population may need medications packaged as unit dose oral liquids. Controlled drugs are usually kept in a controlled room with a pharmacist and one or more technicians assigned to work in the room. Controlled drugs sent to nursing homes are packaged in secure containers to prevent drug diversion. At a prearranged time all medications must be filled, checked by the pharmacist, and packed for delivery to each individual home. The technician may be the person who packs the delivery boxes and checks to determine that all ordered items are in the box. The home contracts with the pharmacy for all items ordered daily to be received by the end of the day, so it is important that no item be left out. If a nursing-home patient misses a dose of medication because it is unavailable, that would be considered a medication error for the home.

Depending on the size of the pharmacy, inventory control may be the responsibility of one or several technicians. Often there is a lead technician or technician supervisor responsible for interviewing, hiring, scheduling, and general technician supervision. Many nursing homes use a medication cart system involving the exchange of medication carts every seven days or some other prearranged schedule. In this case, there may be an "exchange technician" who delivers the filled medication carts to the nursing home and returns the empty carts.

Medication carts are filled by technicians using unit dose medications. Many medications are available in unit dose packaging, but if an ordered medication is not available in a unit dose, the technician will package the correct quantity either manually or using a unit dose packaging machine.

Long-term care pharmacies often serve hundreds of nursing homes and fill thousands of orders each day. The technicians' knowledge of medications, convalescent supplies, and the policies and procedures of the facility is crucial for ensuring the smooth operation of the pharmacy and the provision of good pharmaceutical care to the many patients they serve. A position in a long-term care pharmacy can provide a fulfilling opportunity to work in a fast-paced setting where there are many opportunities for advancement and learning.

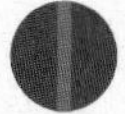

Mail-Order Pharmacy

Mail-order pharmacies are becoming more prevalent because many insurance companies are mandating the use of mail order for maintenance drugs, and some patients appreciate the convenience of receiving their medications through the mail. It is especially helpful for patients who live in rural areas and are unable to drive to a pharmacy. Large mail-order pharmacies often employ hundreds of registered pharmacists and pharmacy technicians, and process thousands of prescriptions each day.

Technician positions are delineated into the various functions required to process prescriptions. Often there is a complete department of technicians responsible for answering phones and either transferring the call to a pharmacist or, if it is a refill order, recording the order and sending it to data entry to begin processing. The data-entry technicians receive the mail, the refill orders that have been called into the order line, and the new prescriptions that have been called in to the pharmacists. The prescriptions are evaluated for completeness and if there are any concerns about content dose or legibility, the prescription in question is sent to the phone area where a pharmacist completes the evaluation process and calls the prescriber for clarification if necessary. The phone-clarification area is staffed by pharmacists and technicians. The technicians call prescribers for refill authorization and missing prescriber identification, and a pharmacist is available if other medication verification is necessary.

When the prescription information is complete and accurate, the data-entry technicians process them and produce labels and paper work for each prescription. The technicians who prepare and label the medications continue the prescription processing and send the completed prescriptions and paper work to a pharmacist for the final check and transfer to the packaging and shipping area. This process must be completed in a timely manner so that patients can receive their medications promptly. To ensure an efficient process, technicians also perform inventory control, handle insurance processing, and help to stock and maintain the automated machines involved in dispensing. All technicians work under the direct supervision of pharmacists; however, there may also be a technician supervisor to handle scheduling and other technician issues.

A relative newcomer to the scene of pharmacy practice settings is the Internet pharmacy. Before accepting a position, the technician should be certain that the pharmacy has a valid license and is operating legally in the states it serves. The technician's duties can vary from gathering data from the computer to verifying prescription information, entering data into a patient's profile, counting and labeling medications, and packaging the order for delivery to the patient. The technician should be supervised by a licensed pharmacist who can verify that the prescriptions are legitimate orders prescribed by a licensed physician.

Common Aspects of Technician Training

This chapter has given an overview of the more common practice settings and some of the technician responsibilities associated with them. Technician education and training should not be specific to a given practice setting. All technicians must be educated in all aspects of their profession. This will cultivate a sense of pride, confidence, and professionalism that will be visible to all who are served by technicians. Certainly, there must always be a period of orientation when one begins a position in a new setting, but the basic skills must be present. There should be national educational standards so that an employer can be assured that a technician will possess certain basic skills when hired. In our society, respect as a professional is earned, not arbitrarily granted. There are many technicians who have elevated their duties to a professional level by their diligence in continuing education and training. But the time has come for the professionalism of a technician to be validated by educational institutions and training standards that are standardized across the country. The remaining chapters will continue to provide information to help you embark on a fulfilling career as a pharmacy technician professional.

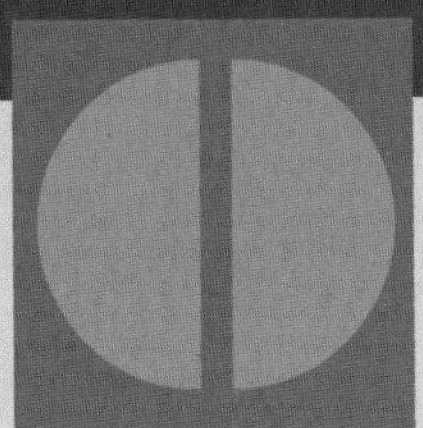

Case Study 2.1

Eric has decided to begin a new career. His work in the mail room of a large hospital has given him the opportunity to visit all the departments in the hospital and observe employees at work. He has been impressed by the professional atmosphere in the inpatient pharmacy and begins to ask some of the technicians questions about their position. As he delivers the mail to Jim one day, he asks, "Jim, you seem to be doing something different every time I see you. How were you able to learn all the different tasks?"

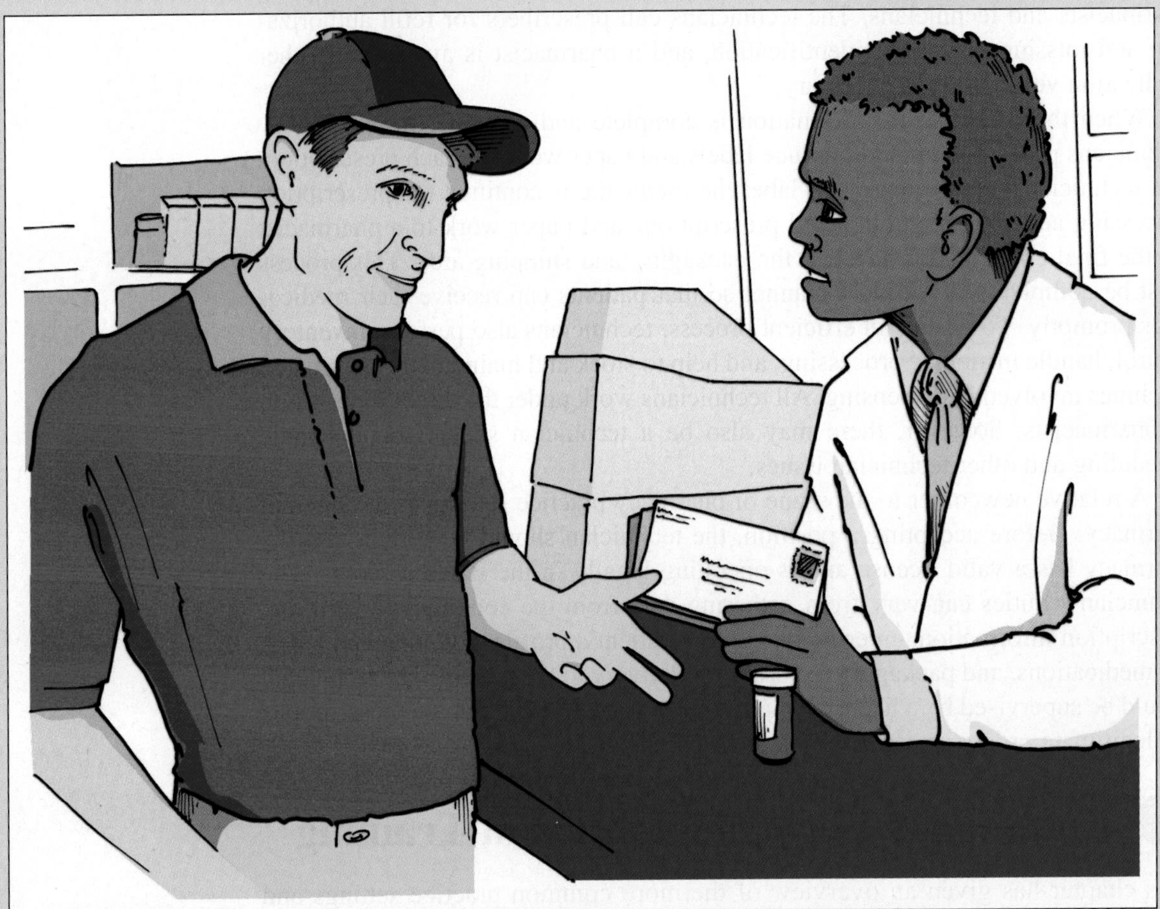

"Well, Eric, I began by attending a pharmacy technician education program. There I learned the background knowledge to understand why certain procedures are so important," Jim replied. "During the program, I trained here as a student with a preceptor to supervise me. That helped me turn my classroom learning into practical application."

Eric thought for a moment and then responded, "Jim, you seem so happy and sure of yourself. I wonder if I could become a pharmacy technician, but I don't know how to begin. It all seems so complicated."

"Eric, I was pretty scared at first, but my education and training have given me the confidence I need to perform well. Knowing that I am a qualified health professional having a positive impact on the lives of patients is very fulfilling."

"Well, Jim, I'd better be on my way so the mail gets delivered on time. See you tomorrow."

As Eric completed his work day, he continued to think about the pharmacy and wonder whether that would be a good fit for him. After work, he searched the Internet for more information on the pharmacy technician profession. He hadn't realized that it was actually a profession and not just a job. The more he learned about it, the more enthused he became. The next day when he delivered the mail to the pharmacy, Jim introduced him to the technician supervisor, who invited him to return on his day off to shadow Jim. When the day arrived, Eric followed Jim through his work day. He was impressed by the many tasks that Jim performed with such confidence. Jim gave Eric the phone number of the pharmacy technician program he had attended, and Eric applied the next day.

1. Describe the process you went through as you researched the pharmacy technician profession to be sure it would be a good career for you.
2. Use the Internet and speak with experienced technicians to add to your information.

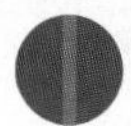

Chapter Summary

- Pharmacy technicians must prepare for a new model of practice to meet the growing needs of the profession.
- A technician's responsibilities in a community pharmacy include inventory control, prioritizing phone calls, receiving and verifying prescriptions, data entry, preparing prescriptions for dispensing, assisting with third-party billing, and completing the sale of prescriptions.
- Technicians must develop and utilize the professional judgment of a technician to make competent decisions to delineate a technician's duties from those that require a pharmacist.
- Communication skills are important when serving the pharmacy needs of patients.
- Specialty pharmacies offer unique settings for a technician to specialize and develop career opportunities.
- Preparation for a career in a specialty pharmacy begins with basic technician education and training, but may require additional education and training either on the job or in a formal certification program.
- Large chain pharmacies with a high prescription volume require competent technicians who are capable of multitasking while maintaining their concentration.
- Workflow models vary according to the practice setting, prescription volume, and number of employees.
- Pharmacy software will provide drug interaction alerts during the data entry process. These alerts must be brought to the attention of the pharmacist.
- Technology in the outpatient pharmacy depends on the size and prescription volume of the pharmacy. It is important for the technician to be knowledgeable about the maintenance and operation of any technology in use.

- Minimum education requirements for technicians should include medical terminology, anatomy and physiology, law and ethics for the allied health professional, communication skills, pharmacy math, basic computer skills, a pharmacy practice course and laboratory, and a pharmacology course.
- Technicians working in an inpatient pharmacy must complete the basic technician education courses and gain an understanding of microbiology and the infection process. A thorough education in aseptic technique, including hands-on practice, is essential for patient safety.
- Home infusion pharmacies send IV medications to the patient's home for administration, so the strictest aseptic guidelines must be followed.
- Compounding pharmacies must follow good manufacturing practices to ensure the quality of the compounds dispensed to patients.
- Nuclear pharmacy is a unique setting that requires a technician to complete a certification program in addition to basic technician education and training. Working with radiopharmaceuticals requires site-specific terminology and knowledge about radioactive drugs and their hazards.
- Telepharmacy involves a pharmacist at a central site supervising technicians at several remote sites through the use of audio, video, and computer telecommunication systems.
- Long-term care pharmacies supply all the medications and medical supply needs of patients in nursing homes in compliance with the terms of their contract with the home.
- Mail-order pharmacies receive patient prescriptions by phone, fax, and mail. The prescriptions pass through various departments to be processed and shipped to the patient's home. Technicians are an integral part of this process.
- Internet pharmacies are becoming more prevalent, but they must abide by the same regulations as other pharmacies.
- Opportunities for competent, educated technicians are increasing in number and scope, so it is important to be educated and set goals for a rewarding career.

Review Questions

Multiple Choice

Circle the best answer to the following:

1. Inventory control in a retail pharmacy includes all of the following duties except:
   a. ordering medication and supplies
   b. checking expiration dates of medications
   c. updating the patient profile
   d. checking in orders

2. Which of the following duties can the technician perform?
   a. taking a call from a doctor for a new prescription
   b. taking a call from a doctor for a refill prescription
   c. taking a call from a doctor for a refill prescription with different directions
   d. all of the above

3. On-line adjudication means
   a. the pharmacy has a direct line to the prescriber
   b. the prescription is filled using an assembly-line process
   c. the patient faxes the prescription to the pharmacy
   d. the patient's insurance authorizes payment through a computer connection

4. All of the following are supplies that would be found in an asthma clinic, except:
   a. a glucose meter
   b. a spacer
   c. a peak flow meter
   d. an inhaler

5. Patient counseling by the pharmacist is mandated by
   a. the Kefauver Harris amendment
   b. the Pure Food and Drug Act
   c. OBRA '90
   d. state boards of pharmacy

6. A medication has a warning label stating that it should not be used in a patient with high blood pressure. This is an example of:
   a. therapeutic duplication
   b. drug–drug interaction
   c. drug–disease interaction
   d. none of the above

7. An example of a secure automated dispensing cabinet with drawers of various sizes, often used in hospital systems is:
   a. a Pyxis MedStation machine
   b. a unit dose packaging machine
   c. Baker cells
   d. none of the above

8. A stat order should be delivered to the patient:
   a. when convenient
   b. within an hour
   c. the same day
   d. within 15 minutes

9. A parenteral dose may be administered to the patient
   a. subcutaneously
   b. intramuscularly
   c. intravenously
   d. all of the above

10. Microbiology is the study of
    a. plants
    b. insects
    d. microscopic organisms
    e. small animals

Fill in the Blanks

Fill in the blanks with the correct term.

11. A small pharmacy located away from the central pharmacy to serve the needs of a special area in the hospital is called a ______________________ pharmacy.

12. USP Chapter 797 regulations mandated new standards for the preparation of ______________________ medications.

13. TPN stands for ______________________, which is used to provide nutrition for patients who are unable to take oral nourishment.

14. Audio, visual, and computer links between the central pharmacy and remote locations are an essential element in the ______________ practice setting.

15. The practice setting that compounds radioactive materials is called ______________________ pharmacy.

True/False

Mark the following statements True or False. If the statement is false, change it to make it true.

16. ________ Patient medication drawers filled by a pharmacy robot need to be double-checked by a technician and a pharmacist.

17. ________ Mail-order pharmacies provide face-to-face patient counseling to comply with OBRA '90.

18. ________ EDKs contain a small supply of drugs that might be needed quickly in an emergency situation.

19. ________ Long-term care pharmacies send medications to many nursing homes in a given area each day.

20. ________ Inpatient pharmacy technicians spend their entire work day in the central pharmacy.

LEARNING ACTIVITY

1. The following table lists various practice settings and technician responsibilities. Mark an X in each space to indicate technician responsibilities likely to be needed in that practice setting. Discuss the results as they relate to the basic technician education and skills needed in various practice settings.

   Discuss the results as they relate to the basic technician education and skills needed in various practice settings.

Practice setting	Receiving and evaluating	Prioritizing phone calls	Data entry	Filling prescriptions or med orders	Compounding medications	IV admixture
Small retail						
Large chain						
Clinic						
Home infusion						
Hospital inpatient						
Long-term care						

2. Choose a practice setting that you would like to learn more about. Search the Internet to discover job opportunities, qualifications, duties, and salaries in that practice setting. If possible, find a practice setting in your area and request a chance to shadow one of the technicians. Report to the class on your experience.

Suggested Reading

Lacher BE. Pharmaceutical Calculations for the Pharmacy Technician. Baltimore, MD: Lippincott Williams & Wilkins, 2008.

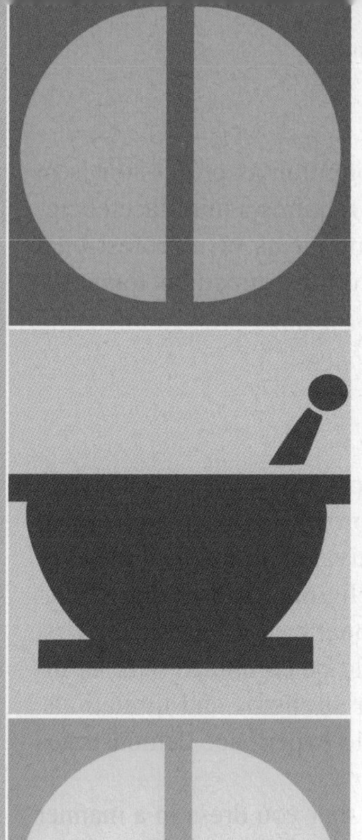

Chapter **3**

Professional Roles in the Pharmacy

OBJECTIVES

After completing this chapter, the student will be able to:

- Define professionalism.
- Demonstrate examples of professional behavior in the pharmacy.
- List steps to gain respect as a pharmacy professional.
- Discuss detriments to being viewed as a professional.
- Define the role of a technician trainer or educator in a hospital pharmacy setting.
- Outline some responsibilities for a technician supervisor in a multi-technician pharmacy setting.
- Explore the role of a warehouse supervisor in a hospital setting.
- Investigate the competencies required of a program director for a pharmacy technician program.
- Discover the responsibilities of a clinical coordinator of a pharmacy technician program.
- Develop a system for technicians to perform medication reconciliation.
- Create a position in a physician's office that involves managing phone triage for patients' prescription refills.

KEY TERMS

- affective behaviors
- clinical coordinator
- drug recalls
- expired drugs
- investigational drugs
- medication reconciliation
- preceptor
- prior authorization
- professionalism
- triage

Pharmacy technicians have long been striving for recognition as professionals in the healthcare field. Attaining respect as a professional requires a multifaceted approach. This chapter will discuss some important components of a professional person, ways in which they can be attained, and some exciting directions for a professional pharmacy technician's career.

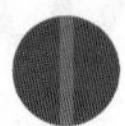 Professionalism

professionalism Term used to describe the conduct of a person who has the knowledge and skills of a profession and incorporates excellent affective behaviors and judgment into his or her daily work.

Let's begin by discussing some of the components of professionalism as they relate to you as an individual. Certain characteristics of professionalism are learned at a very young age and should continue to be cultivated through adulthood. Respecting others regardless of their race, color, sex, religion, national origin, disability, sexual orientation, economic status, or educational background is the first step toward acting in a professional manner. This should be combined with an innate respect for yourself and an understanding of your strengths and limitations. Requesting assistance for a task in which you have little experience demonstrates your ability to make valid decisions.

Respect for yourself and those around you dictates that you dress in a manner appropriate to the situation you are in. Most pharmacies have a dress code—whether that means scrubs, which should be neat and clean, or casual business dress that demonstrates a certain pride in the way you look. Cleanliness is mandatory in the healthcare industry to prevent the spread of disease. Frequent hand washing is the single most important deterrent to the spread of infection. Hair and nails should be neat and clean. Jewelry, if allowed, should be inconspicuous and in no way interfere with the task being performed.

Communication skills are a vital aspect of conveying competence and respect to patients and other healthcare professionals. Tone of voice and body language convey important messages about your attitude. An outstanding attendance record demonstrates to others the importance you attach to your position and your commitment to dependability. A positive attitude even in the most stressful and adverse conditions will help to maintain a professional atmosphere and inspire others to emulate your behavior. These are some individual strengths you can bring to the profession aside from education and training.

As you progress through the education program, a diligence in your study habits will demonstrate your desire to understand all the parameters of your new profession. Couple this with a firm commitment to master the skills required for your position and a personal pledge to always perform to the best of your ability, and you will be on your way to an exemplary career as a pharmacy technician professional.

The completion of a comprehensive course as a pharmacy technician will allow you to gain a sense of confidence that you can successfully perform the tasks required of you. As you grow in knowledge and competence, as you communicate respectfully with patients and coworkers, you will develop an air of professionalism that is obvious to all you meet. The pharmacists will not need to be reminded that you are a professional, because they will have learned that you are knowledgeable and dependable. Most importantly, the pharmacists and patients will develop a sense of trust in your ability to perform competently and handle difficult situations, and your critical thinking skills, which direct your professional judgment as a technician. This professional judgment dictates when a skill or question is within the scope of your practice and when the professional judgment of a pharmacist is required. Pharmacists and technicians are not in competition. There should be no reason for conflict between them and they should support each other. A knowledgeable, competent technician who can be trusted to make accurate decisions will enhance the pharmacist's capacity to pursue clinical and patient counseling roles that are vital to excellent pharmaceutical care. However, true professionalism has another component. This component is a love of your profession and a true passion to serve your patients. The single most important aspect of your daily work is to provide outstanding care to the patient at all times. This will set you apart as a leader dedicated to excellence.

Professional Judgment Scenario 3.1

Terri is a pharmacy technician student and is working in a retail pharmacy as part of her clinical rotations for the program. She really doesn't like this setting and hopes they won't offer her a job, but she wants to get a passing grade in the class. She decides that if she just does enough to "get by," she will pass and can look for a job elsewhere.

Her friends stop by often to chat, but she does stop to wait on customers when they approach the pharmacy counter. If no one else answers the phone after several rings, Terri will answer, but her greeting sometimes sounds irritated. She does any task she is asked to perform but takes no initiative to do anything extra. Occasionally, she is a few minutes late but doesn't offer any explanation. When she arrives during the second week wearing jeans and a sweatshirt, the pharmacist decides it's time for a discussion.

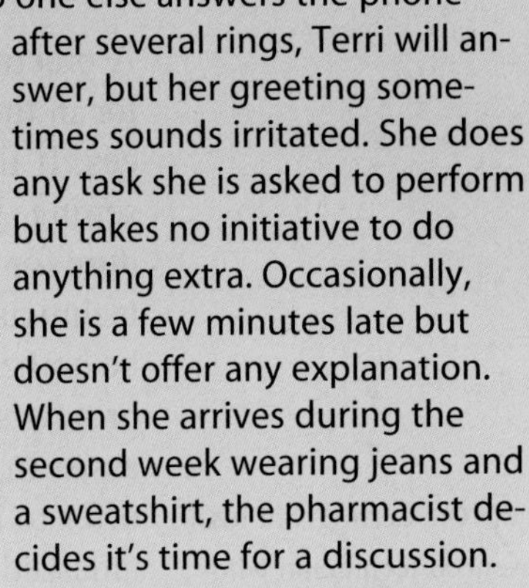

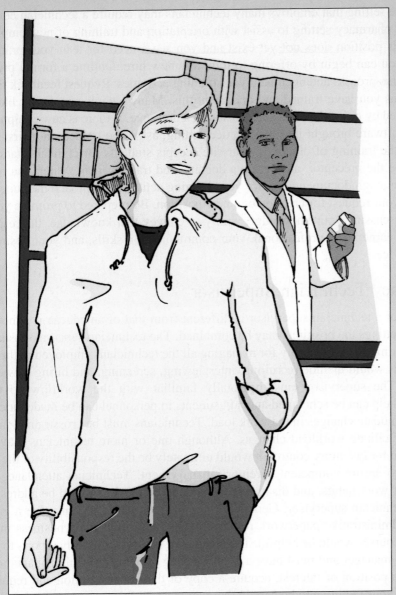

1. Create a dialogue that might take place between the pharmacist and Terri. What obstacles is she creating to being respected as a professional? Does she understand that even though she doesn't want a position in this pharmacy, this pharmacist will have input to her file and may be asked for a recommendation when she applies for another position? What responses might she make in her defense?
2. Discuss a resolution to this problem that might be acceptable to Terri and the pharmacist.

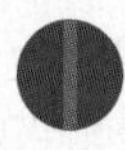 Positions Available for Pharmacy Technicians

On completion of an educational and training program, technicians will find that positions as a staff pharmacy technician are available in a number of practice settings. These positions offer valuable experience and continued opportunities for learning about the many facets of the profession. Continuing education is also available to increase knowledge. National certification provides a verification of your knowledge. As you continue to develop expertise in your profession, you should continue to be alert for opportunities for advancement. Keep a log documenting all aspects of your education, training, certifications, and job responsibilities in preparation for any opportunity that arises. Continue to explore all related horizons to find that perfect position that will open the door to a fulfilling career.

Pharmacy Technician Educator

A practice setting that employs many technicians may require a technician educator in the pharmacy setting to assist with orientation and training of new employees. If this position does not yet exist and you see a need for it in your practice setting, you can begin by offering to train any new hire. Outline a formal procedure for this process and document your training activities. Request feedback from technicians you have trained and document this. Many technicians do not like to be bothered by training others and consider it a nuisance. If there is new equipment or new software brought into the practice setting, ask to be trained on it first and assist in the training of others. If your site accepts students for clinical rotations, offer to be the preceptor, and set up a documented training plan. When you have amassed enough documentation for your training activities, approach the supervisor with your request for creation of a new position. Be prepared to promote yourself by discussing your knowledge, ability to convey that knowledge, the respect you have earned as a professional, your communication skills, and your desire to be of service.

preceptor Term given to an experienced technician who helps to supervise and mentor a student during clinical experience.

Pharmacy Technician Supervisor

The role of a technician supervisor is different from that of an educator, although in some settings the positions may be combined. The technician supervisor usually has the ultimate responsibility for managing all the technicians employed in the facility. This would include recruiting, interviewing, screening, and hiring new employees. The supervisor must be totally familiar with the workflow so that adequate help can be scheduled and adjustments in personnel can be made quickly to accommodate changes in the work load. Technicians must be crosstrained in all areas to facilitate workload changes. Although one or more technicians may be designated for inventory control, it would ultimately be the responsibility of the supervisor to ensure competent inventory management. Technician attendance issues, poor work habits, and disagreements among employees would be addressed by the technician supervisor. Generally, this position would also involve a great deal of administrative paperwork responsibilities, and often some business management courses would be helpful. The technician supervisor usually reports to the pharmacy manager and must have a good working relationship with management. If this is a position of interest, acquire a copy of the job description and requirements for your facility and be certain that you meet all the requirements.

Pharmacy Warehouse Supervisor

A large hospital facility will require a pharmacy warehouse separate from the hospital warehouse facility so that medications can be more closely monitored. There may be an opportunity for a qualified technician to assume the role of pharmacy warehouse supervisor. This position would require good computer skills, proficiency in using the ordering system, and great organizational skills. A systematic approach to receiving orders, accurately stocking the shelves, and distributing medications to other areas is essential. Adequate procedures for the handling of controlled drugs will prevent the chaos that accompanies discrepancies. This person would also be responsible for handling expired drugs and drug recalls. Interviewing, hiring, and training other technicians working in the pharmacy warehouse would also be parts of the responsibilities of the supervisor, along with scheduling, monitoring attendance, and assigning job duties. Good communication skills will aid in motivating other warehouse technicians and conveying warehouse procedures to other health professionals.

expired drugs Drugs that have passed the date printed on the bottle indicating the manufacturer's guarantee of safety and potency. They must be removed from the shelf according to the protocols of the pharmacy.

drug recalls Official notices (warnings) issued by the manufacturer or the FDA that a drug must be removed from the shelf and returned to the manufacturer. They are classified according to the seriousness of the problem.

Clinical Coordinator for a Pharmacy Technician Program

Pharmacy technician education programs are becoming increasingly prevalent across the country as the need for more competent, educated technicians in the workforce is recognized. Education can be a very rewarding pathway to a fulfilling career as a professional. A logical next step up the career ladder for a technician educator would be a position as clinical coordinator for a formal education program. Classroom instruction about extemporaneous compounding and handling of sterile products may be the responsibility of the clinical coordinator. Supervising laboratory experiences to prepare students for actual experiential time in a pharmacy setting is an important responsibility of the clinical coordinator. Maintaining an inventory of laboratory supplies and placing equipment and supply orders would also be duties of the coordinator. Teaching other classes in the curriculum might be included in the job description, depending on the expertise and credentials of the technician.

clinical coordinator The faculty member who manages the laboratory skills and onsite experience of students in a pharmacy technician education and training program.

The coordinator also serves as a liaison with experiential practice sites and cultivates a relationship with possible preceptors, assisting in their understanding of the important role they play in the education and training of the student. The coordinator meets with the students for discussions about their goals and decides on the practice settings that would be the most productive for the training of each individual student. A booklet is prepared for each student and each clinical rotation. The competencies required of the student will vary depending on whether the setting is inpatient or outpatient. Contained in the booklet will be daily logs to document hours worked by the student and a brief description by the student of the work day. Each student should also fill out an evaluation of the site and the preceptor. For the preceptor there will be a checklist of competencies to be mastered by the student during the rotation, and an evaluation form for the affective behaviors observed in the student.

affective behaviors An important aspect of professionalism. They convey attitude, cooperation, and initiative apart from knowledge and skills.

The clinical coordinator will make regular visits to each site on a predetermined schedule and meet briefly with the preceptor and the student to assess the learning and deal with any concerns. Any serious concerns should be directed to the program director for assessment and resolution. Often the clinical coordinator will also facilitate preparation for job interviews, assist in resumé writing, and help the technician supervisor place students for employment after they complete the educational program. This position requires great organizational skills, outstanding clinical skills, an ability to teach effectively, and good communication skills to develop effective relationships with experiential sites.

Director of the Pharmacy Technician Program

The director of a formal education program is ultimately responsible for the quality and viability of the program. Program directors often have an associate's or a bachelor's degree, and in some cases may have a master's degree and/or may be a pharmacist. In some cases the program director is responsible for developing and implementing every aspect of the program, but often some of the core courses are already in place and provide a foundation for pharmacy technician-specific courses. The total curriculum for the program must be decided and the faculty hired. The Model Curriculum for Pharmacy Technician Training Programs developed by the American Society of Health-System Pharmacists (ASHP) provides a great guideline for this process. Textbooks must be chosen for each course. Admission requirements must be established, keeping in mind the state board of pharmacy guidelines for pharmacy technicians. Depending on the expertise of the program director and the number of faculty available, some courses may be taught by the program director. Other duties could include advertising the program, recruiting students, accepting applications, and selecting students for the program. Advising students can be very time-consuming but also rewarding, as the students share their dreams and goals with you and you help them map out a plan to realize those goals. Advising can also be very difficult when a student has developed an attendance problem or his or her grades have fallen below acceptable standards and an improvement plan must be implemented. The ability to maintain confidentiality about student issues is extremely important in this position, as are organizational, managerial, and teaching skills.

Investigational Drug Pharmacy Technician

investigational drug A drug for which the manufacturer has submitted a New Drug Application to the Federal Drug Administration and received approval to begin trials in humans.

Some large hospital systems are very involved in investigational drug studies and have a department devoted to record-keeping and dispensing of investigational drugs. Skilled technicians are vital to this important aspect of the pharmacy profession. Each study drug has hundreds of protocols outlining everything from the specifications for the patients admitted to the study to the way the drug is labeled and dispensed to patients. The technician is responsible for documenting the many protocols used to validate the study. Confidentiality and accurate documentation are important because the pharmacy personnel may be the only ones who know which patients are taking the actual drug and which are taking placebos in the case of a double-blind study. An ability to read and understand the protocols enables the technician to set up the proper documentation for the various phases of the studies. Exact records of medications must be kept, and any medication not used by a patient must be retrieved because it is not an FDA-approved drug. All of these tasks are performed under the supervision of a pharmacist, but the technician has great responsibilities in a rewarding and professional setting.

Refill Triage Pharmacy Technician

triage A process in which the urgency of each situation is determined and the most urgent problems are resolved first.

In a busy physician's office, the phone rings incessantly and the fax machine continually prints requests from pharmacies for refill authorizations. The office personnel are busy taking care of patients and their immediate needs. A pharmacy technician can be invaluable, especially in a multi-physician office, to organize and triage the requests so that patients can receive their medications in a timely manner. The technician documents all the information from the phone request, along with the call-back number and the pharmacy name. The patient charts are then retrieved and the refill request is checked against the documentation in the chart. The technician should learn the established protocols for refill authorization for patients and note when the patient was last seen in the office. The prescription refills to be called into the pharmacies should be written up on the appropriate form. A similar procedure is followed for requests that are faxed to the office. The prepared forms are placed along with the patient chart in the appropriate place for the prescribers to sign off on the refills. The authorizations can then be faxed back to the pharmacy and the designated person can return the calls for the phoned-in requests. The charts can then be refiled. To be qualified for this position, a technician must have good organizational skills, be fluent in medical terminology and experienced in reading patient charts, and be able to communicate well with the prescribers and work cooperatively with the other office personnel. A strong background in pharmacology, emphasizing brand and generic names and drug uses, will help the technician check the chart for similar drugs that have been prescribed and others that may have been discontinued. If a fast-paced physician's office appeals to you as a possible place to work, prepare yourself educationally, decide whether your personality type fits with this type of work, and contact some physicians and let them know what you are capable of doing for them.

Medication Reconciliation Pharmacy Technician

The Joint Commission Accrediting Healthcare Organizations (JCAHO) has mandated that all patient medications go through a verification process each time the patient is moved from one facility to another or from one unit to another. The medication reconciliation process is designed to prevent duplication of medications ordered by different physicians or by the same physician at different times.

medication reconciliation Process of evaluating the list of drugs a patient is taking against any admission or discharge orders to check for interactions or duplications.

When a patient first enters a healthcare facility, an accurate listing of all medications the patient is currently taking is compiled with information from the patient or a caregiver. This list is compared with the physician admission orders to check for any duplications or discrepancies. The professional judgment of the technician is invaluable at this step and aids in the decision to alert the pharmacist about a medication concern. Discrepancies are then evaluated by a pharmacist using knowledge-based professional judgment to decide whether a medication adjustment is within the pharmacist's scope and standards of practice, or whether a consultation with the physician is required to resolve the issue. Any changes in the physician's orders are documented, and the reconciliation form should become a part of the patient's chart. This form should follow the patients each time they are moved to another unit in the facility and continue with them if they are transferred to another facility or discharged to home.

Each of these steps should be documented according to a previously designed set of protocols established by the institution involved. The institution should have an official reconciliation form to be utilized and guidelines for the qualifications of the staff members allowed to participate in this process. A staff education process should be put into place for all staff involved in this process. In some institutions, this process may be performed by the nursing staff or by pharmacists. This is a process that requires a considerable commitment of time to be effective. An educated pharmacy technician has more knowledge about pharmacology and a better understanding of the medication process, especially concerning brand and generic drug names, drug classes, adverse effects, and interactions, than the nursing staff. A competent pharmacy technician understands the scope of practice and standards of practice, and how they relate to the professional judgment of a technician. A competent, educated, and certified pharmacy technician is trained to exercise the professional judgment of a technician to alert the pharmacist to any discrepancies that require evaluation by the pharmacist. If this position interests you, prepare yourself by excelling in your educational requirements, demonstrating your skills as a staff technician, building a sense of trust with the pharmacists, and consistently proving your professionalism. Then you must make a formal request to train for this position.

TIP **Don't be deterred if someone tells you that pharmacy technicians don't perform that role in a particular facility. Be prepared to demonstrate your ability and desire to be a part of the reconciliation team.**

The increase in third-party insurance companies offering a multitude of plans for prescription coverage has created a need for pharmacy benefit managers (PBMs). PBMs use the formulary specifications of the insurance programs and evaluate prescription drug claims that are received from pharmacies to determine the amount of coverage the plan participant will receive from the insurance company. According to protocols established by the individual companies, with the assistance of clinical pharmacists, the technician will process the claim, refer it for prior authorization by the physician, or recommend that the patient request a similar formulary drug from the prescriber. This process generally takes place during on-line adjudication. The technician will need excellent computer skills; comprehensive knowledge of brand and generic drug names, drug uses, and adverse effects; and a working knowledge of the formularies of each insurance benefit plan, including the quantities allowed. The technician must also have excellent organizational and interpersonal communication skills to assist in answering questions from pharmacies.

prior authorization
Required by insurance companies when a physician prescribes a drug that is not included in the formulary. The physician must call the insurance company or pharmacy benefit manager (PBM) to request coverage.

Computerized Technology Manager

The future of pharmacy depends on the increased use of technology. This will create a vast need for knowledgeable technicians who are qualified to function in the pharmacy environment and can expertly maintain the automated dispensing devices that are becoming a part of every practice setting. A major breakdown in automated equipment can severely compromise patient care in a pharmacy where manual dispensing is not the norm. There may be a great time lag if a technician has to be summoned from the manufacturing company. Having a technician on the premises who is competent in maintenance and repair of all machines will provide a safety net for the practice setting. This may begin as an adjunct to a pharmacy technician staff position. Do personal research on the different systems, especially if the pharmacy is planning to add a new or different system. Offer to serve on the search committee to aid in the decision. Request extra training when the new automated system is added to the pharmacy. Be diligent in learning all you can about pharmacy technology. Pursue any continuing education that will enhance your ability to perform these tasks. Document all training and educational activities, and compile a proposal for the position you seek. Offer to perform these functions in addition to your regular responsibilities until you have proven the need for your services.

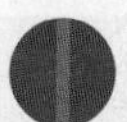

Computer Software Programmer

Pharmacy software programs are becoming more sophisticated as the industry's record-keeping requirements continue to increase. The many specialty practice settings available today have a variety of software specifications and present a great opportunity for the development of software unique to the practice. Large hospital systems and retail chain pharmacies are constantly upgrading their systems to perform added functions to facilitate the daily work load. An educated pharmacy technician with a special interest and some further education in computer programming could be invaluable in developing and evaluating pharmacy software. When the system is installed in the pharmacy, the technician would be well qualified to train all employees on the new system.

Quality Assurance Technician

Medication safety has become a major benchmark for pharmacies everywhere. The technician who is involved with the day-to-day functions performed in the pharmacy is in the best position to observe system problems that may be contributing to medication errors. A quality assurance technician should be familiar with all the established protocols for procedures performed in the pharmacy. These protocols should be evaluated regularly and adapted as needed. The technician in this role should be constantly alert for potential problems that may cause a medication error or a breach of aseptic technique. Documentation of any errors that have occurred and the plan to prevent the error from recurring, along with special training sessions to reinforce skills and education sessions to refresh the memory, would be parts of this role.

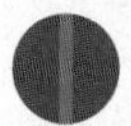

Vision for the Future

This chapter discusses some of the professional duties technicians are performing now or may be performing in the future. That future is in your hands as you begin your journey toward the career goals that are of interest to you. Keep an open mind as you explore this exciting profession because the possibilities are endless. A recent draft of the Long-Range Vision for the Pharmacy Work Force by the ASHP's Council on Education and Work-Force Development described the pharmacy technician of the future with the following role classifications: generalists working in inpatient, ambulatory, chronic, and home care; focused practitioners working in specialty settings; advanced practitioners collecting clinical data for pharmacist evaluation; and managerial roles. Each of these roles would require basic education and training in an accredited pharmacy technician and training program. Each role would require national certification by the Pharmacy Technician Certification Board (PTCB) as soon as possible after completion of the educational program. All pharmacy technicians should be registered by the state BOPs and required to continually update their education. These are the basic requirements of the technician work force of the future according to the vision of the ASHP council. The more advanced roles will require additional experience, education, and credentials. The future is fast approaching! Will you be ready to assume the professional roles awaiting an educated technician?

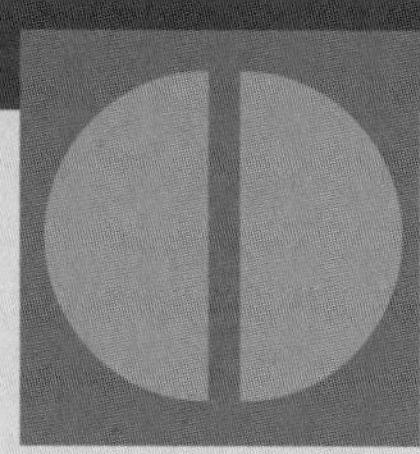

Case Study 3.1

Derek works in the mail-order pharmacy of a large retail establishment. He graduated from an accredited pharmacy technician program and passed the PTCB certification exam last year. He has been working for the past year as a staff technician in a facility where technicians are not considered for any specialty or managerial positions. His profession is very important to him, but he knows he cannot reach his full potential under the current circumstances. Derek requests a conference with Brian, the manager of his department, to see if they can find a solution to his dilemma.

Derek spends the days before the conference assessing his interests and talents, and watching for opportunities to provide a service that would be fulfilling for him and advantageous for the company. The first morning, three different cells in the tablet-dispensing machine jammed and caused a workflow problem in his area. He appeared to be the only person there who was able to remove the cells, clean them, refill them with the correct tablets, and return them to their proper place. Later in the day, when he was on break, he heard that the labeling machine had a label stuck inside and production had to be stopped. He immediately went to the jammed machine and was able to extricate the label. Each time, the technicians were appreciative of his help and he realized this was something he enjoyed. In a large facility such as this, there seemed to be frequent technology problems that frustrated the staff because they interfered with the workflow. Derek began to think about a possible position where he could be responsible for maintaining and repairing the technology and establishing a training program to orient new technicians in the proper use of the machinery. He believed this could save the company a considerable amount of money in terms of lost production hours.

1. Help Derek prepare for his interview with Brian by creating a chart documenting some services he has performed. Include the amount of time he spent, the possible amount of production time he saved (compared with the time involved in calling the company to send a repairman), his ability to set up a regular maintenance schedule to prevent breakdowns, and his willingness to set up a schedule for training other technicians to care for the machinery.
2. Create a dialogue between Derek and Brian as Derek sells his idea to management.

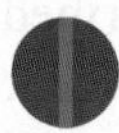

Chapter Summary

- Professionalism involves knowledge and understanding of the pharmacy technician's responsibilities, outstanding skills to perform the required tasks, written and verbal communication skills, and well-developed affective behaviors, including attitude, respect for others, and confidence in one's ability and judgment.
- Professionalism will command the respect of pharmacists, coworkers, and patients.
- Dedication to patient care is the most important aspect of a pharmacy technician's practice.
- Basic pharmacy technician education and training followed by national certification by the PTCB should be the minimum requirements for practicing as a staff technician.

- Responsibilities that are more focused in specialty areas may require additional education and training to meet qualifications.
- Pharmacy technician education programs are increasing in number, mandating an increase in faculty to teach the curriculum.
- With the expansion of the pharmacist's scope of practice, technicians are being promoted to more administrative and managerial positions.
- Specialty practice settings are utilizing the services of pharmacy technicians in more innovative ways.
- New JCAHO requirements are opening the door for technicians to train in new positions.
- Third-party insurance coverage has become so complicated that it often requires a specialist to sort out the details.
- Technology is the wave of the future in pharmacies and requires a technician that is knowledgeable and skillful in the proper maintenance and repair of machines.
- Medication error reduction or elimination is a major benchmark for all pharmacies, and a quality assurance technician can have a great impact on progress.
- Technicians must constantly search for the professional role that will bring them fulfillment, and then prepare educationally by enhancing their skills and demonstrating professional behavior and the professional judgment of a technician in carrying out the responsibilities of their practice.

Review Questions

Multiple Choice

Choose the best answer to the following questions:

1. Investigational drugs are
   a. drugs that have been recalled because of an adverse effect
   b. drugs that are near the expiration date
   c. new drugs that are being tested in humans
   d. drugs that can be manufactured by generic companies

2. Comparing a patient's current drug list on admission to a healthcare facility with the admission orders of the physician is an important part of
   a. on-line adjudication
   b. medication reconciliation
   c. prior authorization
   d. none of the above

3. A pharmacy benefit manager
   a. administers employee benefits
   b. works in the pharmacy
   c. evaluates prescription claims for insurance companies
   d. must be a pharmacist

4. Quality assurance involves
   a. dispensing the right drug
   b. dispensing to the right patient
   c. removing expired drugs from the shelf
   d. all of the above

5. Telephone triage involves
   a. prioritizing phone calls according to their urgency
   b. establishing a communication link between the pharmacy, the patient, and the physician
   c. using a cellular phone, a land line, and a fax machine at the same time for refill call-backs
   d. none of the above

Fill in the Blanks

Fill in the blanks with the correct word or words.

6. The single most important way to reduce infection in a hospital setting is ______________________.

7. The ______________________ of a technician education program is responsible for teaching the laboratory skills and supervising the experience in the pharmacy.

8. A manager of computerized technology would be responsible for the ______________________ of the automated dispensing machines in the pharmacy.

9. National certification is available through the following organization: ______________________.

10. List two detriments to being viewed as a professional
    a. ______________________
    b. ______________________

True/False

Mark the following statements True or False. If the statement is false, change it to make it correct.

11. ________ Mixing intravenous medicine is an example of an affective behavior.

12. ________ Respect as a professional is automatically granted when you complete an educational program.

13. ________ A pharmacy technician can be a director of a pharmacy technician education program.

14. ________ Patient care is the most important part of a technician's job.

15. ________ A preceptor mentors a technician student in the practice setting.

LEARNING ACTIVITY

Jim has been working in the hospital pharmacy for several years and tries to improve his knowledge by continuing his education and reading about new regulations that affect the hospital setting. He reads that the JCAHO now requires medication reconciliation, and the hospital has decided that the pharmacy should be responsible for this task. The pharmacy director is concerned about the time required for this task because his pharmacists are very busy with the clinical care of patients.

Jim believes this is a task that can be performed by certified technicians under the supervision of a pharmacist. He decides to create a form that would facilitate this task and help him present his case to the pharmacy director.

Help Jim by creating a form that would list all the pertinent information for a patient's current medication and any new medications that have been prescribed. Include columns listing the date of admission, current brand name of meds, generic names of drugs, drug class, and directions for use. Include columns for the same information about any new drugs prescribed, and a space for the pharmacist to make notations during the evaluation of the medication regimen. Work individually or in groups to design the form and then compare all forms created by the class for efficiency and clarity. Why do you think this task can be performed by a knowledgeable technician?

UNIT II

Pharmacy Law, Ethics, and Confidentiality

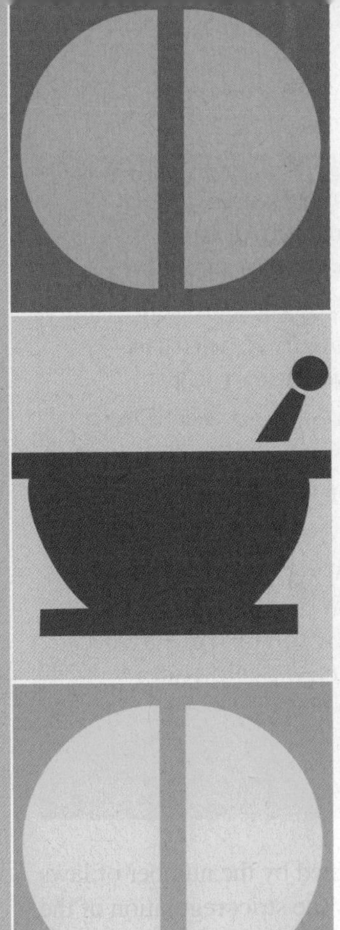

Chapter **4**

Pharmacy Law

OBJECTIVES

After completing this chapter, the student will be able to:

- Discuss reasons for the strict legal regulation of pharmacy operations.
- Explain some common legal terminology pertinent to healthcare.
- Relate some episodes that prompted the passing of the Pure Food and Drug Act of 1906 and the Food, Drug and Cosmetic Act of 1938.
- Describe the differentiation of drugs mandated by the Durham-Humphrey Amendment of 1951.
- Explain the purpose of the Kefauver-Harris Amendment of 1962.
- Outline the phases of the clinical trials for investigational new drugs and differentiate between an NDA, an ANDA, and an SNDA.
- Describe some rights and responsibilities of manufacturers when marketing an FDA-approved drug.
- Demonstrate using the professional judgment of a technician to alert the pharmacist to the possible need for a Medwatch report.
- List important requirements for ordering, storing, and dispensing drugs regulated by the Controlled Substances Act.
- Apply legal regulations to labeling, filling, and dispensing prescriptions.
- Explain laws affecting the labeling and sale of nonprescription drugs, insulin syringes, and exempt narcotics.
- Discuss the new federal law concerning the sale of pseudoephedrine products.

KEY TERMS

- Abbreviated New Drug Application (ANDA)
- adulterated drugs
- black box warning
- brand name
- breach of duty
- burden of proof
- child-resistant cap
- contributory negligence
- Controlled Substances Act
- DEA form 222
- defendant
- direct cause
- drug recalls
- Durham-Humphrey Amendment
- exempt narcotics

- expiration date
- Food, Drug and Cosmetic Act
- four D's of negligence (duty, dereliction of duty, damages, and direct cause)
- generic name
- Good Manufacturing Practices (GMP)
- indication
- institutional review board
- Investigational New Drug Application (INDA)
- Kefauver-Harris Amendment
- malpractice
- Medwatch
- misbranded
- NDC number
- New Drug Application (NDA)
- Omnibus Budget Reduction Act of 1990 (OBRA '90)
- Orphan Drug Act
- patent protection
- package insert
- patient package insert
- plaintiff
- Poison Prevention Packaging Act
- Prescription Drug Marketing Act
- Protected Health Information (PHI)
- pseudoephedrine dispensing law
- Pure Food and Drug Act
- respondeat superior
- standard of care
- State Boards of Pharmacy (BOPs)
- Supplemental New Drug Application (SNDA)
- tort

As a new pharmacy professional, you may be overwhelmed by the number of laws governing your profession. There are several reasons for the strict regulation of the practice of pharmacy. The most important component of every aspect of the practice of pharmacy is the health and safety of the patient. The nature of our profession requires that patients must be able to trust that their medication needs will be met by knowledgeable, competent professionals who are practicing with excellent skills and using the best judgment. Another reason for strict regulation is that pharmacies dispense many dangerous and addictive drugs that may result in drug abuse and the many adverse effects that accompany such abuse. Although the laws may seem restrictive at first, they also provide guidelines to aid and protect pharmacy professionals and patients. The scope of practice and standards of practice for pharmacy technicians are based on laws governing the profession. Understanding and complying with these laws will enhance your professional judgment as a technician and protect you from malpractice issues.

malpractice A form of professional negligence, a careless mistake, breach of confidentiality, or an error in judgment.

Pure Food and Drug Act Act passed in 1906 to regulate the quality, strength, and purity of drugs being marketed in the United States.

Food, Drug and Cosmetic Act Act passed by Congress in 1938 requiring new drugs to be proven safe before marketing. It also extended controls to cosmetics and therapeutic devices.

New Drug Application (NDA) An application that must be filed by a company before marketing a new drug.

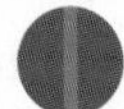 20th-Century Regulation of Drugs

By the end of the 19th century, a number of conditions mandated that the federal government establish some legal regulation of the food and drug industry. Drugs were being manufactured in unsanitary conditions, there were no safeguards in place to ensure that the products being sold were safe for use or effective for the conditions for which they were marketed. Traveling drug salesmen were going from town to town making preposterous claims for their products, which generally had a high alcohol content and sometimes made people feel better temporarily but were often harmful. In 1906 the Pure Food and Drug Act was passed to regulate the strength, quality, and purity of drugs being marketed in this country. This began an attempt to establish stricter oversight by the federal government, but it proved to be ineffective. Several decades later, after sulfanilamide had demonstrated such great success with streptococcal infections during World War I, an oral formulation was marketed that used diethylene glycol to mask the bitter taste of the drug. One hundred and seven people subsequently died from ingesting the poisonous substance, which is often used today as automobile antifreeze. This prompted the passage of the Food, Drug and Cosmetic Act of 1938, which required a premarketing approval process before a new drug could be marketed. Manufacturers were now required to file a New Drug Application (NDA) with the FDA before marketing a new drug. The Food and Drug Administration (FDA) was established to administer these laws and formulate a process for obtaining premarketing approval of a new drug. In 1962 the Kefauver Harris Amendment was passed, which requires drug manufacturers to file an Investigational New Drug Application (INDA) to prove that a product is both safe and effective before filing an NDA for approval to market a product. This process will be discussed later in the chapter.

Kefauver-Harris Amendment Amendment passed in 1962 that requires manufacturers to prove the effectiveness of products before marketing them.

Investigational New Drug Application (INDA) Application that must be filed before a new drug is approved for human testing.

Durham-Humphrey Amendment Law mandating that certain drugs require a prescription written by a licensed practitioner.

state boards of pharmacy (BOPs) Groups of pharmacists, usually appointed by the governor of each state, who convene on a regular basis to govern and direct the practice of pharmacy in that state.

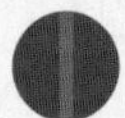

Legal Guidelines for Filling Prescriptions

The Durham-Humphrey Amendment of 1951 mandated that certain drugs would be considered safe for use only under the supervision of a licensed practitioner. Such drugs must be prescribed in writing or transmitted orally to a pharmacist by the prescriber or his or her agent. Prescriptions can only be filled and dispensed under the supervision of a licensed pharmacist. A written prescription must contain certain information about the patient, the prescriber, and the medication and its use. See Figure 4.1 for the required information and the usual location on a prescription. This information should be committed to memory because it is vital to the technician's responsibility for receiving and evaluating prescriptions. Some regulations regarding the requirements for processing prescriptions are governed by the state boards of pharmacy (BOPs). Be sure to learn the rules established by the BOP in the state of your practice.

TIP

Tips for evaluating written prescriptions:

1. **The required information may be in different locations on the prescription.**
2. **Patient information, if missing, may be obtained from the patient.**
3. **Prescriber information, if missing, may be obtained by a call to the prescriber. The technician may call and document the information with the permission of the supervising pharmacist.**
4. **Missing or inaccurate information pertaining to the drug, dosage, or directions must be verified by the pharmacist.**

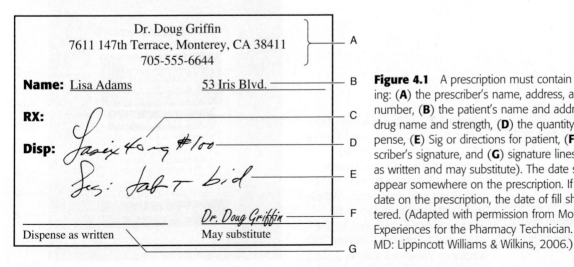

Figure 4.1 A prescription must contain the following: (**A**) the prescriber's name, address, and phone number, (**B**) the patient's name and address, (**C**) the drug name and strength, (**D**) the quantity to dispense, (**E**) Sig or directions for patient, (**F**) the prescriber's signature, and (**G**) signature lines (dispense as written and may substitute). The date should also appear somewhere on the prescription. If there is no date on the prescription, the date of fill should be entered. (Adapted with permission from Mohr ME. Lab Experiences for the Pharmacy Technician. Baltimore, MD: Lippincott Williams & Wilkins, 2006.)

A — PHARMACY TECHNICIAN PHARMACY
5015 S. CAMILLA WAY
317-861-5432

B — RX: 765423 | PRESCRIBER: MAXIM, RICHARD — C

D — PATIENT: MORGAN SPAMBERGER | 1801 S. MERIDIAN WAY

TAKE ONE CAPSULE THREE TIMES A DAY AS DIRECTED BY YOUR PHYSICIAN. — H

F — AMOXICILLIN 250 MG CAPSULES | QUANTITY: 40 CAPSULES — I

G — Ace Pharmaceuticals | 12-20-08 — E

J — NO REFILLS

DISCARD AFTER 12-20-09

Figure 4.2 A prescription label shows the following information: (**A**) pharmacy name, address, and phone number; (**B**) prescription number; (**C**) prescriber's name; (**D**) patient's name; (**E**), date of fill; (**F**) drug name and strength; (**G**) manufacturer's name; (**H**) patient directions; (**I**) quantity dispensed; and (**J**) refills.

Prescription Labels

After the prescription has been evaluated and the information completed, there are laws dictating the information that is required on the prescription label affixed to the vial dispensed to the patient. See Figure 4.2 for an example of a prescription label and the required information. Most pharmacy software systems will prompt you for the required information. Auxiliary labels should be attached with care so that pertinent information on the label is not covered up.

Medications requiring a prescription must be labeled by the manufacturer with the words "Rx only according to the FDA Modernization Act to replace the older statement 'Federal Law Prohibits Dispensing Without a Prescription.'" The law requires other information to be on the label, as shown in Figure 4.3. It is important

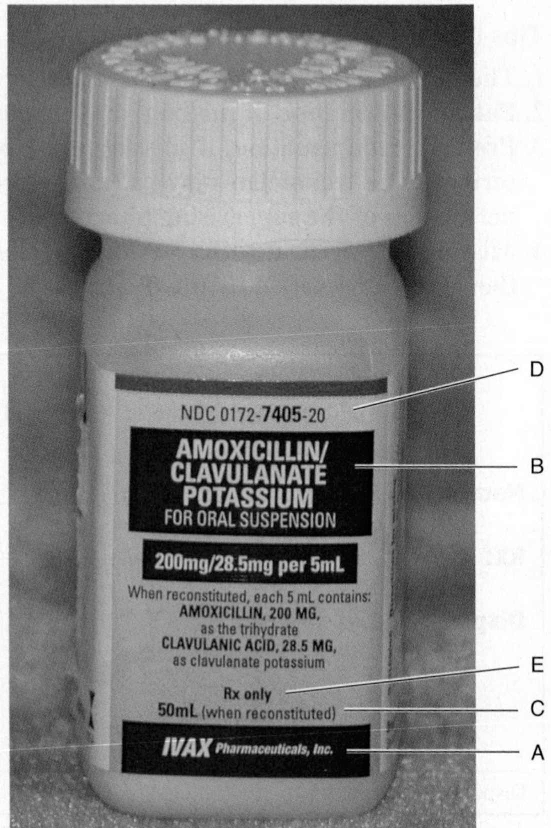

Figure 4.3 A label of a manufacturer's product contains the following: (**A**) manufacturer's name, (**B**) generic name, (**C**) total volume after reconstitution, (**D**) NDC number, and (**E**) Rx only designation. (Adapted with permission from Lacher BE. Pharmaceutical Calculations for the Pharmacy Technician. Baltimore, MD: Lippincott Williams & Wilkins, 2008.)

generic name Specific name given to a drug by the United States Adopted Names (USAN) Council; official name of a drug listed in the USP along with the standards that must be met to make it official regardless of the manufacturer.

for the technician to accurately check the information on the bottle to determine that it is the correct drug, strength, and dosage form, and is not expired. The NDC number is a drug identifier that will assist in verifying the correct drug. The NDC number is a 10- or 11-digit number. The first four or five digits are a number assigned to the manufacturer by the FDA and will be the same for all drug products manufactured by that company; the second four digits are a number assigned by the manufacturer to identify a specific drug, dosage form, and strength; and the last two digits signify the package size of the product. Notice the NDC number on the label in Figure 4.3.

NDC number Identifying number given to each prescription drug before it is marketed.

package insert Informational sheet required to be included by the manufacturer in drug packaging intended for health professionals.

black box warning Warning included by the manufacturer at the beginning of the package insert concerning a serious adverse effect.

indication Condition for which a drug has been approved by the FDA.

patient package insert (PPI) Patient information sheet that is required to be given to the patient for certain drugs before the first dose is taken.

Package Inserts

Valuable information about a drug is included in the package insert. Included in the insert will be any black box warning, information about the chemical structure of the drug, the indication, minimum and maximum doses, and adverse effects and contraindications of the drug. Package inserts are being redesigned by manufacturers to make pertinent information more readily available. In addition to the package insert, which is written in technical language and intended as information for the health professional, many drugs require a patient package insert (PPI). The patient must receive the insert before administration of the first dose of the drug (if the patient is in an institution) or before receiving the original prescription in an outpatient setting. The technician should be aware of medications that require a PPI and place it with the filled prescription. Some drugs that require a PPI are listed below:

- Accutane or isotretinoin
- antidepressants
- Cytotec
- NSAIDs
- oral cancer meds
- products containing estrogen
- products containing progesterone
- "statin" drugs used to lower cholesterol

Caps

When the correct product has been secured from the shelf and the label accurately printed, the technician may count or pour the prescribed amount of medication into an appropriate container and apply a child-resistant cap. Child-resistant caps are mandated by the Poison Prevention Packaging Act; however, the following drugs are exempt from the requirement:

- sublingual nitroglycerin
- sublingual and chewable isosorbide dinitrate <10 mg
- cholestyramine and colestipol powder packs
- inhalation aerosols
- Mebendazole with <600 mg/package
- Prednisone <105 mg per package
- Methylprednisolone <84 mg per package
- Pancrelipase preparations
- oral contraceptives in dialpaks

child-resistant cap Special safety caps required on prescription vials by the Poison Prevention Packaging Act to reduce poisoning in children.

Poison Prevention Packaging Act Act that requires the use of safety closures on all prescription drugs and most over-the-counter drugs to protect children from accidental poisoning.

- potassium supplements in unit dose packaging
- aspirin and acetaminophen effervescent tabs
- sodium fluoride <264 mg per pack

The patient or the prescriber may request in writing that non-child-resistant caps be used on a prescription, and this request should be documented on the prescription and in the computer for future reference. This should be done for each new prescription.

CAUTION **Remember, these caps are child-resistant, not child-proof.**

The prescription container may then be labeled, including any necessary auxiliary labels, and left with the medication bottle and paperwork for the final check by the pharmacist.

TIP **If the patient makes an OTC purchase that may cause an interaction with the prescription(s), politely excuse yourself before completing the sale and alert the pharmacist to your concern.**

Additional Legal Requirements for Controlled Drug Prescriptions

Controlled Substances Act Legislation by Congress to regulate the sale of habit-forming and addictive drugs.

The Controlled Substances Act (CSA) of 1970 classified drugs into five schedules according to their potential for abuse. Dispensing, handling, and storage requirements vary according to the schedule, so it is imperative for the technician to be cognizant of the classification of controlled drugs. Commercial containers of controlled drugs are required to have the schedule stamped on the label (such as C-II for a schedule II drug). These drugs can only be prescribed by a prescriber who is registered under the CSA and possesses a Drug Enforcement Administration (DEA) number, and must be filled in a pharmacy or institution with a valid DEA number. Some institutions, such as hospitals, allow prescribers working in their institution who have not yet received a DEA number (interns and residents) to use the DEA number of the institution with a numerical suffix, such as the last four digits of their Social Security number. This number is only valid while they are actually working in the institution and cannot be used for prescribing at another facility.

Schedule I drugs have a high potential for abuse and no accepted use in the United States. Included in this schedule are heroin, marijuana, peyote, and other hallucinogens.

Schedule II drugs also have a high abuse potential, but are considered to have a legitimate use in this country. Some general categories of drugs in this class are opium and opium derivatives, amphetamines, some barbiturates, and other drugs predicted to cause extreme physical or psychological dependence if abused. Schedule II drugs require a new written prescription each time they are filled. The physician may write refills on the prescription but they cannot be legally refilled, so the refills should not be entered into the computer. The prescription must be written in indelible ink or typewritten and have the actual written signature of the prescriber. The prescriber's DEA number must be on the prescription. The prescriber may not call or fax a prescription for a schedule II drug into the pharmacy unless it is an emergency situation. If it is an oral prescription, the pharmacist must immediately reduce it to writing, and "authorization for emergency dispensing" must be written on the face of the prescription. Within seven days the physician must supply a written prescription to the pharmacy. Some states have more stringent requirements, such as requiring the prescription to be written on safety paper or a duplicate form to be sent to the DEA office. Be sure to learn the special laws of your state. When state and federal laws differ, the stricter of the two must be followed. A schedule II prescription may be partially filled when the total amount is not in stock. The quantity dispensed and the dispensing date must be recorded on the face of the prescription, and the remainder must be dispensed within 72 hours of the original fill or the remaining quantity must be voided and the physician informed of the partial fill.

All prescriptions for controlled drugs must bear on the prescription label the following statement: "Caution: Federal law prohibits the transfer of this drug to any person other than the patient for whom it was prescribed." The prescription label must also contain the name and address of the pharmacy; the name of the prescriber; the name of the patient; the prescription number; the name, strength, and quantity of the medication; the directions for use; and the date filled. It is helpful to indicate the number of refills (if any) and the expiration date of the refills (e.g., five refills by May 5, 2008).

expiration date Refills for controlled drugs expire after 6 months.

Schedules III, IV, and V prescriptions also must be written or typed in indelible ink or typewritten and signed by the prescriber. (Some states require that controlled-drug prescriptions be handwritten.) These prescriptions may be refilled up to five times in a six-month period. The prescription expires after six months regardless of the number of refills left. The drugs may be called in orally or faxed to the pharmacy directly from the prescriber's office. No new prescription may be faxed or called in to the pharmacy by the patient.

CAUTION

Patients often will call and ask that a prescription on file be refilled even though there are no refills available, because they will be bringing in a new prescription from the doctor. This is very risky because the doctor may have changed the dose or directions on the updated prescription. These changes may be overlooked if the prescription has been prepared before the new prescription is evaluated.

Schedules III and IV drugs have accepted medical uses and a proportionately lower potential for abuse. Schedule III drugs are often compounds with limited quantities of narcotics, and schedule IV drugs include tranquilizers and minor hypnotics. The dispensing regulations are the same for both of these schedules.

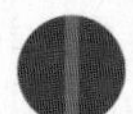

Exempt Narcotics

Schedule V drugs contain very small amounts of narcotics. They are generally products used as antitussives or antidiarrheals. Some may require a prescription, but many are considered exempt narcotics. Exempt narcotics may be sold without a prescription, except in states where prohibited, when special regulations are followed. Such medications can be sold only by a pharmacist, although the actual transaction may be carried out by the technician after the pharmacist has performed his or her professional responsibilities. The purchaser of an exempt narcotic must be at least 18 years old and present identification (if not personally known to the pharmacist). The purchaser's name and address, and the drug, quantity, and date purchased must be placed on record in an exempt-narcotics record book. This book must be kept in the pharmacy for a period of 2 years after the last dated entry, and be readily available for inspection by the state BOP or federal inspectors when requested. The quantities purchased are limited to 240 mL (8 oz) or 48 solid dosage units of any substance containing opium products, and 120 mL (4 oz) or 24 solid

exempt narcotics Controlled drugs that can be sold in limited quantities without a prescription.

dosage units of any other schedule V product in a 48-hour period to the same purchaser without a prescription.

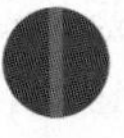

Storage, Theft, and Mailing Requirements for Controlled Drugs

Schedules II, III, IV, and V drugs must either be stored in a locked cabinet or dispersed among the noncontrolled drugs on the shelves. They cannot be kept together in one section on an open shelf. A combination of these two storage methods may be used, such as storing schedule II drugs in a safe or locked cabinet and dispersing the other controlled drugs through the stock. Any theft or loss of controlled substances must be reported to the DEA. Likewise, the theft or loss of schedule II order forms must be reported to the DEA.

Controlled substances can be mailed to a patient's home in reasonable quantities pursuant to a valid prescription and for the personal use of the patient. They should be packaged in a plain box or wrapper that gives no indication of the contents.

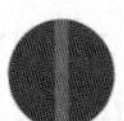

Record-Keeping for Controlled Drugs

Records of all receiving and dispensing of controlled drugs must be kept in a place separate from other records for a period of at least 2 years (state regulations may require longer periods of time). These records must include a biennial inventory of all controlled substances in stock at the time. During this inventory, all schedule II drugs must be counted exactly. The count of schedule III, IV, or V drugs can be estimated unless the container holds 1000 or more tablets or capsules. In this case, an exact count must be made. Although the DEA does not require a copy of this inventory, some states require pharmacies to send the agency a copy. The records for schedule II drugs should be separated from the other schedules. Many pharmacies keep a daily schedule of C-IIs and enter each dispensing transaction as it occurs. This helps to verify the transactions on a daily basis, and if a discrepancy occurs, it can be more easily tracked.

Prescription files can be organized in several ways to manage the record-keeping requirements. A three-file system would require C-IIs to be filed in one file; C-III, -IV, and -V drugs in another file; and all noncontrolled drugs in a third file. A two-file system would require all C-IIs to be filed in a separate file, and all C-III, -IV, and -V drugs would be filed with all the noncontrolled drugs. Each controlled drug would be required to have a large red C, not less than one inch high, stamped on the face of the prescription in the lower-right corner. Another form of a two-file system would have all the noncontrolled drugs in one file and all the controlled drugs in a second file. This would also require that drugs in schedules III, IV, and V have the red C stamped in the lower-right corner unless the pharmacy uses a computerized system that indicates controlled drugs. State regulations may vary, so be sure to check the requirements of your state.

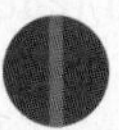

Ordering Controlled Drugs

Schedules III, IV, and V drugs may be ordered along with noncontrolled items either by phone or by computer entry. The ordering pharmacy must have a valid DEA number on file with the wholesaler filling the order. When the order is delivered, the controlled drugs will be in a separate tote (usually locked), and will be listed on an invoice separate from the noncontrolled drugs. The delivering driver may require the signature of the pharmacist verifying that the order was received. The contents of the tote should be carefully checked against the invoice and/or packing list, and any discrepancies reported immediately to the pharmacist. The invoice should be dated and initialed by the person checking the order. A copy of the invoice and/or packing slip should be stored in a special file so that it can be readily available if an inspector needs to see it.

Schedule II drugs must be ordered using DEA form 222. This form can be obtained from the regional DEA office nearest the pharmacy. It can also be ordered on-line by registered applicants. It will be preprinted with the name, address, and registration number of the pharmacy. Only the authorized registrant or an agent who has been given power of attorney may sign the order form to place an order. The order forms are in triplicate and come in books of seven forms each. They must be completed in triplicate on a typewriter or with an indelible-ink pen. There are 10 item lines on each form and each line may contain only one product. For instance, if the same drug is available in both capsules and tablets in the same strength, they must be listed on two separate lines. If less than 10 items are ordered, the remaining lines must be voided and the total number of lines indicated at the bottom of the form. The wholesaler cannot make any changes on the form, so if there is an error, the form must be voided and returned to the pharmacy. This can present a problem if a patient needs pain medication and must wait several more days to receive the medication. When the form is complete, it must be dated and signed by the authorized purchaser and separated. Copies 1 and 2 must remain intact with the carbon between them. The purchaser retains copy 3 in the file until the order is received and sends the order to the distributor. When the order is received, the purchaser documents the items received on the order form copy and files it in the schedule II file. If a running inventory is being kept, the items received should be entered into the inventory book. A DEA form 222 can only be signed by the registrant or a person who has a power-of-attorney form on file with the DEA. This form must be kept with the controlled-substances inventory and invoice records, and be available for inspection by a state or federal inspector requesting it.

DEA form 222 Order form obtained from DEA and required for ordering schedule II drugs.

Professional Judgment Scenario 4.1

Marjorie is a pharmacy technician working in an outpatient pharmacy. She has been working in this position for several years and is responsible for inventory control in the pharmacy. She orders all the medications, checks in the orders, and puts the orders away. The pharmacist has learned to trust her because she has always maintained the inventory at proper levels. Marjorie realized that it would be easy for her to increase the order for Vicodin by a couple of bottles of 100 tablets each week. Her son had become involved in selling drugs and told her he would split the profits with her if she supplied him with Vicodin. At first Marjorie was apprehensive when she increased the amount of Vicodin ordered. When the order arrived the next day, the pharmacist signed for the tote of controlled drugs and Marjorie took it to the back counter to check the order. She placed the two extra bottles of Vicodin in the pockets of her smock and later transferred them to her purse. She checked in the rest of the order and carefully placed each item on the correct shelf. She initialed and dated the invoice to document that all items were received and placed the controlled drug invoice in the correct file. She was very nervous when she left the pharmacy with the two bottles of Vicodin, but there were no problems and she arrived home safely with the drugs.

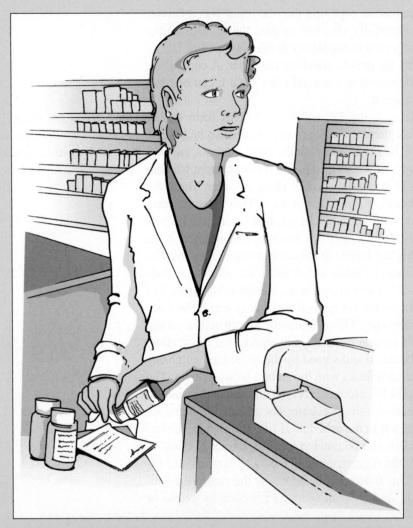

Her son took the bottles that evening and returned home several hours later with $800.00, which he divided evenly with Marjorie. Although Marjorie felt some pangs of guilt, she quickly realized that in a few weeks she could replace her faulty dishwasher with the deluxe model she had been dreaming of for so long. Each week as Marjorie placed the order, it became easier to increase the order. Soon she was bringing home five to six bottles of 100 Vicodin tablets each week, and her son had no problem selling them for $4 to $5 per tablet.

When the inspector from the state BOP arrived for his yearly inspection, he asked to see the file containing the controlled-drug invoices. As he studied the invoices, he noticed that there had been a dramatic increase in the amount of Vicodin purchased during the past year. He asked the pharmacist if there had been an increase in the number of Vicodin prescriptions filled. The pharmacist had not noticed any increase in Vicodin prescriptions, but noted that there was no overstock on the shelf so they must be using the greater quantity. When questioned about the increased orders, Marjorie became very nervous and had difficulty responding to the questions. When they obtained the daily controlled-drug prescription report from the computer, the pharmacist and the state board inspector realized that something was terribly wrong. The DEA was notified and an investigation was launched.

1. What legal and moral issues are involved in this situation?
2. What prompted Marjorie to override her professional judgment and become involved in this crime?
3. Discuss the legal penalties that Marjorie may face as a result of this.
   a. Should she lose her license to practice as a technician?
   b. Will she lose the respect of family and friends?
   c. Will her son also face legal prosecution?
4. How much did the pharmacist's negligence in properly supervising Marjorie contribute to this situation?
5. Will the pharmacist also face prosecution and the possibility of losing his license to practice pharmacy?
6. Discuss the shame and regret Marjorie must deal with as her crime becomes public knowledge and she realizes that she has betrayed the pharmacist who trusted her, and will probably serve time in jail.

Authorized Prescribers for Controlled Drugs

Physicians, dentists, and veterinarians who are registered with the DEA are authorized to prescribe controlled substances in accordance with the CSA regulations. Residents and interns who are working in an institution but have not yet registered with the DEA may be allowed to prescribe controlled substances using the DEA number of the institution followed by a hyphen and an individual code number. In recent years, a number of mid-level practitioners have been allowed to register with the DEA and prescribe or administer controlled substances. This authority varies greatly from state to state, so it is important to be familiar with the laws of your state. Examples of mid-level practitioners are nurse practitioners, physician assistants, and optometrists. Their prescribing authority is limited to their particular scope of practice. DEA numbers are assigned according to the type of registrant. Before October 1985, the DEA numbers of regular practitioners began with the letter A followed by the first letter of the registrant's last name. After this date the registration number began with a B followed by the first letter of the last name. The number for a mid-level provider begins with an M followed by the first letter of the last name. A valid DEA number consists of two letters (the second letter is the first letter of the prescriber's last name) followed by seven digits.

TIP

The following formula will aid in verifying a DEA number: add the first, third, and fifth digits of the number. Add the second, fourth, and sixth digits of the number and multiply this sum by two. Add the results of the first two calculations, and the last digit of the sum should be the same as the last digit of the DEA number.

Professional Judgment Scenario 4.2

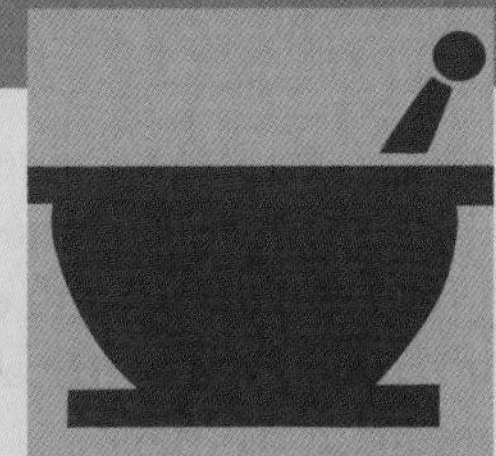

Terri greets a patient she has not met before. He hands her a prescription for Vicodin 5/500 tablets #200 with the directions 1 po q6h prn pain. The prescription was written by Dr. Sam Belden. Dr. Belden's address, phone number, and signature are on the prescription along with the DEA number (BB 6384191). Formulate a case study answering the following questions:

1. What information does Terri need to obtain from the patient?
2. Does this seem to be a valid DEA number for Dr. Belden?
3. Terri has seen Dr. Belden's signature before and this looks like his writing, but she's never known him to write for large quantities of controlled drugs. Does the number "200" on the prescription concern you? If so, what would you do?
4. What action would you expect Marie, the pharmacist, to take after hearing Terri's concern?
5. If the physician's office verifies that the quantity prescribed was 20 tablets and asks that the prescription be voided, how might Marie convey this to the patient?

Sam Belden, M.D.
1206 N. Grant Street
Peoria, IL 54320

(216) 5465-3832 DEA# BB6384191

Name: Collin O'Gara **AGE:** ______
Address: 7043 N. Waston Blvd, Peoria, IL 54326 **DATE:** 7-8-08

RX: Vicodin 5/500

Disp: 200
1 po q6h prn pain

Refills: 0 SBelden MD

Dispense as written May substitute

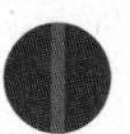

Investigational New Drug Application

The approval process for a new drug is quite lengthy and very costly. The average compound will require 12 to 15 years of testing before it will be approved for marketing to the general public. After up to 70 clinical trials the FDA may consider a drug to be safe, but that does not mean it is risk free. All drugs have adverse effects, but they should be used when the benefits outweigh the risks for a given patient. This is why prescription drugs are only safe for use under the supervision of a qualified health professional who can evaluate the risk-benefit ratio for each patient.

The first part of the process is called the drug discovery process. In this phase, scientists search for compounds with therapeutic benefits. They may be searching for a particular effect or they may discover a therapeutic action by accident while attempting to modify a known drug. The compounds may be formulated synthetically in the laboratory or they may be natural compounds that have existed for many years. When a drug shows a promising therapeutic benefit, the scientists begin to make alterations to increase the benefit and reduce adverse effects. At this point they begin the preclinical testing in the lab using animals such as rats and mice to evaluate toxic effects in both the animals and their offspring, and establish a dose that will be nontoxic. This process usually takes 6 to 7 years before they are ready to submit an INDA to the FDA requesting permission to begin clinical trials and outlining a protocol for the trials. This protocol must be prepared with the approval of an institutional review board (IRB) composed of scientists, investigators, and a nonscientific layperson. This board will continue to follow the trials to be sure the protocols are followed and patients' rights are protected.

institutional review board A group of medical professionals and a layperson who oversee clinical trials for a new drug.

Phase I trials are conducted with a small number of healthy human patients to determine the maximum tolerated dose of the drug that will produce no adverse toxicity. These trials typically last 1½ to 2 years.

Phase II focuses on the efficacy of the drug in a group of 100 to 300 volunteer patients who exhibit the indication for which the drug will be marketed. Various dosage regimens may be utilized and any adverse events will be noted along with effectiveness of the drug. Phase II testing will proceed for about 2 years, and if efficacy is shown without significant toxicity, the drug will proceed to phase III trials.

Medwatch Federal reporting process for adverse events of drug therapy.

Phase III trials involve many more patients (often 1000–3000) in some very complex studies that involve many different institutions and last several years. It may be a double-blind study in which neither the researcher nor the patient knows whether the patient is receiving the study drug or another compound. Again, the researcher is searching for efficacy and safety, and may be testing against a similar drug already on the market for the same indication. If these trials are favorable, an NDA will be filed with the FDA and a decision will be made about the approval of the drug. This process usually takes another 1½ to 2 years.

patent protection The manufacturer has the exclusive right to market a drug until the patent expires.

Abbreviated New Drug Application (ANDA) Must be filed by a generic company before it markets its generic version of a brand-name drug to prove its bioequivalence to the brand-name drug.

During phase IV, the postmarketing period, researchers continue to monitor the drug for efficacy and adverse events as it is used in larger populations and in patients with multiple medical problems. It is very important to report serious or unusual adverse events to the FDA through a reporting process called Medwatch. The manufacturer is granted patent protection for a period not to exceed 14 years after the product is approved. This means that the manufacturer has the exclusive right to market that drug until the patent expires. After the patent expires, a generic company can file an Abbreviated New Drug Application (ANDA) demonstrating that its product's properties, bioavailability, and clinical activity are the same as those of the original product. The generic form of the drug can then be marketed by the generic company at a substantially lower price than the brand name drug. If a manufacturer decides to make minor changes in the procedures for making the drug, the company can submit a Supplemental New Drug Application (SNDA), which is considerably shorter than the NDA.

brand name The trade name given to a drug by the manufacturer for marketing purposes.

Supplemental New Drug Application (SNDA) Application for FDA approval for a generic company to make minor changes in manufacturing procedure for a generic drug

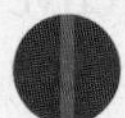 Expiration Dates and Drug Recalls

There are several reasons why drugs may need to be removed from the shelf before they are used. The FDA has published good manufacturing practices (GMP) requiring that an expiration date be placed on the container when it is released for sale. This date must be established by stability testing based on certain storage and packaging conditions. The expiration date is the manufacturer's promise that the drug will retain its potency until this date as long as these conditions are met. If the date is stated as July 2008, the drug will expire on the last day in July 2008. If the expiration date is July 1, 2008, the drug will expire on the first of July. An important responsibility of the technician is to establish a routine for checking expiration dates and removing items from the shelf according to the protocol of the practice setting. Most practice settings will remove drugs from the shelf when they are within 4 to 6 weeks of the manufacturer's expiration date.

good manufacturing practices (GMP) Regulations that set minimum standards to be followed by the manufacturing industry for human and veterinarian drugs. Standards should also be observed for extemporaneous compounds.

When filling a prescription, technicians should make the expiration date a part of the "check three times" process.

TIP

Drugs that are repackaged by the pharmacy should be labeled with an expiration date that is 1 year from the date of repackaging or the expiration date on the original package, whichever is shorter. Most pharmacy software automatically prints an expiration date that is 1 year from the fill date. That expiration date should be changed if the true expiration date is earlier than 1 year.

When a problem is discovered in a drug product after it has been marketed, the manufacturer may issue a drug recall. Drug recalls are divided into three classes according to the seriousness of the problem. The recall may be initiated by the manufacturer or, if the problem may cause serious side effects, the FDA may request a voluntary removal of the product. It is the manufacturer's responsibility to send written recall notices to all wholesalers and retailers. It is the responsibility of the pharmacist and technician to read and act on the recall. Occasionally, the recall will be announced in the news media before the official recall is received. The technician should be alert for any news of this kind and be diligent about removing the products from the shelf. Usually a recall will be accompanied by a form detailing the affected product, with lot numbers and expiration dates. The form should be filled out listing the number of items found, and the directions for return of items should be followed. If none of the affected lot numbers is found, this should be documented on the form and a copy kept in a recall file in the store to verify that a check was conducted for the items. The classes of drug recalls are as follows:

drug recalls Official notices (warnings) issued by the manufacturer or the FDA that a drug must be removed from the shelf and returned to the manufacturer. They are classified according to the seriousness of the problem.

- Class I: may cause serious health problems, even death. Notify patients who have received the drug.
- Class II: no serious effects but may cause temporary or reversible effects.
- Class III: possibly a labeling problem; not likely to cause health problems.

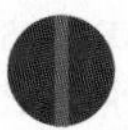 Nonprescription Medications

Drugs that may be legally sold without a prescription are required to have seven items of information on the label: the product name; package contents; name and address of manufacturer, packager, or distributor; list of all active ingredients and some inactive ingredients (such as alcohol); name of any habit-forming ingredient; cautions and warnings for the user; and adequate directions for safe and effective use of the product. A nonprescription medication that is written as a prescription by a prescriber should be relabeled with the information required on a prescription medication label, including the directions for use ordered by the prescriber and any auxiliary labels needed for safe use of the drug. The hard copy should be handled as any other prescription and filed according to protocol. When a prescription drug is changed to nonprescription status, any remaining drug in the manufacturer's original container with the prescription drug labeling must be relabeled to include the expanded OTC information before it can be sold without a prescription. Failure to do this will result in the drug being misbranded. Pharmacies can continue to use the remainder of the drug in the manufacturer's prescription package to fill prescriptions if it is dispensed with a valid prescription label.

misbranded Labeling error or difference between the label information and the actual product.

Some nonprescription items have special restrictions regarding their sale. Many states require that a signature log be maintained for the sale of insulin syringes because they are often purchased for administration of illegal drugs. Also, nonprescription drugs containing ephedrine or pseudoephedrine alone or as an ingredient in a compound are subject to very strict guidelines at both federal and state levels. According to the new federal pseudoephedrine dispensing law, such products must be kept behind the counter or in a locked cabinet. A logbook must be kept identifying the product name, amount sold, name and address of the purchaser, and date and time of sale. All staff members who handle these products are required to undergo training, and purchasers must be 18 years old and provide photo identification at the time of purchase. There are daily and monthly limits on the amounts of these products that can be purchased, but the limits vary by state. Quantity restrictions generally do not apply to medications written as a prescription. These restrictions have been put in place because pseudoephedrine is often used in the illegal manufacture of methamphetamine.

pseudoephedrine dispensing law Federal law regulating the sale of products containing pseudoephedrine.

TIP **A new class of drugs is emerging that can be sold without a prescription but must be obtained in the pharmacy. Cough preparations containing dextromethorphan are being abused, and it is possible that these products will soon be required to be stored in the pharmacy. Plan B, the new product for emergency contraception, requires that the purchaser be at least 18 years of age. Be alert for news of restrictions on OTC products so that your pharmacy will be in compliance with the laws.**

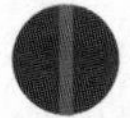 Poisonous Substances

A substance that may be destructive to human life if taken in a quantity of 60 grains or less is classified as a poison. The dispensing rules for these substances vary from state to state, but there are certain guidelines that must be followed regarding labeling. The container must be labeled with the name of the drug and the word "poison," and the name and address of the manufacturer or seller. Most states require the pharmacy to keep a logbook and ascertain that the substance is being purchased for a lawful purpose. Pouring a poisonous substance into a smaller container for sale without adequate labeling is extremely dangerous and illegal.

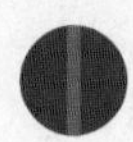

Transferring Prescriptions Between Pharmacies

In our mobile society, it is very common for patients to request that a prescription filled in a particular pharmacy be available for refills at another location. There are set procedures for accomplishing this to accommodate the needs of the patient and still maintain accurate records to fulfill legal requirements. Most major chain pharmacies have their computers linked so that all pertinent information can be obtained electronically, and a phone call will not be necessary. Likewise, all required documentation related to the dispensing and refill calculations can be applied electronically. However, if a prescription is transferred between pharmacies that are not electronically linked, certain information is required at both the transferring and receiving pharmacies to ensure the integrity of the physician's order.

The transferring pharmacy (the pharmacy that originally filled the prescription) must write "void" on the face of the original prescription and record the following information on the back of the original and/or in the computer records for the prescription: the original date the transfer is taking place; the name, address, and DEA number of the receiving pharmacy; and the name of the receiving pharmacist. This part of the information can be legally conveyed between two technicians. The technician at the transferring pharmacy can document this information, but the actual prescription information (drug name, strength, quantity, directions, and refill status) must be transmitted by the pharmacist. The pharmacy receiving the prescription must write "transfer" at the top of the prescription and record the following information on the prescription: the date the prescription was written and the date of the first fill; the name, address, and DEA number of the transferring pharmacy; and the name of the pharmacist. The pharmacist must convey the prescription information, including the drug name, strength, quantity, directions, and refill status, to the receiving pharmacist and document the date of the transfer on the prescription. Both pharmacies must retain these records for at least 2 years. Some of these regulations may vary by state, so be aware of the requirements in your state, especially if a controlled substance is involved. Also, some pharmacists may prefer to perform the entire transfer process themselves. As always, the supervising pharmacist's preference must be respected. As you continue to work with competence and professionalism, you will gain the respect of the pharmacist and be trusted with more responsibility.

This chapter has presented some of the basic pharmacy laws to guide you in your practice as a technician. As you begin your practice, be diligent about staying current with new regulations. Be alert for situations that may present variations of the law and require professional judgment for resolution. Your professional judgment is a skill that will grow with your experience as a technician. If there is any doubt about how a particular situation should be handled, always defer to the professional judgment of the pharmacist, unless you are certain that it will create an illegal situation or cause harm to a patient. In the unlikely event that a pharmacist is making poor decisions or willfully breaking the law, you must use your professional judgment to decide on a course of action. Methods for making these decisions will be discussed in the ensuing chapters.

Torts and Legal Liability

Most laws affecting the practice of pharmacy are classified under the subdivision of civil law called tort law. Torts involve personal injury and the breach of a duty

tort A law concerning personal injury.

breach of duty Not providing a reasonable amount of care in performing a duty that is expected of a technician.

four D's of negligence Duty, dereliction of duty, damages, and direct cause.

direct cause A determination of whether an action or inaction was the reason for the harm done to a patient.

standard of care The quality of care expected from a professional in the practice of his or her profession.

defendant The person against whom a legal complaint has been brought.

plaintiff The party bringing a complaint against a defendant.

burden of proof The person filing the complaint must prove that the defendant committed a violation.

that has been established by law. The breach of duty must have caused some degree of harm to a person or his property. An unintentional tort would be called negligence, and certain factors must be present to constitute professional negligence (also called malpractice). These factors are known as the four D's of negligence:

- Duty: Was there a duty to do something that was not done, or to not do something that was done?
- Dereliction: Was there a breach of that duty?
- Damages: Were damages, such as physical or emotional injury, incurred?
- Direct cause: Did an action that was performed or not performed directly cause the injury?

The question of duty will be decided in a court case by determining what level of action a reasonable person with the same education and in a similar position would have taken or not taken in that situation. This duty is delineated by the scope of practice of the person involved. Often, in the case of a technician, several other technicians will be asked to comment on whether the involved technician acted in a reasonable manner and within the boundaries of the scope of practice of a technician in a similar position. The patient is entitled to a certain standard of care for the practice setting and community where service is rendered. Technicians should be aware of the standard of care in their practice settings and exceed the standard when possible. A civil suit of negligence brought against a defendant by a plaintiff must prove that there was damage and that the damage was a direct result of the action or inaction of the defendant. The burden of proof is on the plaintiff. The defendant may also claim that there was contributory negligence on the part of the plaintiff. For example, if the plaintiff requested non-safety caps on her prescription medicine and left the bottle within reach of her granddaughter, the pharmacy may not be liable for any damages that occurred as a result of the child ingesting the medicine. However, if the plaintiff signed a request for non-safety caps several years ago and there is no documentation for a current update to the request, the pharmacy may at least share in the liability if a child ingests some of the medicine.

CAUTION **Don't forget the importance of documenting and updating requests for non-child-resistant caps on prescriptions each time they are filled.**

contributory negligence An action or inaction on the part of the patient or a family member that caused or increased the risk of harm.

respondeat superior Term holding an employer responsible for contractual agreements made by employee in the name of the company.

A contract is an agreement between two parties that goods or services will be provided in an agreed-on manner. An employee in a business becomes the agent of the employer and enters into contractual agreements that are binding for the employer in the normal course of duty. The Latin term *respondeat superior*, meaning "let the master respond," has been coined to describe this situation. When a technician accepts a prescription, whether it is a refill ordered on the phone or a new prescription brought into the pharmacy, the technician is acting as an agent of the pharmacist and entering into a contract to provide the expected service. This can be extended to helping a patient with OTC products and answering a physician's questions about products. A technician should be very cognizant of the fact that in all their professional functions they are acting as an agent of the supervising pharmacist. The pharmacist will be held liable for the technician's actions, but technicians also assume liability as they become better educated and more respected as professionals. Professionalism demands increased knowledge, skills, and respect, but it also involves an increased risk of liability as the scope of practice of a technician is broadened and the standard of care expected of a technician is increased.

Defamation of character is another tort that is based on a false communication about another person that causes harm to his or her reputation. If it is in the form of a written statement, it is called libel, and if it is an oral statement it is called slander. It may be tempting to make a disparaging comment about a difficult patient after a disagreement, but if it is overheard by the patient or others nearby, it can be grounds for a slander suit. If there is a physician who must be repeatedly contacted regarding omissions on written prescriptions, let the patient know that a phone call is being made to the physician without any comment that might undermine the patient's confidence in the physician. Never place derogatory comments about a patient in his or her computer profile. Often these comments will print on the patient's profile when it is requested for insurance reimbursement. This may result in a lawsuit for libel, and electronic submissions can usually be traced to the person who entered them.

The Orphan Drug Act of 1983 established incentives for drug manufacturers to market drugs that are important to small numbers of individuals with relatively rare conditions. These drugs would otherwise be unprofitable to manufacture, and the patients would be deprived of important drug therapies. The Prescription Drug Marketing Act of 1987 prohibited the reimportation of drugs into this country except by the manufacturer and set restrictions on the distribution of drug samples.

Orphan Drug Act Act that encouraged manufacturers to market drugs for rare conditions by offering financial incentives.

Prescription Drug Marketing Act

The Omnibus Budget Reduction Act of 1990 (OBRA '90) mandated that all Medicaid patients be offered counseling by pharmacists. The state BOPs realized that if counseling were required only for Medicaid patients, it would set up two standards of practice, so they extended the counseling requirement to include all prescription patients. This offer may be made by the technician, but the counseling must be done by the pharmacist. The patient may refuse the offer to receive counseling. If so, the technician must document the refusal and complete the sale, remaining alert for any OTC purchases that may interact with the prescriptions being dispensed. OBRA '90 also mandated a drug utilization review by the pharmacist to screen for any drug or disease interactions or duplication of therapy using the information in the patient profile.

Omnibus Budget Reduction Act of 1990 (OBRA '90) Mandates that patient counseling be performed by the pharmacist for each prescription dispensed.

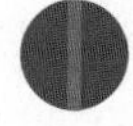

Health Insurance Portability and Accountability Act

The Health Insurance Portability and Accountability Act (HIPAA) of 1996 was created to develop standardized protocols for recording and maintaining protected health information (PHI) for each patient. This law will be discussed in more detail in Chapter 6. As you continue your education, incorporate the legal issues outlined here into your practice. When filling practice prescriptions in class, think through the legal guidelines learned in this chapter and internalize the guidelines and the reasoning associated with them. The law will then become a constant legal assistant to help protect you from incidents involving litigation. Remember that the pharmacist is a licensed professional and your actions may jeopardize that license. You must always be respectful of the fact that your ability to practice your profession is dependent on the pharmacist's license.

protected health information (PHI) Any health information that can be used to identify an individual.

Case Study 4.1

Sally Stoker is a 19-year-old single mother of a 6-month-old baby. She tries to juggle a part-time job, her duties as a mother, and an active social life. She is a pack-a-day smoker and a binge drinker on the weekend, and is taking birth control pills. Patient counseling is difficult because she is constantly talking on her cell phone and generally refuses counseling.

Sally developed a muscle strain during her morning run and was prescribed a muscle relaxer and a schedule IV painkiller to help with the pain. She took the prescriptions to Nickelson's Super Pharmacy and handed them to Jill. Jill gathered information for Sally's patient profile, including her age, allergies, and other medications. Jill then entered the prescriptions into the computer, double-checking the labels with the prescriptions, and proceeded to count out the medication, again checking the medication bottle with the label and the prescription. She poured each medication into a vial, affixed the proper label, and applied auxiliary labels. To the muscle relaxer Jill attached a label stating, "This medication may cause drowsiness. Alcohol may intensify this effect." This label was also attached to the schedule IV painkiller in addition to the warning, "Caution, federal law prohibits the transfer of this prescription to a person other than the patient for whom it was prescribed." After a third check of her work, Jill placed the prescriptions and paperwork in the appropriate place for Marie to check them. Marie called Sally to the counter and began to counsel her regarding the two medications. As usual, Sally seemed irritated and anxious to leave. As her cell phone rang, she turned and headed for the door saying, "I'll call if I have any questions."

Saturday night Sally went drinking and dancing with her friends. She took an extra dose of medicine to be sure her leg wouldn't hurt as she danced. Her friend Sara had a headache, so Sally shared one of her painkillers with her. The next morning Sally was so groggy she could barely get out of bed. She knocked the open medicine bottle on the floor and stumbled in to get her crying baby. As she picked up the baby, she tripped on the rug and fell with the baby, who picked up several tablets and put them in her mouth. Luckily, Sally's mother arrived for a visit and took Sally and the baby to the emergency room for treatment.

The following week, Nickelson's Super Pharmacy received a phone call from an attorney representing Sally. The pharmacy; Marie, the pharmacist; and Jill, the technician, were being charged with malpractice for dispensing such dangerous drugs with no warning about the dangers they might cause.

1. Discuss this case in terms of Jill's actions in filling the prescription, Marie's attempt to counsel the patient, and Sally's interruption of the counseling.
2. Describe some of the defense in terms of contributory negligence.
3. Discuss the seriousness of Sally giving her painkiller to a friend without knowledge of her medical history.
4. What might have happened to her friend as a result of mixing alcohol with the drug? What if she was allergic to one of the ingredients in the drug?
5. If Sally's friend was involved in an accident on her way home, who might be liable for any damages?

Chapter Summary

- The pharmacy profession is regulated by a multitude of laws to protect patients and to monitor the legal and illegal use of controlled drugs.
- Poor manufacturing practices and unscrupulous advertising that caused harm to patients resulted in the passage of the Pure Food and Drug Act and later the Food, Drug and Cosmetic Act.
- The approval process for a new drug is costly and time-consuming, but protects patients from drugs that are not safe and efficacious.

- The investigational new drug process involves four phases of trials to determine safety, dose, efficacy, and adverse events associated with using the drug in larger populations.
- A written prescription must contain required information about the patient, the prescriber, and the medication and its usage.
- The label attached to the prescription vial must contain certain information.
- Package inserts containing important drug information are included in the manufacturer's packaging of prescription medications.
- For some medications a PPI must be given to the patient with the original fill of the prescription.
- The Poison Protection Packaging Act mandated that child-resistant caps be applied to all prescription drugs except those on the exempt list.
- OBRA '90 mandated that patient counseling be offered with each new prescription.
- The Controlled Substances Act administered by the DEA outlines dispensing, storage, and handling requirements for drugs with a potential for abuse.
- Only prescribers that are authorized by the DEA and have a valid DEA number are allowed to prescribe controlled drugs.
- Manufacturers establish an expiration date for medications based on stability testing and storage and packaging requirements.
- There are three classes of drug recalls based on the seriousness of the problem.
- Some nonprescription items have restrictions on the amount and frequency of sale, and a signature log of such purchases must be maintained.
- The transfer of a prescription from one pharmacy to another requires documentation of information by both the receiving and the transferring pharmacies.
- Proving malpractice or professional negligence in a court of law requires that four factors be present: duty, dereliction of duty, damages to the plaintiff, and direct cause.
- The term *respondeat superior* means that when an employee enters into a contract in the name of his employer, the employer is responsible for abiding by the terms of the contract.
- Defamation of character involves libel or slander that damages a person's reputation.
- HIPAA is the Health Insurance Portability and Accountability Act, which sets a national standard establishing protocols for PHI.

Review Questions

Multiple Choice

1. The law that requires manufacturers to prove that a drug is both safe and effective for the condition for which it is marketed is the
   a. Pure Food and Drug Act
   b. Food, Drug and Cosmetic Act
   c. OBRA '90
   d. HIPAA

2. There are ________ categories of drug recalls, and the recall class number that is most serious is __________.
   a. 3 and 1
   b. 3 and 3
   c. 4 and 1
   d. 4 and 4

3. The prime purpose of phase I clinical trials of an investigational drug is to evaluate the
   a. therapeutic index
   b. safety
   c. adverse effects in diseased patients
   d. marketability

4. The level of performance expected of a healthcare professional in carrying out his or her professional duties is called
   a. standard of care
   b. duty of care
   c. ethical behavior
   d. scope of practice

5. Guidelines for activities that can be legally performed by a healthcare professional are called
   a. standard of care
   b. scope of practice
   c. technician standards
   d. none of the above

Fill in the Blanks

Fill in the missing word in the blanks below.

6. The expiration date on a manufacturer's bottle of a prescription medication is June 2007. The actual date this product will expire is ____________________.

7. The form that must be used to order schedule II narcotics is called ______________________.

8. Two drugs that are exempt from the Poison Prevention Packaging Act are ____________________ and __________________________.

9. The middle four digits of an NDC number assigned by the manufacturer identify ____________________________.

10. The statement "Caution: federal law prohibits the transfer of this drug to any person other than the patient for whom it was prescribed" is required to be on the container of any ________________________________ drug that is dispensed.

True/False

Mark the following statements True or False.

11. ______ If a DEA Form 222 has an error on one of the lines, the supplier can cross out that line and fill the remainder of the order.

12. ______ A physician's assistant will have a DEA number that begins with the letter M followed by the first initial of his last name.

13. ______ A schedule III, IV, or V controlled-drug prescription may have the physician's name typewritten on the signature line.

14. ______ All schedule II drugs must be kept in a locked cabinet in the pharmacy.

15. ______ Schedules III, IV, and V drugs may be kept on an open shelf together in one section of the pharmacy as long as they are not in plain view of customers.

Matching

16. ______ Trade name given to a drug by the manufacturer for marketing purposes.

17. ______ Controlled drugs that can be sold in limited quantities without a prescription in some states.

18. ______ Drugs that contain any unclean substance or are prepared in unsanitary conditions.

19. ______ Drugs with a labeling error or any discrepancy between the label and the product.

20. ______ The quality of care expected from a professional in the practice of his or her profession.

21. ______ A law concerning personal injury.

22. ______ The party bringing a complaint against a defendant.

23. ______ A form of professional negligence, a careless mistake, or an error in judgment.

24. ______ An action or inaction on the part of a plaintiff that caused or increased the risk of harm to the patient.

25. ______ Not providing a reasonable amount of care in performing a duty expected of a health professional.

A. Contributory negligence
B. Tort
C. Misbranded
D. Plaintiff
E. Adulterated drugs
F. Standard of care
G. Brand name
H. Malpractice
I. Exempt narcotics
J. Breach of duty

adulterated drugs Drugs that contain any unclean substance, are prepared in unsanitary conditions or containers, or differ in strength, quality, or purity from the official drug standards.

LEARNING ACTIVITIES

1. Eric began working in the hospital pharmacy as a technician in training while he was attending his pharmacy technician training program. He was very excited to be learning and couldn't wait to be fully trained. One day as he was working the front window, he received a stat order for one amp of heparin. It was during the lunch period and the pharmacy was not well staffed. Eric looked for the technician who was precepting him but was unable to find him. The pharmacists all seemed to be very busy in another area of the pharmacy and he knew the floor needed this medication right away. Eric wanted to make a good impression, so he found the heparin amp and brought it to the window. At the window, Eric checked the amp name again to be sure it was correct. It read heparin 10,000 USP units per mL. When the runner from the floor arrived, Eric proudly gave her the amp. She knew it was needed immediately, so she glanced at it to see that it was heparin and returned to the floor. The floor nurse, wanting to help her very ill patient as quickly as possible, administered the heparin to the patient. The patient's condition began to deteriorate quickly and it was discovered too late that the heparin strength should have been 1000 units per mL. The patient bled to death before the antidote could take effect. The patient's family contacted an attorney and the hospital received notification that the hospital, the physician, the administering nurse, the runner, the technician, and the supervising pharmacist were being named in the lawsuit for negligence.

   As a class project, conduct a mock trial to resolve this situation. Assign parts to the attorneys for the defense and the prosecution, each defendant named in the suit, a spokesperson for the hospital system, and any other witnesses, such as family members, who wish to testify. Appoint a judge to learn some basics of courtroom protocols and a jury to decide the verdict. Each person should research his or her position and be prepared for the mock trial.

2. Follow the progression of the development of the pharmacy profession by discussing the legislation introduced.

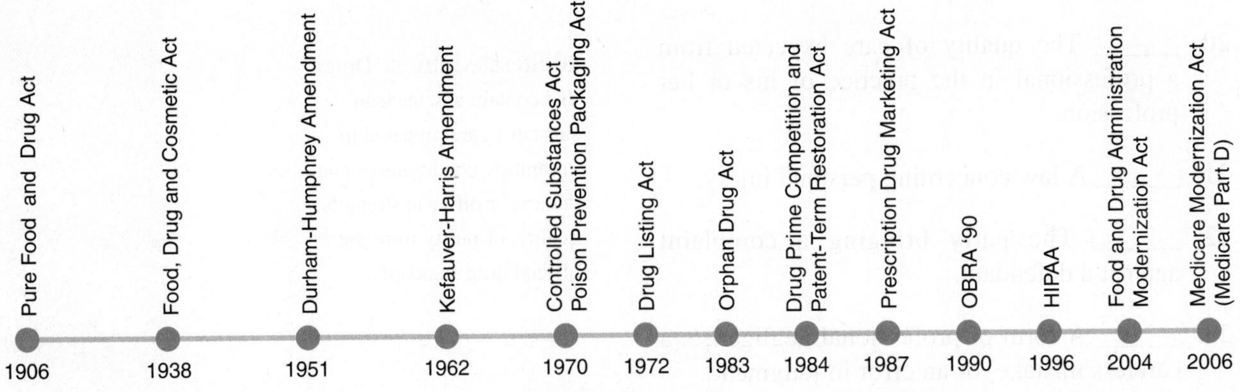

Pharmacy law timeline.

Suggested Readings

Gennaro AR, ed. Remington: The Science and Practice of Pharmacy. Baltimore, MD: Lippincott Williams & Wilkins, 2006.

Lacher BE. Pharmaceutical Calculations for the Pharmacy Technician. Baltimore, MD: Lippincott Williams & Wilkins, 2008.

Mohr ME. Lab Experiences for the Pharmacy Technician. Baltimore, MD: Lippincott Williams & Wilkins, 2006.

Reiss BS, Hall GD. Guide to Federal Pharmacy Law. New York: Apothecary Press, 2003.

Strandberg KM. Essentials of Law and Ethics for Pharmacy Technicians. Boca Raton, FL: CRC Press, 2003.

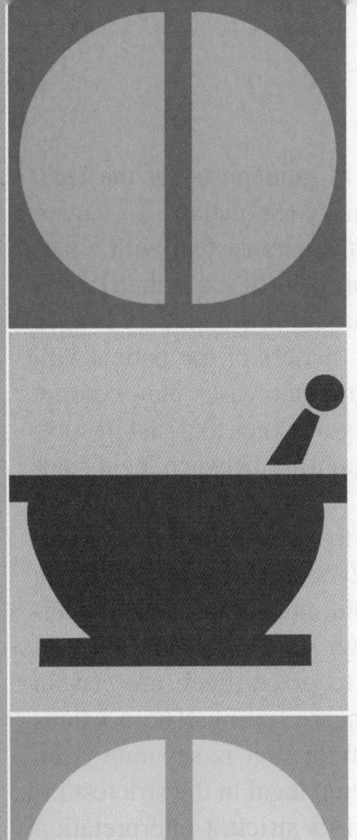

Chapter 5

Differentiating Law and Ethics

OBJECTIVES

After completing this chapter, the student will be able to:

- Define ethics and morality.
- Discuss the importance of ethics in the practice of a pharmacy technician.
- Determine ways to formulate a personal code of ethics.
- Develop a personal code of ethics.
- Differentiate between law and ethics.
- Devise a plan for making decisions when law and ethics conflict.
- Apply decision-making skills to various scenarios.

KEY TERMS

- altruism
- code of ethics
- competence
- consent
- consequential ethics
- disclosure
- ethical
- informed consent
- laws
- medical ethics
- moral standards
- nonconsequential ethics
- understanding
- voluntariness

The laws of each state's pharmacy practice act serve as guideposts for the legal aspect of the scope and standards of practice for pharmacy technicians. However, occasions often arise in which the letter of the law seems inconsistent with a particular situation. Each technician is an individual—a product of his or her family values and religious beliefs, and the environment and culture in which they live. In a diverse patient population, the cultural and religious beliefs of the patient will often conflict with the beliefs of the technician, and in some cases may conflict with the laws of the state. This chapter will offer some guidelines to assist in solving the many dilemmas that may arise when there is a conflict between legal standards and ethical decision-making.

laws Regulations enacted by the federal or local government to guide the actions of people; violations are punishable by fines or prison.

ethical Following a set of principles or values when making moral decisions that affect the care of patients in the community where the practice exists.

medical ethics A set of principles to guide the provision of healthcare by professionals.

Generally, being an ethical person means adhering to a set of standards or values. These standards will often vary from community to community depending on the background of the population. In the healthcare field, making an ethical decision would involve the use of medical ethics. Although standards and values in the healthcare field may vary somewhat from place to place, there are certain basic values that should always be in place in a healthcare setting. These values will form the foundation for developing ethical behavior that is separate from legal issues. What is ethical may or may not be considered legal in the strictest interpretation of the law. Likewise, following the law in its strictest interpretation may not be ethical in some instances. To further complicate matters, a standard that may be legal and ethical to most people may present a moral conflict for some individuals.

Laws, on the other hand, are regulations enacted by a political legislative group (such as Congress or the state legislature). Violation of these rules will result in a punishment consisting of a fine or time in prison. Violation of laws established by a professional regulating body, such as a state board of pharmacy (BOP), may result in suspension or revocation of a license to practice pharmacy or a license to practice as a pharmacy technician.

moral standards Personal beliefs based on cultural, environmental, and religious beliefs.

Moral standards are the most individualized of the three types of standards. Their formation begins very early in life as a result of religious, familial, and cultural beliefs. Enforcement of these standards is governed by the individual conscience of the person involved. If a person violates his or her moral standards, it may result in feelings of guilt and lowered self-esteem as he or she strives to reconcile his or her actions with his or her beliefs. In many cases a situation will require a person to reconcile law, ethics, and morality to reach the best decision possible.

The following moral and ethical standards that should be followed by all technicians in practicing their profession are based on some basic rights of patients:

- The well-being of the patient is the most important aspect of a technician's practice.
- Patients have a right to be treated with dignity regardless of ethnicity, beliefs, economic status, disease state, or sexual orientation.
- Patients have a right to receive accurate information about their health.
- Patients have a right to expect well-educated and competent technicians to be skilled in preparing their medications.
- Patients have a right to expect that technicians will use their knowledge and competence conscientiously to ensure accuracy in the preparation of medications.
- Patients have a right to expect that the technician will listen and respond to their wishes regarding their pharmaceutical care.

As technicians continue to expand their role as pharmacy professionals and increase their knowledge of drugs and drug interactions, their ability and responsibility to exercise professional judgment also increase. The attitude of the technician in a relationship with a patient must be one of altruism. Each decision made in the relationship with the patient should be made with a genuine concern for the well-being of the patient. Each decision must be motivated by what is right for the situation rather than what is easiest for the technician.

altruism True concern for the well-being of the patient.

Pharmacy has always been a profession of trust. This trust between the patient and healthcare professionals is of paramount importance to the exchange of information that must take place to ensure excellent pharmaceutical care. The pharmacist and the technician establish a special commitment of loyalty to the patient. This requires them to always act in the best interest of the patient even if it is not the easiest or most profitable course of action. The technician is usually the first person to greet the patient in a community setting, and that initial conversation lays the foundation for developing that trust relationship. Often a patient will develop a relationship with the technician first and will feel more at ease asking questions of a friendly person they feel can be trusted. This provides a great opportunity for the technician to use his or her professional judgment to involve the pharmacist when a comment or question is beyond the scope of practice of a technician. Any questions or comments directed to or overheard by the technician must be kept in the strictest confidence to continue the trust relationship for the benefit of the patient.

Some ethical situations in healthcare have become widespread issues involving society as a whole, and have been debated by legal authorities. The resolution of some of these issues is legislated by the federal government whereas others are left up to the states to decide, but often those decisions may go against the personal beliefs of the technician. Some common social issues are abortion, assisted suicide, genetic engineering, organ transplants, stem cell research, and in vitro fertilization. Other issues that may be faced on a daily basis include patient confidentiality (e.g., allowing family members to pick up medication, answering questions about medications asked by family members) and deciding how much information to give the patient about his or her medications. If the patient hears about all the side effects, will he or she choose not to take the medication? Should the physician be solely responsible for evaluating the benefit/risk ratio?

The rule of informed consent directs that patients be fully informed about the benefits and risks of taking a medication. Although this creates a dilemma in the day-to-day practice of pharmacy, the problem is compounded when the patient is involved in a clinical trial for an investigational drug. Informed consent is a composite of five different elements. The concept of disclosure requires that the patient receive enough information about the drug and its side effects to make a decision. To ensure understanding, the information the patient receives must be in lay terms and given in a nonthreatening manner so the patient can understand the benefits and make a reasonable decision. Voluntariness means a patient must choose to participate in a drug trial without any coercion. Competence means that a patient has the cognitive ability to assimilate information and make his or her own decision. Consent is the final step in the process, in which the patient makes an informed decision to participate in the trial.

informed consent Consent given by the patient after being provided with adequate information about the positive and negative effects of a medication or treatment.

disclosure Providing the patient with all of the pertinent information needed to make a decision.

understanding Requires that information provided to the patient be presented in lay terms that are clear to the patient so that he or she can assess the benefits and risks.

voluntariness Patients who agree to a course of treatment or drug therapy must do so without the pressure of any coercion.

competence Possessing the education and skills to perform the tasks of the profession.

consent Final step in the process of informed consent, in which the patient makes a final decision to participate in a trial.

 Ethical Codes

The Hippocratic oath has served as a general code of ethics for the medical community for centuries. As health professionals have become more specialized, some professions have established a code of ethics specific to their profession. These codes offer a set of guidelines, but they cannot answer every moral or ethical situ-

code of ethics A list of principles formulated to guide members of a profession in making decisions about matters that are not firmly established by laws.

ation that arises. These codes of ethics must be examined periodically to ensure that they are in keeping with the current scope of practice. The APhA established a code of ethics for pharmacists in 1852 that is still in use today, but it has been modified several times as progress in the profession has mandated changes. For example, the 1952 APhA code of ethics stated that "the pharmacist does not discuss the therapeutic effects or composition of a prescription with a patient." Today this statement would be in violation of OBRA '90, which requires that patients receive counseling from the pharmacist. Every technician should develop a personal formula for ethical behavior that coincides with the standards of practice of a pharmacy technician. The following is an example of professional and ethical standards for pharmacy technicians:

Professional and Ethical Standards for Pharmacy Technicians

The professional pharmacy technician considers the health needs of the patient a top priority.

The professional pharmacy technician understands the importance of a quality education and training program to prepare to serve the needs of the patient.

The professional pharmacy technician continues to update knowledge of new policies, procedures, and technology to assist the pharmacist in providing excellent pharmaceutical care to patients.

The professional pharmacy technician respects the pharmaceutical knowledge and professional judgment of the pharmacist in matters of patient care.

The professional pharmacy technician values diversity among patients and co-workers and treats each individual with the utmost respect.

The professional pharmacy technician assists with quality assurance to dispense medications and devices that meet the highest standards.

The professional pharmacy technician is cognizant of the protocols for maintaining confidentiality of protected health information.

The professional pharmacy technician will uphold the state and federal laws concerning medication dispensing and will report any unlawful activity to the proper authorities.

The professional pharmacy technician uses a wide knowledge base of educational material, journals, and networking with colleagues to establish the foundation for making ethical decisions.

The professional pharmacy technician is fully vested in the profession and demonstrates professionalism by active participation in one or more pharmacy technician organizations.

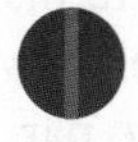

Guidelines For Ethical Decision-Making

Ethics, then, can be a complex issue that often requires a great deal of soul searching. There are some systematic preparation methods that can be used for ethical decision-making. Remember, ethics is doing what you think is right based on your personal experiences and beliefs. Consequential ethics emphasizes the end result. (Does the end justify the means?) Nonconsequential ethics is based on the truth of the situation. (Is the action being taken right now a good and ethical one?)

consequential ethics
Emphasizes the end result. (Does the end result justify the means?)

nonconsequential ethics
A set of principles based on the rightness or wrongness of each action performed regardless of the outcome.

Some preparation tools for ethical decision-making are available. Lifelong learning will enhance your ability to form a knowledge base that will enable you to make accurate decisions. Professional journals provide a wealth of information and descriptions of ethical and legal scenarios and their solutions. Even if you don't agree with the solution presented, it will give you the opportunity to explore other options so that when a similar situation arises, you will be more prepared to make an informed decision. Attend educational seminars, participate in professional organizations, network with colleagues, and be attentive to the media. This will provide you with the opportunity to develop an organized thought process utilizing a vast network of information and the input of many colleagues. Often, when an ethical dilemma arises, you will have already made a decision about your course of action, and this will alleviate some of the stress that arises when you are faced with an unexpected situation.

TIP

If confronted with an unexpected ethical situation, follow these steps to reach a decision:

1. **Gather as much pertinent information about the issue as possible in the amount of time available.**
2. **Carefully identify the problem(s). Do not act in haste. If possible, discuss the problem with the pharmacist or other technicians.**
3. **Analyze the situation and try to identify several possible alternatives.**
4. **Choose the best of the alternatives to solve the problem.**
5. **When time permits, evaluate the solution chosen for future reference.**
6. **Did your solution produce the results desired?**
7. **If not, what could have been done differently?**

Professional Judgment Scenario 5.1

Joan works in a small, independent retail pharmacy. The owner works every day but occasionally takes an evening off to spend time with his family. On these nights he has a retired pharmacist friend who fills in for him. Joan likes and respects her boss, and knows these evenings off are important to him. She agrees to work the nights that he is off so she can help the relief pharmacist, who is not as familiar with the patients. Several times she has been concerned that the pharmacist seemed unsteady on his feet. Occasionally, he seems to slur his speech. Joan watches carefully as he fills prescriptions because he often makes mistakes. Tonight she saw him take a flask from his pocket and take a drink. As she was working closely with him, she smelled alcohol on his breath. Joan knows it will be hard to find another pharmacist to work these nights. She wonders if she can watch him closely enough to prevent mistakes from reaching the patients.

Answer the following questions and discuss them with the class.

1. Discuss the term "loyalty."
2. Has Joan demonstrated loyalty to
   a. her boss?
   b. the patients?
   c. her profession?
   d. the relief pharmacist?
3. Joan wonders if she can be watchful enough to prevent any mistakes from reaching the patients. Is it reasonable for her to assume this risk?
4. Does she have a responsibility to report what she knows to her boss?
5. Help Joan make an ethical decision by using the seven steps listed in the tip box above.

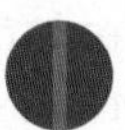

Managing Ethical Dilemmas

Understanding your personal beliefs about issues that may arise in the practice of your profession as a technician will enable you to be proactive on some issues that you feel strongly about. Obviously, if you are morally opposed to abortion, you would not choose to practice in a pharmacy that serves patients from an abortion clinic. If you are opposed to the death penalty or just feel strongly that you would not want to be involved in preparing a medication for a lethal injection, a position in a pharmacy that contracts with a state penitentiary where death by lethal injection is carried out would not be a good choice for you. If you are morally opposed to oral contraception, then a retail or community pharmacy may not be the ideal setting for you because this will be a constant issue.

As you can see, it is important to develop an understanding of the moral issues that may arise so you can be prepared to make an informed decision. As you continue your study of the scope and standards of practice for pharmacy technicians, make note of any moral or ethical dispensing issues that may arise and develop a plan to deal with them. Let your decision about the type of practice setting you choose to practice in be guided by a firm understanding of your beliefs and your comfort zone. If you are constantly faced with ethical dilemmas and feel under pressure to override your feelings and dispense the medication, the stress of going against your beliefs will erode your satisfaction of your profession. Regardless of how carefully you research a practice setting and how thoroughly you understand your personal code of ethics, there will still be occasions when an ethical situation will arise and a decision will be required. If you work in a practice setting where there are several technicians, the easiest solution would be to ask if one of the other technicians would feel comfortable handling the order. Often, if the pharmacist knows of your concerns, he or she will be willing to process the order without any involvement from you. Any serious concerns that you have about ethical dilemmas should be addressed before the situation occurs. During the interview process, if you have a concern about an ethical issue that may arise, have a discussion about the possible alternatives to your being required to dispense certain drugs. Although this may affect your ability to be hired for that position, it would be better to know ahead of time if they are willing to make accommodations for you.

Continue to exercise your professional judgment by using the seven steps outlined above to practice ethical decision-making.

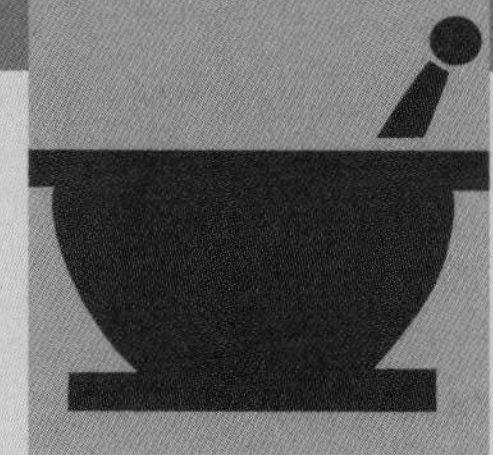

Professional Judgment Scenario 5.2

Jose works as a pharmacy technician in a retail chain pharmacy located near a hospital. The store closes at midnight and there is no other pharmacy near this area. At 11:50 p.m. a man walked into the store and headed straight for the pharmacy counter. The man was wearing a cervical collar and looked somewhat uncomfortable. Jose wasn't sure why, but he felt uneasy as the man approached. "Good evening, sir, how can we help you?" Jose managed to say. "I was in an automobile accident earlier and seemed to have suffered some whiplash," the man responded. "The doc at the emergency room said you could fill this for me. I'm glad I caught you before you closed." Jose looked at the prescription. It was written on a hospital prescription blank and was barely legible, like many he had seen before, but it had all the necessary information, including a valid DEA number. The prescription was written for OxyContin, a class II narcotic. Jose showed the prescription to the pharmacist and they discussed the pros and cons of filling it. After their discussion, Joe began to prepare the prescription, the pharmacist checked it, and Jose completed the sale. Because it was closing time, they turned the lights off and left the store. As the pharmacist was locking the door, they saw the patient toss the prescription bag through the window of a car full of men, take off his cervical collar, and jump into the car as it sped away.

1. Under the circumstances, did Jose and the pharmacist do the right thing by filling the prescription?
2. Would it have been ethical to refuse to fill a prescription that appeared to be legal?
3. What if the patient was truly in pain and was unable to get the pain medicine until morning?
4. What lesson should Joe take away from this incident after evaluating the situation?

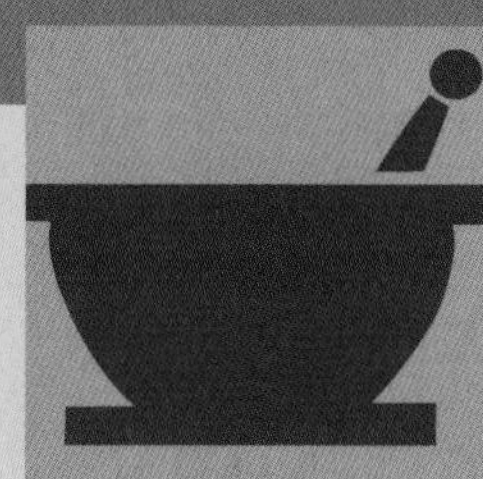

Professional Judgment Scenario 5.3

Mrs. Tam has severe respiratory problems and has been prescribed four different inhalers by her family physician at the outpatient clinic where she is a patient. Susie works in the clinic pharmacy and notices that Mrs. Tam is always early for her inhaler refills. Her inhalers should last her a month according to the directions, but she returns for refills in 2½ weeks. Mrs. Tam has recently arrived from Vietnam and speaks very little English but has brought her teenage daughter to interpret for her. Susie tries to explain that it is too early for refills, but even the daughter can't seem to make her mother understand. Susie checks the inhalers and verifies that they are all empty, but the doctor is not in that day and Susie knows that overuse of inhalers can be dangerous. Susie starts to tell the daughter that she will have to wait at least a week before getting a refill. The pharmacist overhears the conversation and tells Susie to fill the inhalers today and he will have a conference with the physician tomorrow when he returns to the office.

1. Did the pharmacist make a legal decision?
2. Was it an ethical decision?
3. What if Susie had refused to fill the inhalers and the patient had a severe asthma attack and died in the night?
4. What conclusion might Susie reach after evaluating this situation about possible actions in the future?

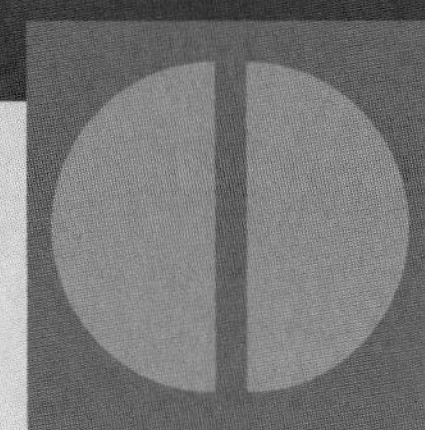

Case Study 5.1

Sally Stoker is a 19-year-old single mother of a 6-month-old baby. She tries to juggle a part-time job, her duties as a mother, and an active social life. She is a pack-a-day smoker, a binge drinker on the weekends, and is taking birth control pills. Patient counseling is difficult because she is constantly talking on her cell phone and generally refuses counseling. On a particularly busy day at Nickelson's Pharmacy, there are many patients waiting for their prescriptions. Marie and Jill are working as quickly and efficiently as possible, but the wait times are long. Sally's baby is buckled into her stroller and Sally is getting impatient. She still needs to stop at the grocery store next door and it is near lunchtime. Suddenly Sally walks away and leaves the baby in the stroller near the pharmacy. Jill looks up as Sally walks out the door and sees that the baby has been left behind.

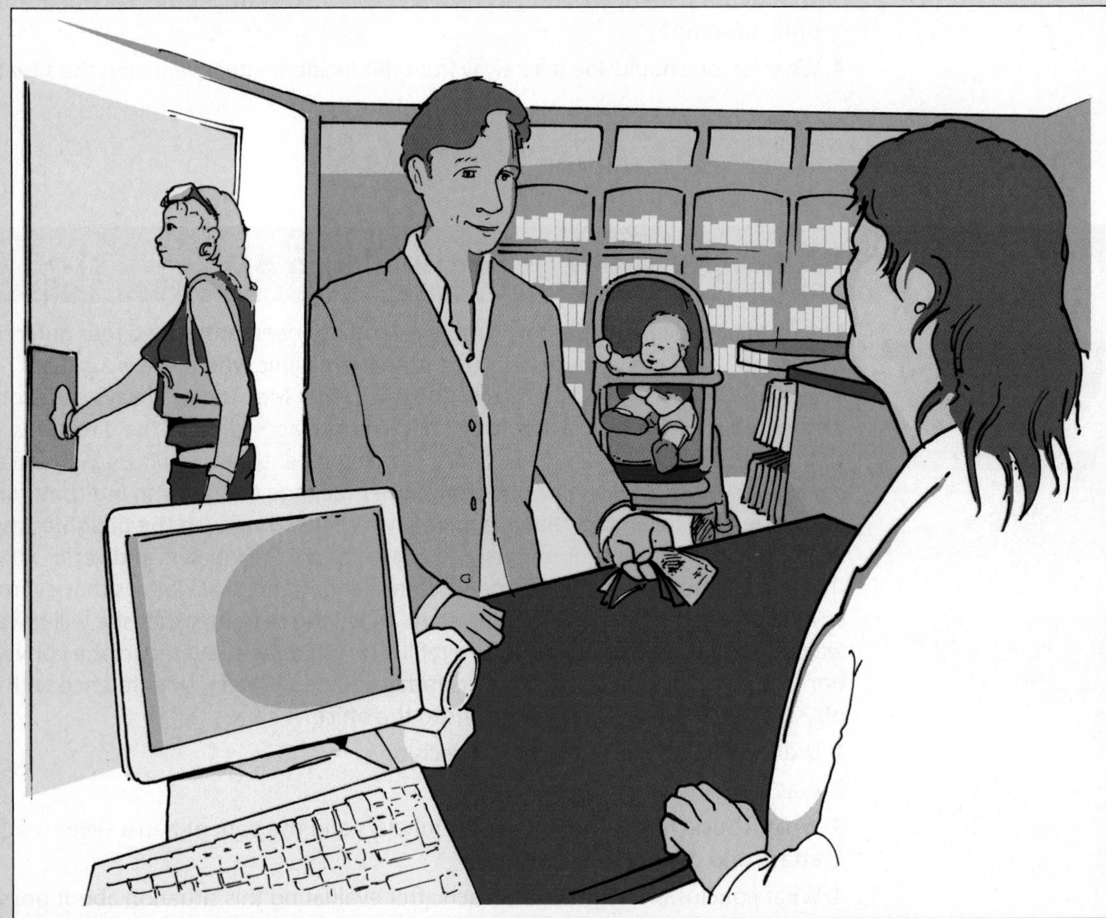

Sally returns in 20 minutes after finishing her grocery shopping.

1. Should Jill have taken some action when she saw the baby unattended?
2. Should she have brought the baby behind the counter and tried to watch her as she worked?
3. Should she have ignored the situation and pretended not to notice?
4. How would Jill feel if she later heard that the baby had been harmed due to parental neglect?
5. Discuss the legal, moral, and ethical issues involved here.

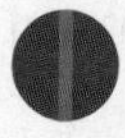

Chapter Summary

- An ethical person is one who adheres to a set of standards or values accepted by the community.
- Medical ethics are principles established by a healthcare profession to aid in decisions pertaining to the medical treatment of the patient.
- Laws are regulations established by a legislative group or the regulating body of a profession.
- Moral standards are the results of cultural, environmental, ethnic, and religious beliefs, and are very individualized.
- All patients have certain basic rights associated with their healthcare.
- The pharmacist and the pharmacy technician must establish a relationship of trust with the patient.
- The technician should exercise professional judgment in communicating with the patient and involve the pharmacist when appropriate.
- Patients should be fully informed about their medications in language they can understand so that they can comprehend the benefits and risks involved with a treatment.
- Technicians should be familiar with the code of ethics for pharmacy technicians and also understand the code of ethics for pharmacists to guide their actions in the pharmacy.
- Lifelong learning, including professional journals, educational seminars, and membership in professional organizations, will provide a knowledge base for making ethical decisions.

Review Questions

Multiple Choice

Choose the correct answer to the following questions:

1. The term describing a genuine concern for the well-being of the patient is
   a. morality
   b. ethics
   c. altruism
   d. competence

2. Consequential ethics means
   a. being concerned that each action taken is right
   b. the end justifies the means
   c. a wrong action results in consequences
   d. none of the above

3. The following are examples of lifelong learning to assist in making ethical decisions:
   a. reading professional journals
   b. attending professional conferences
   c. networking with other technicians
   d. all of the above

4. Ensuring that a patient can give informed consent about a drug treatment can be accomplished by
   a. giving the patient a package insert to read
   b. discussing the advantages of the drug while glossing over the adverse effects
   c. reminding the patient that the physician has decided this is the best course of action
   d. none of the above

5. Which of the following rights is not guaranteed to every patient?
   a. the right to be treated with dignity
   b. the right to expect a prescription to be filled accurately
   c. the right to have a prescription filled with no waiting
   d. the right to receive accurate information about a treatment

Fill in the Blanks

Fill in the blanks with the correct word or words.

6. Personal beliefs based on cultural, environmental, and religious beliefs are called ______________________ standards.

7. The process of providing the patient with all pertinent information needed to make an informed decision about a medical treatment is called ______________________.

8. Violation of regulations in the state pharmacy practice act may result in ______________________ or ______________________ of the pharmacy technician's license to practice.

9. Violation of a federal law governing the dispensing of controlled drugs may result in ______________________ or ______________________.

10. A list of principles that has been formulated to guide members of a profession in making decisions about issues that have not been established by law is called ______________________.

Matching

Match the following with the terms below:

11. ______	Possessing the education and skills to perform the tasks of the profession.	A. Life long learning
12. ______	The patient agrees to participate in a drug trial without any coercion.	B. Ethics
13. ______	Method of enhancing the knowledge base to assist in ethical decision-making.	C. Voluntariness
14. ______	Doing what you think is right based on personal experiences, knowledge, and beliefs.	D. Consent
15. ______	The final decision of the patient, whereby he or she agrees to a treatment after being fully informed about it.	E. Competence

True/False

Answer True or False to the following questions:

16. _____ Following the strict interpretation of the law will always yield an ethical decision.

17. _____ A pharmacy technician should question any conditions or changes in appearance that may affect the quality of the drugs being dispensed.

18. _____ If a technician is opposed to abortion and doesn't want to dispense the "morning after" pill, and is seeking employment in a setting where it may become an issue, he or she should keep his or her opinion to him or herself until after he or she has secured a position.

19. _____ Of the three types of standards (laws, ethics, and morality), the most individualized are the moral standards.

20. _____ Ethical standards are universal and are not affected by the norms of the community.

LEARNING ACTIVITY

Using the information covered in the chapter and suggested readings, write a personal code of ethics for your practice as a technician. Include some ethical and moral issues you feel strongly about. Discuss each code with the class and formulate a class code of ethics.

Suggested Readings

Buerki RA, Vottero LD. Ethical Practices in Pharmacy: A Guidebook for Pharmacy Technicians. Madison, WI: American Institute of the History of Pharmacy, 1997.

Gennaro AR, ed. Remington: The Science and Practice of Pharmacy. Baltimore, MD: Lippincott Williams & Wilkins, 2006.

Reiss BS, Hall GD. Guide to Federal Pharmacy Law. New York: Apothecary Press, 2003.

Strandberg KM. Essentials of Law and Ethics for Pharmacy Technicians. Boca Raton, FL: CRC Press, 2003.

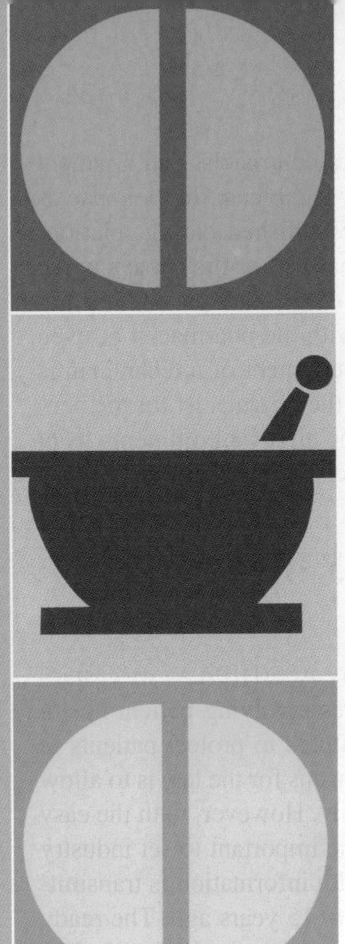

Chapter **6**

Confidentiality and HIPAA

OBJECTIVES

After completing this chapter, the student will be able to:

- Define confidentiality as it applies to healthcare.
- Discuss the importance of confidentiality.
- List examples of protected health information (PHI).
- Define HIPAA.
- Outline the important regulations included in HIPAA.
- Discuss confidentiality as it relates to morality, ethics, and the law.
- Describe common situations in a technician's practice that may violate patient confidentiality.

KEY TERMS

- confidentiality
- Health Insurance Portability and Accountability Act (HIPAA)
- patient authorization
- protected health information (PHI)
- privacy notice

The trust relationship that has always existed between a pharmacist and a patient has now, in many cases, been extended to the pharmacy technician. In their role as pharmacy professionals, pharmacy technicians have established caring relationships with patients and are usually the first to greet the patients as they arrive in the pharmacy. As a result of this trust relationship, patients often share personal health information with a technician that hasn't been shared with the pharmacist or even their physician. An important part of the professional judgment of a technician is to realize when such information should be shared with the pharmacist for the benefit of the patient. Use your education and training to be alert for comments from a patient that may signal a problem requiring a pharmacist's intervention.

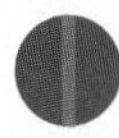

Health Insurance Portability and Accountability Act

Health Insurance Portability and Accountability Act (HIPAA) Federal law passed in April 2003 to set standards for the healthcare industry for sharing and transmitting health information.

After the Health Insurance Portability and Accountability Act (HIPAA) was established as a federal law in 2003, many routine procedures involving patient health information needed to be redesigned. The law was instituted to protect patients in several ways. As the title suggests, one of the primary reasons for the law is to allow patients to transfer their health insurance plans more easily. However, with the easy availability of electronic access to information, it became important to set industry standards for electronic transfers to ensure privacy. Health information is transmitted electronically in various forms that did not exist 10 to 15 years ago. The ready availability of e-mail over the Internet, fax machines, and the trend toward electronic medical-record systems have increased the ease of access to health information for health professionals, but they also allow for easier access by persons who have no right or need to know such information, and may use it improperly.

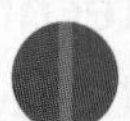

Protected Health Information Protocols

protected health information (PHI) Any health information that can be used to identify an individual.

confidentiality Accessing only the patient information that is required for the specific task being performed and extending the information only to those who have a genuine need to know.

Protected health information (PHI) is any information related to a person's past or present health conditions, healthcare, or payment for care. Included is any name or number that may identify an individual, such as the medical record number, social security number, address or telephone number, diagnosis, medical history, and history of medication use. The law requires HIPAA training for all individuals who work with PHI. Patient confidentiality should be a constant consideration throughout your education and training, and should become an integral component of your professional judgment as a technician. Access to PHI must be on a "need to know" basis. This means that you should not access patient information out of curiosity about an unusual situation or look up a friend's records to see how he or she is recovering. You should search only for required information to assist in patient care. Never divulge any PHI to another person without clearance from the pharmacist.

TIP **Learn the HIPAA protocols established for your practice setting and abide by them.**

All businesses that deal with PHI must offer a notice of privacy to patients detailing how their information will be used. Some particular concerns for the technician include discussing a patient's prescription within earshot of other people, leaving protected information on the computer screen where others may see it, or leaving phone messages on an answering machine accessed by others. No patient information may be placed in the regular trash containers unless it is rendered unreadable. Be cautious when preparing medication printouts for tax purposes. Third-party insurance companies require a certain amount of personal information about their clients. The patient should sign a permission ledger for each prescription billed to the insurance. Care should be taken to prevent unauthorized viewing of the signature log containing protected information. When there is any doubt about the disclosure of PHI, consult the pharmacist for a decision.

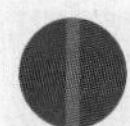

Procedures for Protecting Health Information in the Pharmacy

Aside from the professional responsibility to maintain patient confidentiality, there are civil and criminal penalties for releasing PHI to the wrong person. Because HIPAA is now a law, there can be substantial fines and prison sentences for knowingly obtaining or disclosing patient information for malicious uses. Even for accidental disclosures there can be civil fines.

Some routine ways that PHI is utilized in the pharmacy settings include evaluating and dispensing prescriptions, entering data into the patient profile, and being present as the pharmacist counsels the patient about his or her prescriptions. When you receive a new prescription that is missing required patient information, request the information from the patient in a discreet manner so that it is not overheard by others in the pharmacy area. The pharmacy counter should be designed so that only one patient can be at the window at any given time. When updating the patient profile, do not ask, "Mrs. Jones, do you have any other health conditions besides high blood pressure?" Instead, use a lower tone of voice to ask, "Mrs. Jones, has there been any change in your health condition since you were last here?" Protect information that is visible on the computer screen from being viewed by unauthorized people. Log out of the patient profile immediately after the prescriptions are completed. If the patient brings a refill bottle to the pharmacy, after obtaining the required information, either return the empty bottle to the patient or discard it in an appropriate container designed to destroy PHI. Do not place it in a regular trash container where it might be accessed by an unauthorized person.

The fax machine has become a quick and efficient method for transmitting information. There are several safety factors that must be considered to ensure privacy when faxing PHI. Use a fax machine that is located in a secure place in the pharmacy. Remove incoming faxes promptly and place them in the proper location. When faxing refill authorization requests to a physician's office, be certain that the fax number being utilized accesses a machine in a secure location in the office. Call the office personnel to alert them that a fax is being sent so it can be properly handled.

Promptly report any concern about unauthorized access to PHI to the pharmacist. CAUTION

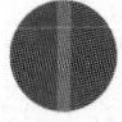

Verbal Health Information

Any health information expressed to the technician by the patient, or any information overheard by the technician during the pharmacist's consultation with the patient is to be kept strictly confidential. Even seemingly good news, such as a patient telling the pharmacist she is pregnant as she inquires about drug interactions and adverse effects, must be kept in the strictest confidence. If the patient is a friend or neighbor, it is inappropriate to call her and congratulate her on her pregnancy unless she shares this news with you outside of the pharmacy setting. If, however, you have overheard that a patient is pregnant and you see her purchasing over-the-counter (OTC) medications that may be harmful to the fetus, it is appropriate to mention this purchase to the pharmacist for a possible follow-up consultation.

Professional Judgment Scenario 6.1

Jim, a pharmacy technician in a retail pharmacy, overheard a patient discussing his struggle with alcoholism and the fact that he had joined Alcoholics Anonymous with the pharmacist. After leaving the consultation area, the patient brought his prescriptions and a few OTC items to the checkout counter and Jim began to complete the sale. Among the OTC items was a large bottle of a night-time cough medicine that Jim remembered from his classes contained a high alcohol content.

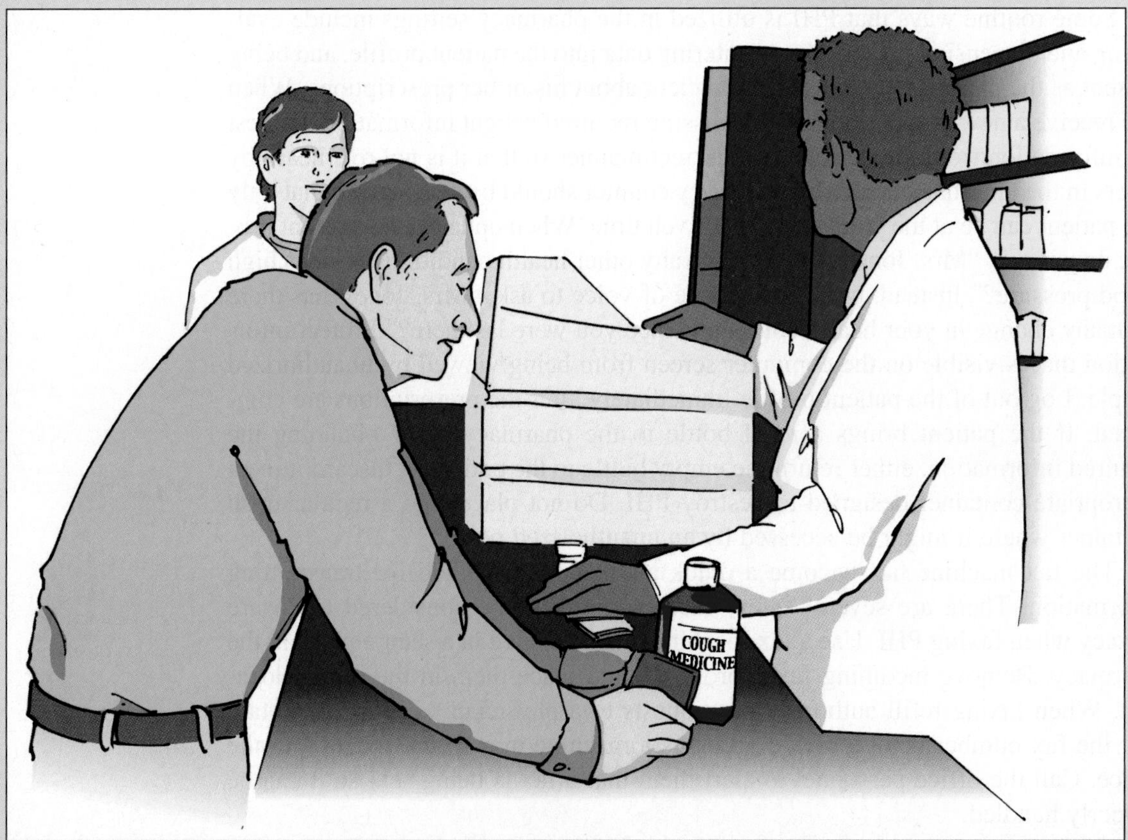

Help Jim decide the proper course of action, keeping in mind the HIPAA rules and the need to put the patient's health first.

1. Should Jim point out the alcohol content to the patient and risk embarrassing the patient and violating confidentiality in an area where others may hear?
2. To preserve confidentiality, should Jim ignore what he knows about the medicine and ring up the sale as if nothing were wrong?
3. Discuss possible solutions using the professional judgment of an educated technician.

Proper handling of PHI and using professional judgment to guide your actions will set you apart as a professional pharmacy technician who understands and follows the scope and standards of practice of a pharmacy technician.

Frequently during the year, especially during tax preparation time, patients will call and request a printout of their prescriptions for the year. This is a service provided by most retail pharmacies and a task that is often delegated to the technician.

Be certain about the identity of the person making the request and the person who will be picking up the printout. CAUTION

If someone other than the patient will be picking up the printout, obtain permission from the patient to release it and ask the person for identification. Keep social e-mail separate from work e-mail to ensure that no PHI will be accidentally attached to a personal e-mail. When sending health information over the Internet, double check the e-mail address of the recipient and be certain that you are using a secure network. Never share your password with another employee because it can and will be used to trace every computer transaction back to you. Any errors, intentional or accidental, made under your password will be attributed to you. Likewise, never request a fellow employee's password to log in and perform a task. Your computer password is your computer signature and verifies that you have performed a task.

Access to the pharmacy should be limited to authorized pharmacy personnel. Any maintenance, housekeeping, or repair personnel should be supervised at all times when in the pharmacy. They should have identification and work only in the area specified. Only computer technicians who have been called to the pharmacy should be allowed to touch the computer systems. Patient health information should be diligently protected from nonpharmacy workers in the pharmacy.

Conversations in the break room about a patient's unusual health situation are a tempting way to spend the lunch break. Although there are not likely to be any legal repercussions for discussing PHI with other healthcare workers, it is a violation of the spirit of the law. Unless the discussion is required because that healthcare worker will be following up on the care of that patient and therefore has a need to know the information, it should not be shared. These types of chatty conversations are certainly a violation of the moral and ethical behaviors expected of a professional pharmacy technician. Even more damaging are comments made to coworkers in the halls and elevators of a hospital. Discussing the particulars of a patient's situation, even though the patient is not identified, can be extremely disconcerting to the family members of a patient who may recognize their loved one by hearing certain health or diagnosis details as they ride the elevator.

The ability to handle PHI in a legal, ethical, and moral way is the mark of a true professional. It will set you apart as a person of trust who demonstrates the professional judgment of an educated technician. As you proceed through your practice, learn appropriate techniques from your mentors and preceptors, and develop a personal confidentiality standard as part of your personal code of ethics.

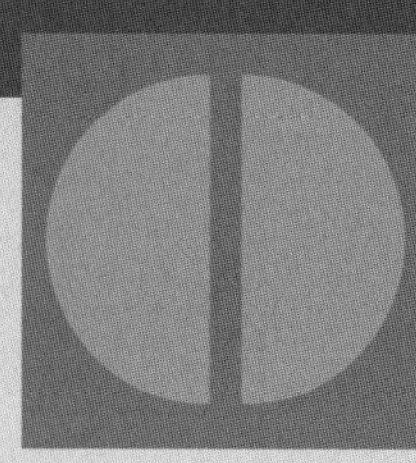

Case Study 6.1

"Nickelson's Super Pharmacy, Jill the technician speaking, how may I help you?"

"Hi, Jill, this is Bill Sands. My wife Betty gets her prescriptions filled at your pharmacy. I'm working on my taxes and I need a printout of her prescriptions for last year. Can I come over and pick it up this afternoon?"

"Sure, Mr. Sands. I'll have it ready for you by 3:00," replied Jill. Last week Marie, the pharmacist, had trained Jill on producing computer printouts because it was nearing tax time and there would be many requests for this service. Jill was happy that she could perform this task without asking for Marie's help. As she prepared the printout she noticed that Mrs. Sands had several prescriptions for antidepressant and antipsychotic drugs. She seemed to remember hearing Mrs. Sands tell Marie that she and her husband were getting a divorce.

This situation or a similar one may occur frequently in a retail pharmacy. Put yourself in Jill's place and answer the following questions:

1. Can Jill legally prepare printouts of patient medications for tax or insurance purposes?
2. Is there cause for concern if Jill makes this printout available?
3. What action should Jill take before making the printout available to Mr. Sands?
4. If Jill consults Marie about the situation, how might Marie resolve the issue?
5. Discuss HIPAA and how its guidelines for handling PHI can assist the technician in reaching a resolution to this scenario.

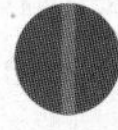

Chapter Summary

- HIPAA is a law instituted to facilitate a patient's ability to transfer healthcare plans and to set industry standards for the protection of health information.
- PHI is any individually identifiable information related to a person's past or present health conditions, healthcare, or payment for care.
- Healthcare organizations are required to give a copy of their privacy notice to patients.
- Electronic transfers of PHI must be carefully monitored to avoid a breach of confidentiality.
- Technicians should guard their computer password from unauthorized use by another person.
- Pharmacy security should restrict access to the pharmacy by unauthorized persons.
- Maintenance and housekeeping personnel with identification may be allowed in the pharmacy but should be supervised at all times to protect patient confidentiality.
- Conversations concerning patients should be restricted to those who "need to know" and not be discussed in the halls and elevators of the hospital.

privacy notice Patients must receive a copy of the organization's privacy policy, and the pharmacy should make an effort to get a signed acknowledgment of the notice from the patient.

patient authorization Written consent to share health information, signed by the patient, if possible with specific instructions about the content of the material shared.

Review Questions

Multiple Choice

Choose the best answer to the following questions:

1. The document given to each patient detailing how a healthcare facility will handle patient information is called
   a. HIPAA
   b. patient authorization
   c. privacy notice
   d. consent form

2. Which of the following should be allowed unsupervised access to the pharmacy?
   a. the pharmacist
   b. the technician
   c. a drug salesman
   d. a physician

3. Which of the following should be allowed *unsupervised* access to the pharmacy?
   a. housekeeping personnel with identification
   b. repairman with identification
   c. computer technician with identification
   d. police officer with identification
   e. none of the above

4. PHI can include the
   a. patient's name
   b. medical record number
   c. diagnosis
   d. refill history
   e. all of the above

5. Deliberate violation of confidentiality rules may result in
   a. fines
   b. jail sentences
   c. suspension or revocation of the pharmacy technician's license
   d. loss of job
   e. all of the above

Fill in the Blanks

Fill in the blanks with the correct word or words.

6. The federal law passed to set standards for transmitting patient health information is ______________________________.

7. Health information that contains individually identifiable information is classified as ______________________________.

8. ______________________ in a healthcare setting refers to accessing only the patient information required for the specific task being performed and sharing the information only with those who need to know.

9. Access to the pharmacy should be limited to ______________ personnel.

10. Housekeeping and repair personnel with proper identification should be ______________________ at all times while in the pharmacy.

Matching

Match the following with the terms below:

11. ______ The type of relationship that exists between a pharmacy technician and a patient.

12. ______ Information related to a person's past or present health conditions, healthcare, or payment for care.

13. ______ Access to PHI must be for this reason.

14. ______ Written consent to share health information signed by the patient.

15. ______ Computer signature verifying that a person performed a task.

A. PHI
B. Patient authorization
C. Password
D. Need to know
E. Trust

True/False

Mark the following statements True or False.

16. _____ HIPAA protocols will be standardized in every practice setting.

17. _____ Faxing PHI to a patient's office fax number is an efficient use of technology.

18. _____ Each pharmacy must present patients with a notice of privacy to describe its handling of PHI.

19. _____ Patient confidentiality regulations only apply to information discussed during the consultation with the pharmacist.

20. _____ Pharmacy technicians are exposed to PHI as a routine part of their practice.

LEARNING ACTIVITY

Design an internal form to be used as a warning for incidents that might breach patient confidentiality. Include a checklist of common infractions (such as leaving patient information on the computer screen, discussing patient information during breaks, etc.), a plan for corrective action, and a timetable for review of the employee's progress. Begin using the form during lab time to reinforce the confidentiality issues pertinent to a technician's practice.

Suggested Reading

Health Insurance Portability and Accountability Act . Available online at http://www.HIPAA.org. Accessed July 7, 2008.

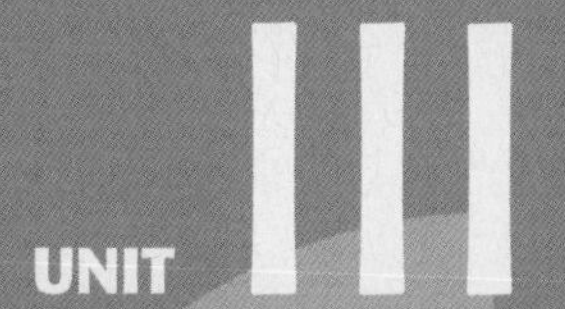

UNIT III

Technician's Role in Ensuring Patient Rights

Chapter 7

The Right Medication to the Right Patient at the Right Time: Communicating Clearly

KEY TERMS

- unapproved abbreviations and symbols
- brand name
- chemical name
- generic name
- inpatient prescription
- medication order
- outpatient prescription
- patient profile
- stat orders

OBJECTIVES

After completing this chapter the student will be able to:

- Evaluate an outpatient prescription for completeness.
- Evaluate an inpatient prescription for accuracy.
- Gather information for a patient profile.
- Explain the meanings of the terms "brand name," "generic name," and "chemical name."
- Communicate effectively with patients and healthcare professionals.
- Communicate effectively with special-needs patients.
- Describe the expected turnaround time for medication orders.
- Develop a procedure for verifying unacceptable abbreviations.
- Use professional judgment to determine which communications require a pharmacist's intervention.

One of the most important roles of a pharmacy technician is to ensure effective communication with patients and other healthcare professionals. The medical field has a language of its own that is familiar to healthcare professionals but is often very confusing to the patient. An experienced technician with a background in medical terminology can help to bridge the communication gap and provide a comfort zone for patients, paving the way for more effective communication with the pharmacist. Although it is important for the technician to speak in understandable terms to the patient, it is equally important to utilize the language of medicine when speaking with other health professionals. The initial encounter with a patient often involves accepting a prescription and evaluating it for completeness and accuracy. This chapter will provide information to facilitate that process.

Outpatient Prescription

outpatient prescription A medication ordered by a prescriber on a prescription blank intended to be dispensed in a pharmacy outside the hospital, with instructions for the patient to take the doses at home.

medication order Any drug ordered by a qualified prescriber, but usually considered to be an inpatient order.

An outpatient prescription is a written or oral medication order from an authorized prescriber for a specific medication to be dispensed to a specific patient pursuant to the diagnosis of a condition or a risk factor. It is generally intended to provide a cure, slow the progression of disease, treat the symptoms, or prevent a risk factor from developing into a health problem. There are several ways in which an outpatient prescription can reach the pharmacy. When the patient arrives at the pharmacy counter with a new prescription, the technician greets the patient and begins the very important task of evaluating the prescription for completeness and accuracy. As the patient is greeted, the technician should carefully observe the patient for any concerns that might create a communication or special-needs challenge. Most prescriptions are written in the format shown in Figure 7.1. This format helps the technician quickly locate the required information and request any additional information needed from the patient. The following information refers to the labels in Figure 7.1:

A. Name, address, and phone number of the prescriber or the hospital or clinic where the prescriber practices.

B. Full name and address of the patient (verify the spelling).

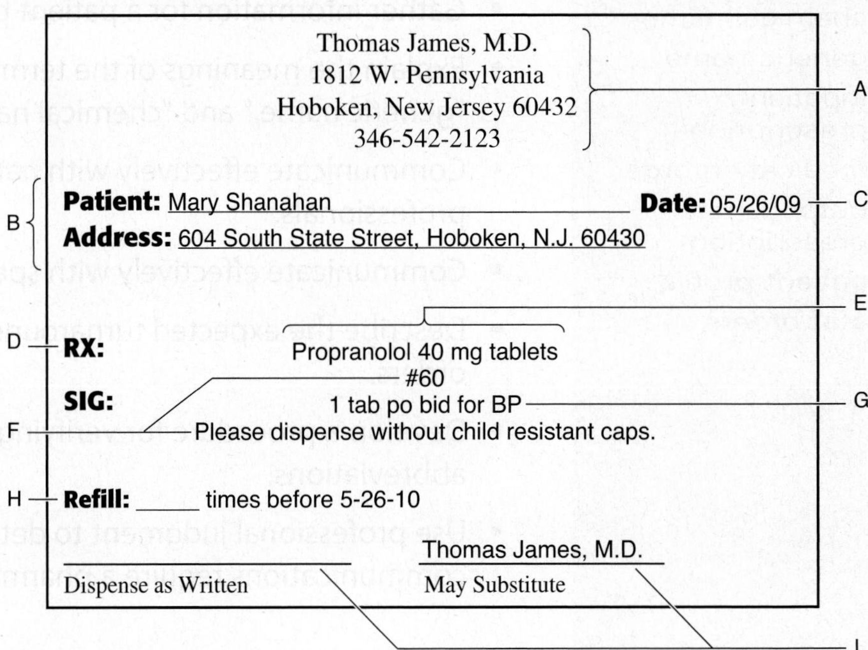

Thomas James, M.D.
1812 W. Pennsylvania
Hoboken, New Jersey 60432
346-542-2123

Patient: Mary Shanahan **Date:** 05/26/09
Address: 604 South State Street, Hoboken, N.J. 60430

RX: Propranolol 40 mg tablets
#60
SIG: 1 tab po bid for BP
Please dispense without child resistant caps.

Refill: _____ times before 5-26-10

Dispense as Written ______ Thomas James, M.D. May Substitute

Figure 7.1 A typical outpatient prescription includes the (**A**) prescriber's contact information, (**B**) name and address of the patient, (**C**) date written, (**D**) Rx symbol, (**E**) drug name or inscription, (**F**) dispensing directions, (**G**) Signa, (**H**) refill instructions from the prescriber, and (**I**) prescriber signature line.

C. Date written, if known. The date written is especially important for controlled substances because they can only be filled within 6 months after the prescription was written. For a noncontrolled substance, unless there is serious concern about the length of time elapsed, the date the prescription is filled can be used if there is no date entered.

D. Rx symbol (also called the superscription) preceding the drug name.

E. Drug name or inscription—includes the medication, strength, and dosage form. Be certain to check each of these for legibility and accuracy. As you grow in knowledge, unusual doses will prompt you to check the literature for acceptable dose ranges.

F. Dispensing directions, including the quantity to dispense (also called the subscription). The quantity should be reasonable for the course of therapy.

TIP

A prescription written for 60 capsules with directions to take one capsule four times a day for 10 days with no refills should prompt a phone call to the prescriber's office.

G. Signa or Sig: directions to a patient, often using abbreviations that must be clearly typed on the label in fully understandable text. The directions should coincide with the drug name, dose range, and route of administration.

CAUTION

Caution: Labeling a suppository with orders to "take by mouth" is an obvious error.

H. Any special instructions from the prescriber concerning refill authorization or expiration date of prescription. A prescriber may give a patient a prescription for pain in case he or she needs it immediately after a procedure, and put a 7-day expiration date on the prescription so the patient does not hold the prescription and try to fill it later for another problem.

I. Prescriber signature line: may contain two lines labeled "Dispense as Written" or "May Substitute" to indicate the prescriber's authorization for generic substitution.

Prescription blanks for controlled substances require the physician's DEA number, and some states require a special prescription blank written on security paper that will print "void" across the blank if it is reproduced by a copy machine. Any missing patient information can be obtained from the patient. The patient should be asked as each new prescription is presented if he or she has any drug allergies, and the response(s) should be noted on the prescription. If the patient gives a positive response, the question should be repeated (any others?) until a negative response is received. If the patient indicates no allergies, the letters "NKA" (no known allergies) should be documented on the prescription and in the patient profile.

patient profile Computer file that lists a patient's medication history, including allergies, diagnoses, age, weight, and all medications ordered.

Many pharmacies have a patient profile form for new patients to document and update information for the patient profile. If there is no written form, use the computer software to request and document patient information. Each new medication dispensed to the patient then becomes a part of the patient profile to assist the pharmacist in the drug utilization review (DUR) to assess the appropriateness of the new medication for this patient. It is extremely important for the patient profile to be accurate and current because the computerized drug interaction alerts that warn of medication concerns during data entry are based on the drugs, allergies, and diagnoses listed in the patient profile. Another important factor to consider when receiving a new prescription is the patient's method of payment. Third-party insurance information must be entered into the patient profile before the prescription is entered. This will be discussed more fully in Chapter 9. Figure 7.2 shows an example of patient profile information that should be entered into a software program. All of the patient's information is helpful in preventing adverse events, but some of the information is not legally required and some patients may refuse to give additional information. The technician must be sensitive to the patient's reluctance to provide more information than is legally required. If the prescription is written for a brand name drug and the physician has authorized a generic substitution, the patient should be asked if he or she prefers brand-name or generic drugs, keeping in mind the cost difference and the fact that a third-party insurance plan may mandate the use of a generic drug.

brand name The trade name given to a drug by the manufacturer for marketing purposes.

TIP **A drug will have three different names; the brand name which is a trade name assigned by the manufacturer for marketing; a generic name given to the drug by The United States Adopted Names; and a chemical name derived from the exact chemical formula of the drug.**

The prescription evaluation process may take only a few minutes or it may be much more complicated, but the time spent communicating with the patient during this initial process begins the establishment of a trust relationship between the

Name________ D.O.B.________ Sex ____

Address ________ Phone ________

Diagnoses ________

Allergies ________

Primary Insurance ________ Group Number ________

Plan Number ________ Subscriber ________

Subscriber ID Number ________ Patient Code ________

Secondary Insurance ________ Group Number ________

Plan Number ________ Subscriber ________

Subscriber ID Number ________ Patient Code ________

MEDICATION LIST

RX NUMBER	DRUG	QUANTITY	DATE FILLED	RPH COMMENTS

Figure 7.2 Patient profile.

patient and the pharmacy professionals. On the most difficult day, when every patient has presented challenges and it's almost closing time, as the last patient of the day walks up to the pharmacy counter with six new prescriptions and an insurance card you have never seen before, take a deep breath and put that friendly smile on your face and greet the patient.

Professional Judgment Scenario 7.1

On a Sunday evening as the pharmacy is about to close, Mrs. Jones, a new patient, arrives at the pharmacy with six new prescriptions for her husband from the nearby hospital emergency room and presents an insurance card. Jill, the pharmacy technician, gathers the pertinent patient information and creates a new patient profile, being careful to note any allergies or drug interactions reported by the patient. She enters the third-party information from the patient's insurance card and begins to enter the prescriptions into the computer. With each prescription entered, the software returns a message that insurance coverage is denied. After double checking that all numbers were entered correctly, Jill informs Mrs. Jones that her insurance has denied coverage and she will need to pay cash for the prescriptions and submit them to her insurance company for reimbursement. The insurance company cannot be contacted by phone until Monday morning. Mrs. Jones becomes irate and insists that her insurance is valid and should cover all of the medicine, and Jill must have made a mistake. It is now past closing time, Jill is very tired, and her family is holding dinner for her.

The pharmacist is finishing some of the closing paperwork and waiting to check the prescriptions so she can go home after a long weekend of work. Mrs. Jones has changed from yelling to pleading with Jill to fill the medications because her husband needs to begin them immediately and she has no money to pay for them. Discuss the following resolutions to the situation and decide which would be the most appropriate action for Jill to take:

1. Tell Mrs. Jones that it is past closing time and she needs to either pay for her prescriptions or take them elsewhere.
2. Fill the six prescriptions and tell Mrs. Jones the insurance company will be contacted in the morning.
3. Consult with the pharmacist about possible solutions, such as:
   a. Fill each prescription with enough medication to last until the morning when Mrs. Jones can call her insurance company.
   b. Apologize to Mrs. Jones and direct her to a 24-hour pharmacy in the next block.

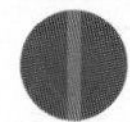

Inpatient Prescriptions

An inpatient prescription is written in a different format compared with an outpatient prescription and some of the required information is different. These orders are written for a patient in a hospital, nursing home, or some other institutional setting where the medication will be administered by a healthcare professional. The labeling requirements also differ from those for outpatient prescriptions. Each institution usually has a certain form that is used by the prescriber. Often the form is in triplicate and one page is sent to the pharmacy. In some cases the medication orders may be written into the patient chart and transcribed by a nurse or another healthcare

inpatient prescription A medication order written by a prescriber for a patient who is in an institution; the order is intended to be dispensed by the hospital pharmacy and administered to the patient by a healthcare professional.

Date/ Time	Orders	Progress Notes
3/15/04	Admit: GMF	54 y/o ♀ c̄ h/o HTN, DM, ↑lipids
1300	Dx: pyelonephritis	presents c̄ 2 days of worsening
	HTN	Ⓛ side low back pain, dysuria
	Type 2 DM	and fever. She does have a
	hyperlipidemia	h/o frequent UTIs; last one
	Condition: good	several months ago. She
	V/S: q shift	states she also has lower Abd
	Activity: up ad lib	pain and some nausea s̄ emesis
	Nursing: I+O's, Accu✓ qAC+HS	pt notes blood in urine
	Diet: ADA 2000 calorie	PMH: HTN, DM, ↑lipids
	Allergies: Sulfa	PSHx: hysterectomy
	meds: Rocephin 1gm IV q24°	FHx: CAD, HTN, CVA
	Accupril 20mg p.o. qd	SocHx: Divorced - receptionist
	glucophage 500mg p.o. BID	⊕ Tob 1ppd soc ETOH ∅ illicits
	Lipitor 40mg p.o. qd	All: Sulfa meds: Accupril 20 qd
	Demerol 50mg IM q4-6° PRN pain	glucophage 500 BID
	Pyridium 200mg p.o. TID x 2 days	Ⓞ gen A/Ox3 NAD Lipitor 40 qd
	Tylenol 500mg p.o. BID PRN fever	VSS T-100°
	Restoril 15mg p.o. q HS PRN insomnia	CV - RRR Lungs - CTA
	Compazine 25mg p.o. q8° PRN nausea	Abd - soft tender suprapubic +BS
	Labs:	⊕ CVAT
	CBC, Chem 22, KUB	Ext - ∅ CCE
	Renal Ultrasound	A/P 1) Pyelonephritis 2) DM 3) HTN
		4) ↑lipids
		Admit, IV antibx, pain control
		IVF - continue current meds

PATIENT INFORMATION

Jane Doe 54 y/o

2-23-50

MEDICAL ORDERS AND PROGRESS NOTES

EL-FR-NR-1001-1101

CHART COPY

Figure 7.3 Admission orders with SOAP notes. (Reprinted with permission from Mohr ME. Lab Experiences for the Pharmacy Technician. Philadelphia: Lippincott Williams & Wilkins, 2006.)

professional trained for this task. Many hospitals have pharmacists on the floors to verify medication orders and enter them into the computer for the pharmacy to fill. Some medication orders may be entered into an automated dispensing system so the nurse can retrieve the medication and administer it to the patient. The institution may use a medication cart system that can be filled by a robotic system. These automated systems will be discussed in a later chapter. Some smaller hospitals may use a manual fill cart system whereby the pharmacy fills the medications for a predetermined day's supply and exchanges the drawers when empty. Learning to work with each of the different systems will be a continuing part of your education and orientation in different practice settings because reading and evaluating the medication order is an important responsibility of technicians in many institutional settings.

Three types of medication orders are usually seen in an institutional setting:

- **Admission orders:** medication orders and nursing instructions written by a physician when a patient is first admitted to a facility. See Figure 7.3 for an example of an inpatient admission order.
- **Routine medication orders:** written after a routine physician's visit with the patient, indicating any change or addition to the medication regimen. See Figure 7.4 for an example of a routine medication order.
- **Discharge orders:** orders written by the physician when the patient leaves the facility and returns home. See Figure 7.5 for an example of a discharge order.

All of these orders usually include nursing instructions, diagnosis, treatment plans, and/or other information that may not be applicable to the pharmacy. It is important for the technician to understand the format for the orders and choose the items that the pharmacy needs to fill so that patient care is not compromised. Admission orders often include information written in the form of a SOAP note:

- **Subjective:** the patient's description of the problem.
- **Objective:** the physician's observations and questioning of the patient.
- **Assessment:** the physician's examination results and diagnosis of the problem(s).
- **Plan:** the treatment plan ordered by the physician.

Date/Time 05-03-06 Medication Orders

Lasix 40mg / D5W 100ml

Infuse over 30 minutes once daily

M Amado MD

Medical Orders

Pharmacy Copy

Patient Information

Sandra Smithson 45 yo female

Figure 7.4 Routine medication orders (Reprinted with permission from Mohr ME. Lab Experiences for the Pharmacy Technician. Philadelphia: Lippincott Williams & Wilkins, 2006.)

Date/Time 05/05/06	Discharge Orders	
D/C Lasix 40 mg/D5W		
D/C IV Heparin		
D/C Vasotec 5 mg		
Losarten 50 mg	#30 1 po qd am	Refill X6
Lasix 40 mg	#30 1 po qd am	Refill X6
Coumadin 5 mg	#30 1 po qd am	Refill X6
Have regular checks at Coumadin Clinic each month Call office for follow-up appointment.		Dr. M. Amado
General Hospital 1204 E. Grant Green Mountain, Wisconsin	Sandra Smithson 6800 Westfield Boulevard Green Mountain, Wisconsin	

Figure 7.5 Discharge orders.

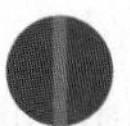

Communicating with the Patient

Counseling patients about their medications is the right and responsibility of the pharmacist, who has spent years studying to become a medication expert. This is a vital part of excellent pharmaceutical care that will give the patients the knowledge to make informed decisions about their health. The patient is more likely to be compliant with his or her dosage regimen if all his or her questions and concerns have been addressed. In the busy world we live in, there are many impediments to the provision of patient counseling. The patient may have taken time off from work to see a doctor and needs to return to work after procuring the prescription.

The patient may be ill or be the caregiver of an ill child or adult and need to return home quickly. When asked if he or she has any questions for the pharmacist, the patient will often not know what questions to ask and refuse counseling. The pharmacist has many demands on his or her time and may seem too busy to be bothered with questions.

The technician's role in facilitating patient counseling can make all the difference in whether effective counseling takes place. This role begins when the technician greets the patient and accepts the prescription. A friendly, welcoming greeting will help put the patient at ease and demonstrate a caring attitude. Remember that patients may be facing many different challenges that interfere with their ability to respond in an agreeable manner. If the patient has just been released from the hospital, he or she may be concerned about taking care of his or her health needs without the assistance of the nurses at the hospital. He or she may be nervous about returning to a situation where he or she is expected to look and act normal when he or she still feels ill. If the patient has just been diagnosed with a disease that will require major lifestyle changes, such as diabetes, he or she may be feeling overwhelmed. A patient living with a chronic condition that requires intervention by healthcare workers coming to the home for therapy, or by frequent visits to a hospital or clinic, may be upset by the intrusions into his or her life and the constant expense of his or her condition. A person with a terminal illness may be going through one of the various grief stages of denial, anger, bargaining, and acceptance. One or more of these challenges may be facing each patient who arrives at the pharmacy counter, and the technician's ability to communicate in a professional manner will set the stage for the patient's willingness to accept patient counseling from the pharmacist. As the patient approaches the counter, the technician should be alert for any special needs the patient might have. Following are some problems you might encounter and some possible solutions:

- The patient speaks a different language.
  - Ask if the patient brought a family member who speaks English.
  - Ask if anyone in the pharmacy speaks the patient's language.
  - Have a translation dictionary available.
  - Some pharmacy software will print prescriptions in several languages.
- The patient is hearing-impaired.
  - Do not yell, but speak distinctly in a moderately loud voice.
  - Look at the patient as you speak, because hearing-impaired people often can read lips.
  - Ask if anyone knows American sign language (consider adding sign language as one of your skills).
  - Keep a pencil and paper to write notes to patients and have them respond in writing.
- The patient is visually impaired.
  - Greet the patient as he or she walks up to help him or her locate the counter.
  - Introduce yourself as the pharmacy technician because he or she may not be able to read your name tag.
  - Make a note to place items on the prescription vials (if there are more than one) to help the patient differentiate the medications at home. Tape a rubber band to one vial and a paper clip to another so the patient can feel the difference. Be sure to explain to the patient how each vial is marked.
- The patient is angry or upset.
  - Do not enter into a shouting match with a patient.
  - Do not take the patient's anger personally; you just happened to be the one in front of him or her at the time his or her anger exploded.
  - Speak in a calm voice and ask the patient to explain the problem so you can help find a solution.
  - If you are unable to defuse the situation, excuse yourself, step away from the patient, and enlist the help of another technician or a pharmacist.
  - If the patient seems distraught, ask if there is anything you can do to help.
  - Listen if he or she chooses to describe his or her health problem, because sometimes a patient just needs to verbalize his or her fears to someone who will understand.
  - Remember that any information heard during this encounter is privileged and highly confidential unless there is a serious concern that needs to be addressed with the pharmacist.

Your experience and your professionalism will enable you to become adept at gathering needed patient information during this initial encounter. The technician's ability to gather important data and gain the patient's trust will create an environment where the patient will feel safe and be willing to accept counseling from the pharmacist and ask any questions that need to be addressed. See Preparation Method 7-1 for step-by-step instructions for greeting the patient, evaluating the prescription, and gathering needed information for the patient profile.

Telephone Protocols

Answering the telephone in a busy pharmacy is traditionally the technician's responsibility and one that requires a professional attitude and good judgment. The technician must decide quickly whether the caller should be directed to the pharmacist or whether a technician can provide the requested information. The technician should answer the phone by saying the name of the pharmacy and identifying themselves as a technician. "Good afternoon, this is Nickelson's Pharmacy, Jill the technician speaking." This is especially important if a physician is calling in a prescription, because many times when someone answers a pharmacy phone, the physician will immediately begin to give the oral prescription for a patient. The technician must speak in a very professional manner and ask the physician to hold for a pharmacist. At the present time, it is not legal in most states for a technician to take an oral prescription from a prescriber. If, as sometimes happens, the physi-

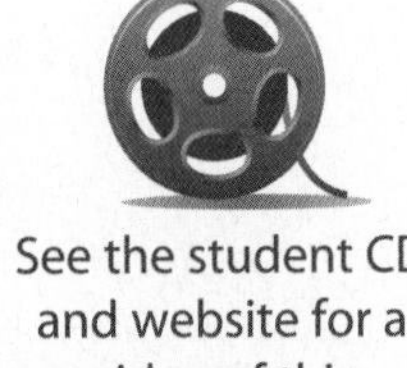

See the student CD and website for a video of this procedure.

Preparation Method 7.1
Instructions for Greeting the Patient, Evaluating the Prescription, and Gathering Needed Information for the Patient Profile

1. Observe as the patient approaches the counter for any special health needs the patient may have and for clues to the patient's demeanor.
2. Make eye contact as the patient nears the counter and smile pleasantly. Don't overwhelm the patient with exuberance until you assess his or her mood.
3. Speak clearly and distinctly. "Hello, Mrs. Smith, how can I help you today?"
4. As the patient hands you the prescription, quickly examine it for any missing patient information.
5. "Have you had prescriptions filled here before, Mrs. Smith?" If so, use the patient identifier that will bring up the patient profile in the computer (usually a date of birth or phone number).
6. Verify that the demographic information is still the same.
7. Verify that the third-party insurance information is current.
8. If allergies are listed in the computer profile, ask the patient if there are any additional allergies.
9. If no allergies are listed, ask the patient if he or she has any allergies. If the patient gives a positive response, document the allergy on the prescription and in the computer profile, and continue to ask if there are any others until a negative response is received.
10. Ask if the patient will wait for the prescription or pick it up later. If he or she says he or she will wait, give the patient an approximate wait time. If the patient prefers to pick the prescription up later, ask when he or she will return.

cian speaks so quickly that you are unable to interrupt, write as clearly as you can the physician's order, including the patient's name, and get a contact number from the physician so the pharmacist can call back and verify the prescription. Technicians should practice taking oral prescriptions from other students even though this is not currently a technician's responsibility. There is reason to believe that at some time in the future, qualified, educated technicians will be allowed to perform this function, and education should prepare you for the future as well as the present.

If a patient is calling in to check on refills, to order a refill, or to ask if the doctor's office has called in a new prescription, the technician can usually respond without interrupting the pharmacist. If a patient calls with concerns that he or she may have received the wrong medication, the technician may take all the pertinent information, including the patient's name, the prescription number, drug name, date of fill, description of the tablet, and why he or she believes there is an error. The technician can look up the prescription and any other needed information to verify the issue, but must then take the information to the pharmacist, who will probably want to speak to the patient personally. Likewise, if the patient calls to report he or she is having an adverse effect or allergic reaction from a medication, the call should be immediately referred to a pharmacist. The technician should let the pharmacist know the nature of the call instead of just saying, "Pharmacist: call on line one." When a patient calls with questions about his or her medication or asks for a recommendation for an over-the-counter product, this call should also be referred to a pharmacist for patient counseling.

Communicating With Health Professionals

Frequently in a pharmacy, a health professional will either call or stop by for various reasons. It is important for technicians to identify themselves by wearing a name tag or informing a caller of their position. Technicians must always be cognizant of the types of questions they are qualified to answer. In a teaching hospital there will be many students from various health professions who may stop by the pharmacy with questions. They will assume that any information you give them is correct and will act on it, so it is important to use professional judgment in deciding which questions should be referred to the pharmacist.

As you grow in knowledge and experience, you will also grow in the confidence to communicate in a professional manner with other health professionals. It is important to use correct terminology and speak with dignity and respect. Remember that the fact that you are speaking with another health professional does not allow you to breach a patient's confidentiality. Be aware of the difference between idle gossip about a patient and the health professional's need to know. Communicating with other health professionals is a rewarding aspect of a technician's career and will increase your knowledge and enhance the respect you receive from others.

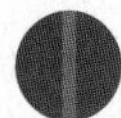

Evaluating the Prescription

After the initial communication with the patient and gathering of the profile information, the prescription can be evaluated, entered into the computer, and prepared for the pharmacist to check. Gathering patient and physician information involves the components shown in Figure 7.1 A–C. Evaluating the prescription for data entry involves a close examination of parts D–I in Figure 7.1. This prescription format should be committed to memory so that missing information will be obvious when you examine the prescription. Keep in mind that a prescriber may use a different format, but as long as all of the required information is present, the prescription is valid. First examine the drug name line to be certain that all of the required information is listed to ensure that the exact drug, strength, and dosage form will be dispensed to the patient. If the medication prescribed is available in only one strength, the prescriber may not include the strength. If the strength is missing and more than one strength is commercially available, a call to the prescriber's office is required to verify the correct strength. Check the entire body of the prescription for any information that needs to be verified before the call is placed. Check the quantity and the directions to be sure they are legible and coincide with the drug and dosage form in the medication line. (More details about dosage form and route of administration are discussed in Chapter 8.) The route of administration may or may not be indicated in either the medication line or the Signa line, but in many cases the dosage form and route of administration can be deduced by analyzing the whole prescription.

Professional Judgment Scenario 7.2

A patient presents a prescription to Jill, the technician in a retail pharmacy. After gathering the patient's information, Jill evaluates the body of the prescription to begin data entry.

The prescription reads: Lasix 40 mg #30 1 bid. Lasix is available in liquid oral solutions (10 mg/mL and 40 mg/5 mL), oral tablets (20 mg, 40 mg, and 80 mg), and an IV or IM solution for injection at 10 mg/mL.

All of these dosage forms may be listed in the computer databank. Using the professional judgment of a technician, help Jill decide which dosage form and strength should be chosen for this prescription and give reasons for your choice.

Any information obtained in a phone call to the prescriber that will result in a change in the body of the prescription must be transmitted to a pharmacist by the prescriber (or his agent). The pharmacist will then document the change on the prescription. As you grow in experience and knowledge, you will be able to use your professional judgment to determine which aspects of the prescription can be ascertained and when the prescriber must be contacted for verification by utilizing available clues. Remember, if there is any doubt about the correctness of the information, always check with the pharmacist. As the pharmacist begins to trust that you will bring any uncertainty to him or her, you will begin to feel a mutual professional respect developing, and you will be trusted with increased responsibilities that will result in a fulfilling career path.

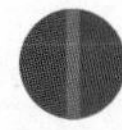 Prescription Turnaround Time

There are various ways to manage the prescription workflow in an outpatient pharmacy to prevent long wait times for patients. Patients should be encouraged to call in refills a day early or order them on the Internet so that wait times can be reduced for patients with new prescriptions. The patient cannot call in a new prescription or fax it to the pharmacy using a personal or commercial fax machine. A new prescription can only be faxed directly from the prescriber's office or a hospital fax machine to the pharmacy. A patient presenting a new prescription at the pharmacy counter should always be offered the opportunity to drop it off and return later to pick up the completed prescription. This will enable the pharmacy to quickly assist patients who have a need to begin medication immediately. The ability to prioritize prescriptions will increase with experience. A patient who is obviously ill or in pain, or a mother with a child crying from the pain of an ear infection should be assisted as quickly as possible without upsetting other patients who are waiting. A technician with excellent communication skills and a good rapport with patients can facilitate this process.

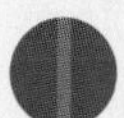

Medication Order Turnaround Time

Inpatient medication orders should be filled as soon as possible. Most institutions have regular administration times for routine medications, and new patients should begin receiving their medications at the next regular administration time. An order marked "asap" should generally be returned to the floor within the hour. Stat orders should be filled immediately and are expected on the floor within 15 minutes. Each institution will have protocols concerning medication administration times, and the technician should be familiar with these and follow them as closely as possible for the well-being of the patient.

stat orders Medication orders written in a hospital setting that should be delivered within 15 minutes.

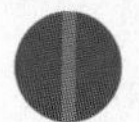

Pharmaceutical Abbreviations

The medical and pharmaceutical professions have traditionally used many abbreviations, which often lead to medication errors. It is important for the technician to recognize and correctly interpret abbreviations that are still in common use today. In recent years, the Institute for Safe Medication Practices (ISMP) and the Joint Commission on Accreditation of Healthcare Organizations (JCAHO) have compiled lists of problematic abbreviations. The JCAHO has instituted a list of unapproved abbreviations for institutions seeking accreditation, and requires institutions to add abbreviations to the do-not-use list that are a concern in their facility. An expanded list of problematic abbreviations will be listed in Appendix B and this topic will be further discussed in Chapter 10, but is important to note as a vital issue in the evaluation of a prescription. The technician should verify any abbreviation or symbol that is not clear before continuing with data entry. Each institution must have in place protocols for verifying abbreviations and symbols that appear on the do-not-use list even if their meaning seems clear. This frequently may be the responsibility of the technician and is another area where the technician must use professional judgment and appropriate communication skills.

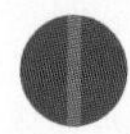

Overcoming the "Halo Effect"

A recurring theme in this book is the importance of developing your knowledge and skills and learning to trust your own professional judgment as a technician as you build that trust with the pharmacists and other health professionals you encounter in your work. When you see an error or something that seems questionable and may cause harm to a patient, you must speak up! Even if the pharmacist or physician is the most outstanding person in his field, even if you will be severely chastised for questioning him or her, even if you may be wrong, you must question him or her! Many patients are dead because technicians didn't feel that it was "their place" to question a pharmacist or a physician. The best pharmacists and the best physicians are still human and human error is always a possibility, especially in the busy world of healthcare.

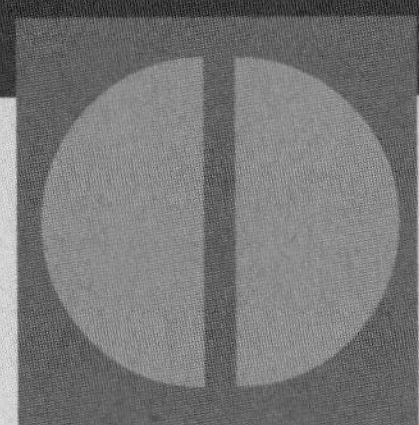

Case Study 7.1

Tamara has been working as a technician in the Medical Arts Building Clinic Pharmacy for several years and has become acquainted with all the other health professionals in the building. The patients see one of the physicians in the clinic and also visit the dental clinic. It is a full-service clinic with laboratory and X-ray facilities, and a nutritionist. The clinic operates with a true team atmosphere and provides excellent holistic care to its patients. Tamara has developed a trusting relationship with the patients as a result of her outstanding communication skills. One morning, Mrs. Eads arrived at the pharmacy counter to pick up some refills she had called in earlier. Tamara noticed that her speech was slurred. She knew that Mrs. Eads did not drink alcohol and that her speech had never been this way before.

"Mrs. Eads, are you feeling well this morning?" Tamara asked.

"I feel fine, Tamara," stated Mrs. Eads, "but for some strange reason I don't seem to be able to speak clearly. I woke up this morning and my face felt a little droopy, and I just can't seem to talk correctly."

"Mrs. Eads, would you like me to call an ambulance? I think you need to be checked at the hospital."

"Oh heavens no, I feel fine and I have lots to do today. I'll just take my prescriptions and be on my way."

Tamara was extremely worried that Mrs. Eads might have had a stroke and didn't want her to leave. As Tamara went to get the prescriptions, she picked up the phone and buzzed the nurse across the hall. "Nancy," she said, "please come over and check on Mrs. Eads. Her speech is slurred and I am concerned about her."

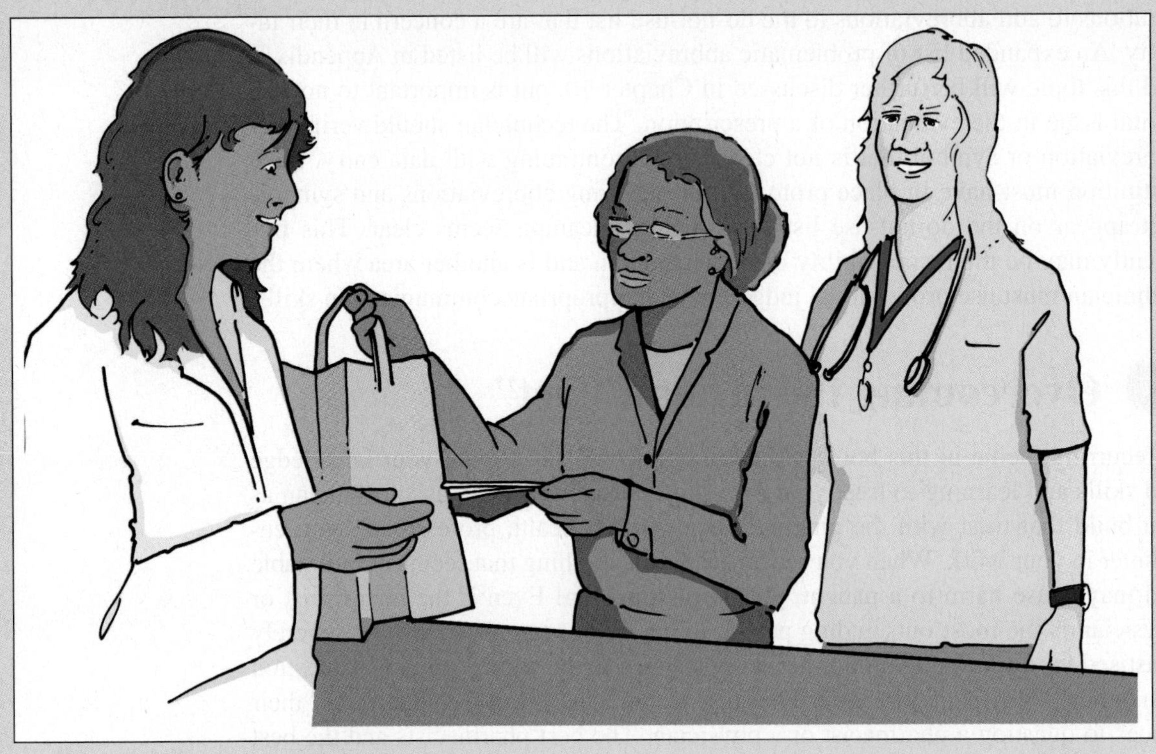

After speaking with Mrs. Eads, Nancy was able to persuade her to at least take a cab to the hospital to be checked out. Later in the day Tamara received a call from Mr. Eads saying his wife had been admitted to the hospital; she did indeed have a stroke, but arrived at the hospital early enough for them to initiate treatment and prevent serious damage.

1. Did Tamara breach Mrs. Eads's confidentiality by calling the nurse without her permission?
2. How important was the previous relationship established by Tamara with her patient?
3. If the pharmacist was busy on the other phone, should Tamara have waited to ask her advice before calling the nurse?
4. Should an ambulance have been called even though the patient refused?
5. Was this an occasion where Tamara needed to trust her professional judgment to save precious time?

Chapter Summary

- The technician's role in greeting and communicating with patients is essential for developing a trust relationship with the pharmacy personnel.
- An accurate drug utilization review performed by the pharmacist depends on the proper patient information being entered in the patient profile.
- Learning the general format for required information on an outpatient prescription will enable the technician to quickly determine if required information is missing.
- Each time a patient presents a new prescription, the technician should ask if the patient has any new drug allergies.
- Evaluate the body of the prescription for legibility, dosage form, route of administration, compatibility, and the use of unapproved abbreviations.
- Medication orders will have a different format than an outpatient prescription and require different information.
- The technician must be familiar with terminology to read and understand an admission order and choose the items that pertain to the pharmacy to dispense in the proper manner for the practice setting.
- The technician should be alert for any special challenges the patient may have that would require special consideration.
- Telephone protocols will vary according to the practice setting and the nature of the call.
- All patient information is strictly confidential unless there is a need to share it with another healthcare professional.
- Time and workflow management will decrease the wait times for outpatient prescriptions, but some prescriptions may still need to be prioritized because of the condition of the patient.

- Medication orders may be routinely dispensed to accommodate the next medication administration time, marked "asap" to be sent within the hour, or designated stat orders, which should reach the floor in 15 minutes or less, if possible.
- Some medication abbreviations should no longer be used because they have resulted in an increased error rate.
- Technicians must always question any situation they believe might cause harm to a patient.

Review Questions

Multiple Choice

Choose the correct answer to the following questions:

1. All of the following information is required to be on an outpatient prescription except the
   a. patient name
   b. patient address
   c. patient date of birth
   d. prescriber name and address
2. The drug name or inscription on an outpatient prescription includes all of the following except the
   a. medication name
   b. quantity to dispense
   c. drug strength
   d. dosage form
3. An inpatient medication order would include all of the following except the
   a. patient name
   b. patient address
   c. physician signature
   d. patient diagnosis
4. All of the following are effective ways to communicate with a hearing-impaired patient except:
   a. Look at the patient as you speak.
   b. Use sign language.
   c. Write notes on a pad and let the patient respond in writing.
   d. Yell as loudly as you can to see if they can hear you.
5. All of the following can be considered a technician's responsibility except:
   a. answering the pharmacy telephone
   b. greeting the patient
   c. counseling the patient
   d. evaluating the prescription for missing information

Fill in the Blanks

Fill the blank(s) with the missing word or words.

6. The SOAP note written by the physician with the admission orders contains four parts: subjective, ________, assessment, and ________.
7. The medication orders written when a patient leaves an inpatient facility are called ________________________.
8. A stat order should be delivered to the hospital floor within ________ minutes.
9. If a patient responds that he or she does not have any allergies, the letters ____________ should be written on the prescription.
10. The patient profile screen in the computer includes the patient ______________ and the list of ______________.

Matching

Match the following statements with a T for technician or a P for pharmacist to indicate whether the function can be performed by a technician or requires a pharmacist.

11. ______ Answering a physician's question about whether a drug is in the hospital formulary.
12. ______ Helping a patient choose a suitable OTC cough syrup for her child.
13. ______ Helping a patient find an OTC fever reducer recommended by her physician.
14. ______ Calling the physician's office for refill authorization on a patient's prescription.
15. ______ Taking a call from the physician's office and accepting a new oral prescription.

True/False

Place a T or an F in the blanks below to indicate if the statement is true or false.

16. ______ If the physician writes the brand name of a drug on the prescription, the brand name drug must always be dispensed.
17. ______ The technician should never question the pharmacist about a possible medication error because the pharmacist has years of education.
18. ______ If a physician calls in a refill authorization to the technician but then changes the dose or directions on the prescription, the call must be transferred to a pharmacist for verification.
19. ______ A new prescription faxed from a fax line in the patient's home or place of work can be filled.
20. ______ If the pharmacist leaves the pharmacy for lunch, it is okay for the technician to remain in the pharmacy as long as no new prescriptions are filled.

LEARNING ACTIVITIES

1. Re-read the case study in Chapter 1 about Terri and Mr. Laker (Case Study 1.3) and discuss how the different actions of Terri with Mr. Laker, and Tamara with Mrs. Eads resulted in different outcomes for the patients. Create a dialogue for Terri in the situation with Mr. Laker that might have created a better outcome for him. Discuss the phone call Tamara might have received from Mr. Eads if she had not intervened and had allowed Mrs. Eads to leave the clinic alone.

2. Use the information in Figures 7.3, 7.4, and 7.5, and the abbreviations in Table 7.1 to answer the following questions.

   Questions related to Figure 7.3:

   a. If Jane Doe is a new patient, list the information that would be entered into her patient profile.

   b. What medications was the patient taking before entering the hospital?

   c. List the new medications that have been ordered.

   d. Who is the prescribing physician?

   Questions related to Figure 7.4:

   e. What other patient identification would be helpful to ensure that the order is administered to the correct patient?

   f. Will this order replace another order or be added to the orders already in place?

   g. Will this order be administered IV, IM, or PO?

   Questions related to Figure 7.5:

   h. What does the abbreviation D/C mean in this order?

   i. Why is it important to D/C these orders before the patient leaves the hospital?

   j. Discuss how these orders will be entered into the patient profile.

Table 7.1 Abbreviation List for Figure 7.3

ATSO GMF	Admit to service of ____________ on General Medical Floor.
ADA diet	American Diabetic Association diet
Abd	abdomen soft and tender with positive bowel sounds
A + O X 3	alert and oriented to person, place, and time.
CAD	coronary artery disease
CTA	lungs clear to auscultation
CVA	cerebral vascular accident—stroke
CV-RRR	heart—regular rate and rhythm
CBC	complete blood count
Chem. 22	lab profile of blood
DM	diabetes mellitus
Ext-No CCE	no cyanosis, clubbing, or edema of extremities
FHx	family history
HTN	hypertension
I + O's	measure fluids in and out
KUB	kidney-ureter-bladder ultrasound
NAD	no apparent distress
PMH	past medical history
PSHx	previous surgical history
Social ETOH	social alcohol drinker
SocHx	social history
VSS	vital signs stable

Suggested Readings

Allen L, Popovich N, Ansel H. Ansel's Pharmaceutical Dosage Forms and Drug Delivery Systems. 8th ed. Baltimore, MD: Lippincott Williams & Wilkins, 2005

Genarro AR, ed. Remington: The Science and Practice of Pharmacy. Baltimore, MD: Lippincott Williams & Wilkins, 2006.

Mohr ME. Lab Experiences for the Pharmacy Technician. Philadelphia: Lippincott Williams & Wilkins, 2006.

Thompson J. A Practical Guide to Contemporary Pharmacy Practice. 3rd ed. Baltimore, MD: Lippincott Williams & Wilkins, 2004.

Chapter **8**

The Right Dosage Form and the Right Route of Administration: Working With Accuracy

KEY TERMS

- alcoholic solution
- angina
- anhydrous absorption bases
- aseptic technique
- binders
- bioavailability
- bolus dose
- buccal tablets
- compressed tablets
- continuous infusion
- controlled-release tablets
- diluents
- disintegrates
- effervescent tablets
- elixirs
- enteric-coated tablets

OBJECTIVES

After completing this chapter, the student will be able to:

- Describe the various dosage forms available for medications.
- Define the routes of administration for medications.
- Correlate the dosage forms with the appropriate route of administration.
- Apply the dosage form and administration route to prescription evaluation.
- Utilize appropriate reference books to verify prescription information.
- Adapt the dosage form and administration route for special-needs patients.

- excipients
- fast-dissolving tablets
- film-coated tablets
- glycerite
- granules
- hydroalcoholic solution
- hydrocarbon bases
- hydrophobic
- implant
- inhalation
- intra-arterial administration
- intra-articular administration
- intracardiac administration
- intradermal injection
- intramuscular (IM) administration
- intraperitoneal administration
- intrapleural administration
- intravenous (IV) administration
- lubricants
- occlusive
- oleaginous
- orally disintegrating tablets
- parenteral
- percutaneous absorption
- stability
- subcutaneous (SQ) administration
- sublingual tablets
- tincture
- transdermal route of administration
- vehicle
- viscous aqueous solutions

diluents Usually inert powders added to a drug to increase the volume.

binders Materials added to a tablet formulation to hold the powders together.

lubricants Topical compounds that are intended to sooth and moisturize dry irritated skin.

disintegrates Compounds added to a tablet formulation to ensure that the tablet will break apart and be available for absorption into the system.

compressed tablets Tablets that are produced by a tablet press exerting great pressure on powders, and shaped by punches and dies of various sizes.

film-coated tablets Tablets covered with a thin layer of polymer designed to dissolve at the desired place in the gastrointestinal tract.

enteric-coated tablets Tablets formulated to pass through the stomach unchanged and dissolve in the intestine.

Medication can be administered in a variety of forms to accommodate the special needs of the patient, to facilitate delivery to the indicated site, or to control the rate of absorption. The available dosage form will determine the route of administration, although some dosage forms can be administered by more than one route. An important aspect of the prescription evaluation process performed by the technician involves matching the dosage form ordered with the route of administration prescribed in the directions to the patient. Any discrepancy should be verified before the prescription is entered into the patient profile.

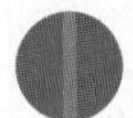

Solid Oral Dosage Forms

Tablets

One of the oldest and most common dosage forms is the oral tablet. The tablet is a solid dosage form that contains an active ingredient (the drug) and may or may not have additional diluents, binders, lubricants, colorings, flavorings, and/or disintegrates. Most commercial tablets on the market today are compressed tablets formed by using pressure and some type of punch machine to create the desired size and shape. Compressed tablets may be sugar-coated and the coatings may be flavored and colored (see Fig. 8.1). This coating process has little therapeutic effect but increases patient acceptance and creates a pharmaceutically elegant tablet. Film-coated tablets are similar in appearance to sugar-coated tablets but the film is a thin layer of water-soluble material. See Figure 8.2 for an example of a film-coated tablet. Enteric-coated tablets are useful for drugs that may be irritating to the mucosa of the stomach or will be inactivated by the gastric fluid in the stomach. The coating is formulated to resist dissolving in the stomach but will disintegrate in the intestine. Figure 8.3 shows an example of an enteric-coated tablet.

Figure 8.1 The most common tablet form is the compressed tablet.

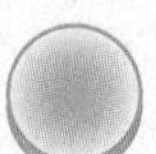

Figure 8.2 Compressed tablets may be coated with a thin layer of water-soluble material to form a film-coated tablet.

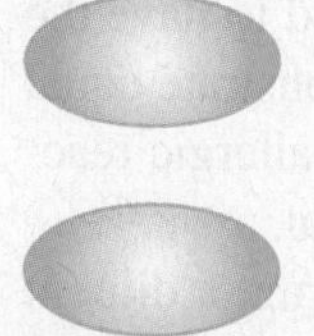

Figure 8.3 Enteric-coated tablets are coated with a substance that will resist dissolving in the stomach but will readily dissolve in the intestine.

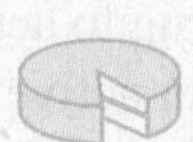

Figure 8.4 Controlled-release tablets release the drug over a period of time.

Controlled-release tablets are formulated to release the drug over a predetermined period of time to provide more constant levels of the drug in the bloodstream (see Fig. 8.4 for a controlled-release tablet). This may be accomplished in several ways. The drug may be encapsulated into beads or granules of various sizes and thicknesses to dissolve at different times. The tablet may have two or more layers formulated to release the drug at different times. The drug may be embedded in an inert wax matrix that allows the drug to leach out through a small hole. With this type of tablet the wax coating may be eliminated in the feces of the patient, causing him or her to think the drug did not have any effect. The patient may need reassurance that the drug was released and exerted the proper therapeutic effect.

Effervescent tablets combine the drug with sodium bicarbonate and an acid so that when water is added the tablet will disintegrate, releasing bubbles of carbon dioxide and forming an effervescent solution. An effervescent tablet is pictured in Figure 8.5. Buccal tablets are small, flat tablets that are placed between the lip or cheek and gum, and dissolve slowly into the oral mucosa. Sublingual tablets are similarly formulated to dissolve and be rapidly absorbed through the oral mucosa, but are placed under the tongue. Orally disintegrating tablets are manufactured by means of numerous technologies to formulate a powder into a tablet that will quickly dissolve when placed in the mouth. This dosage form originated to prevent psychiatric patients from storing tablets in a pouch in the cheek (a process known as "cheeking") and removing them after the nurse leaves the room. This would interfere with their medication therapy. A number of products have emerged from the use of this technology to create a convenient tablet that does not require water to facilitate swallowing. Figure 8.6 shows an orally disintegrating tablet.

Tablet Ingredients

Because most tablets on the market today are compressed tablets produced by compression with a punch and die machine, the ingredients added to the drug are important for producing a uniform tablet that has the correct amount of hardness, will not stick to the machine, and will disintegrate and dissolve in the correct amount of time to release the drug for absorption into the system. These added ingredients are called excipients; they are considered to be inert, but research has shown that they do affect the stability and bioavailability of the dosage form. It is important for the technician to be aware of the excipients used because they may vary when a brand-name drug

controlled-release tablets Tablets that have been formulated to release a drug slowly over a predetermined period of time.

granules Powders that have been wetted and broken into coarse particles to increase stability.

effervescent tablets Tablets that are compounded with an effervescent salt that releases a gas when placed in water, causing the medication to dissolve rapidly.

buccal tablets Tablets designed to be placed in the cheek so that the drug can be absorbed through the oral mucosa.

sublingual tablets Small, fast-dissolving tablets that are administered under the tongue and absorbed through the oral mucosa.

excipients Ingredients added to a drug in a solid dosage form to create an acceptable tablet or capsule.

stability The amount of time a drug or compound retains its stated potency.

bioavailability The ability of a drug to exert its therapeutic effect on the body.

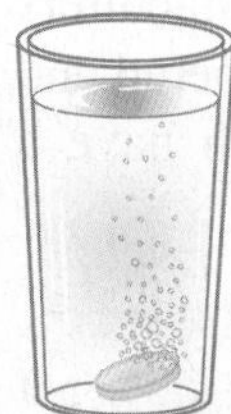

Figure 8.5 Effervescent tablets have sodium bicarbonate and an acid added to the drug so that when they are placed in water they form a bubbling solution.

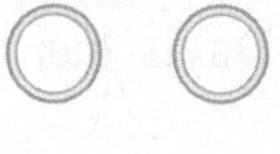

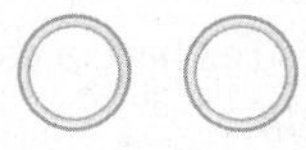

Figure 8.6 Orally disintegrating tablets will dissolve quickly when placed in the mouth.

is reformulated as a generic. The generic version of the drug is required to have the same amount of active ingredient as the brand-name product and demonstrate equal bioavailability, but a change in one or more excipients could cause an allergic reaction in a patient or cause the drug to act differently in a given individual.

When the single dose of an active ingredient is small, such as 1 mg, a diluent must be added to improve accuracy in the dose and to make a tablet of a reasonable size. Sometimes the diluent can impart other properties to the tablet, such as increasing the rate of disintegration to make the tablet acceptable for a chewable dosage form. Binders are used to increase the cohesiveness of the powders so that the tablet will not crumble during or after compression. Care must be taken to use the proper amount of binder so that the finished tablet will not be so hard that dissolution will be affected.

lubricants Topical compounds that are intended to sooth and moisturize dry irritated skin.

disintegrants Compounds added to a tablet formulation to ensure that the tablet will break apart and be available for absorption into the system.

Lubricants are added to prevent the tablet from sticking to the machine and affecting the appearance and strength of the dosage form. Disintegrants are added to the tablet formulation to ensure that the tablet will break up and release the active ingredient in a reasonable amount of time so that it may be absorbed into the system. Coloring agents serve several purposes. They add pharmaceutical elegance to the finished product, can serve as a quality control factor during product manufacture, and aid the patient in product identification. Flavoring agents are especially important in the formulation of chewable tablets to improve palatability.

Advantages of Tablets

- formulated to give an exact dose
- convenient to carry
- long shelf life
- usually tasteless
- can be formulated for controlled release

Disadvantages of Tablets

- may need a liquid to take dose
- difficult to adjust dose
- may be hard to swallow
- impossible for unconscious patients
- time delay for dissolution and absorption into the bloodstream

Capsules

Another common solid oral dosage form is the capsule, which consists of either a hard or soft gelatin container with the drug and any excipients enclosed inside. A hard-shell gelatin capsule consists of the body, which contains the drug and any additives, and the cap that slips over the body to form an oblong shape. See Figure 8.7 for a picture of a hard-shell gelatin capsule. Some manufacturers have patented capsule shapes, such as Lilly's pulvules, which have a tapered end similar to a bullet. Parke-Davis has trademarked its Kapseals, which have a

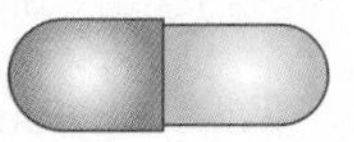

Figure 8.7 Hard gelatin capsules have a cap that slips over the body of the capsule to enclose the drug.

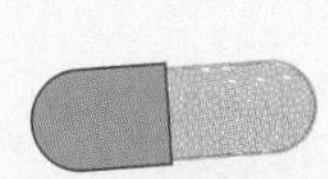

Figure 8.8 Some capsules contain the medication in small pellets that have been coated to release the medication over a period of time.

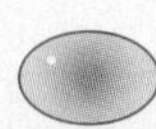

Figure 8.9 Soft gelatin capsules may contain a paste, liquid, or powder, and have a seam that opens in the stomach to release the medication.

colored gelatin band around the center to secure the capsule. Manufacturers have had to utilize many creative sealing methods for capsules and locking devices for bottles to provide tamper-resistant packages because there have been a number of tampering incidents involving capsules. Also available are capsules containing small pellets of medication. These capsules can be opened and the medication pellets sprinkled on applesauce for children or other patients who are unable to swallow the capsule. It is important to ensure that the child does not chew the pellets because this will adversely affect the release of the medication. Some capsules are formulated to release a drug over a controlled period of time. This may be accomplished by enclosing the active ingredient in various coatings that will release small amounts of the drug at different times to maintain a more constant blood level. These coated pellets are then enclosed in the capsule. See Figure 8.8 for a picture of a controlled-release capsule.

Soft gelatin capsules may contain liquid, paste, or powder, and have a seam at the middle that opens to release medication in the stomach within 5 minutes of ingestion. They are available in a wide variety of shapes, sizes, and colors. Soft gelatin capsules are often used for oils, such as vitamin E, and for cough preparations containing a liquid cough suppressant. Figure 8.9 shows an example of a soft-shell capsule.

Lozenges, Troches, and Lollipops

Lozenges and troches are oral medication dosage forms. They are usually round in shape and contain a drug in a hard candy or suitably flavored base designed to dissolve slowly in the mouth. They release the drug as they dissolve. They are commonly used as an oral anesthetic, antiseptic, antibiotic, antitussive, analgesic, or decongestant. Many are available commercially, but they are often compounded extemporaneously by the pharmacy using either a hard candy base or an acacia and powdered sugar compound that can be molded or kneaded into a pipe form and cut into equal-sized lozenges. Lozenges have the advantages of being easily transported, requiring no liquid to consume, being premeasured, and providing a topical therapy in addition to the systemic action of the drug. Several drugs are formulated as lollipops to facilitate administration to children and elderly patients who have difficulty swallowing traditional tablets. Figure 8.10 shows an example of a lozenge, and Figure 8.11 shows a lollipop that contains a drug.

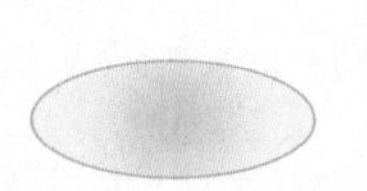

Figure 8.10 A lozenge is usually a small, disc-shaped dosage form that may contain a medication and is intended to be placed in the mouth and sucked to dissolve.

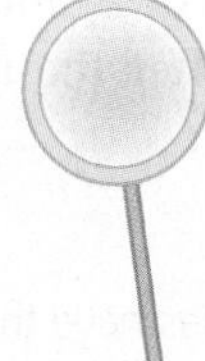

Figure 8.11 Lollipops contain the medication in a hard candy base to be dissolved in the mouth and release the medication.

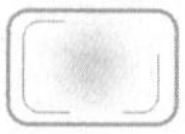

Figure 8.12 Chewing gum can be a vehicle for medication. A common example is nicotine chewing gum for smoking cessation.

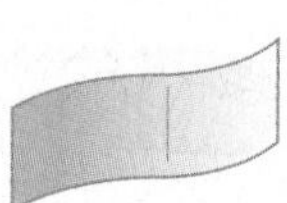

Figure 8.13 Medicated thin strips are a novel dosage form. They offer the convenience of easy portability and require no water or dosing device to provide an accurate dose.

Medicated Chewing Gum

Recently the use of chewing gum as a delivery system for medications has increased. For many years aspirin has been available as a gum, offering the advantage of a topical effect—especially for throat and mouth discomfort. Nicotine gum has been utilized as an aid in smoking cessation. The gum is easily portable and aids in the oral fixation of smoking as well as nicotine withdrawal. Chewing gums are being evaluated for other uses as topical medication delivery systems. Figure 8.12 shows an example of a medicated chewing gum.

Medicated Thin Strips

A novel dosage form has emerged to provide a convenient dosing mechanism for the mobile world in which we live. The medication is formulated in a thin flavored strip that dissolves when placed in the mouth. Cough suppressants and analgesics for children, and breath fresheners and anti-gas medications for adults are available in this palatable and portable dosage form. It is important to store these strips in a cool place or they may melt and stick together or to the packaging. Figure 8.13 shows an example of a medicated thin strip.

CAUTION **Keep out of the reach of children because they may consider them a treat.**

Other Solid Dosage Forms

Suppositories—Rectal, Vaginal, and Urethral

Suppositories are solid dosage forms that are commonly made with a cocoa butter base that allows for the inclusion of a medication and the molding of the suppository into a product tapered at one end for easy insertion into the designated body cavity. The most common type is a rectal suppository that is designed for insertion into the rectum and is often used as a topical remedy for hemorrhoids. The heat of the body will cause the suppository to melt, releasing the drug. An adult rectal suppository should weigh about 2 grams, and an infant suppository about 1 gram. Suppositories may contain sedatives, analgesics, tranquilizers, or other medications administered for their systemic effects. The medication is quickly absorbed into the rectal mucosa and delivered to the bloodstream. See Figure 8.14 for a picture of a rectal suppository.

In vaginal suppositories the medication may be encapsulated in a soft gelatin base or it may be in the form of a tablet. Such tablets are often ovoid in shape and may weigh 2 to 5 grams. After the tablet is inserted into the vaginal canal, the

Figure 8.14 Rectal suppositories have the advantage of quickly dissolving and releasing the drug into the bloodstream.

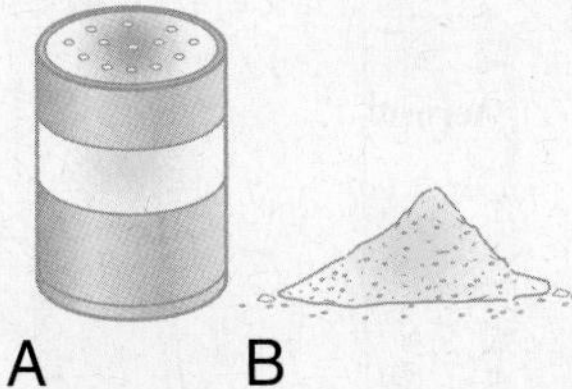

Figure 8.15 (**A**) Topical powders are conveniently packaged in a canister shaker. (**B**) Topical powders must be finely ground for smooth application.

medication is released and absorbed into the vaginal mucosa for either a topical or systemic effect.

A urethral insert used for erectile dysfunction in a male weighs 4 grams and is in the form of a micropellet that is designed to be inserted with an applicator. A urethral suppository for a female weighs only about 2 grams and can be used to treat urethritis or inflammation of the urethra.

Powders, Granules, and Aerosols

Powders are mixtures of drugs and inactive ingredients that can be either sprinkled on an external area for a topical effect or dissolved in liquid prior to ingestion for a systemic effect. External powders should be finely ground into a smooth, homogenous mixture to prevent irritation at the site of application. If an active ingredient is present, the smaller the particle size of the drug the greater the effect, because there will be more surface area of the drug to contact the affected area. See Figures 8.15 and 8.16 for the different textures of a powder and a granule.

Granules are powders that have been wetted and allowed to dry in coarse particles. Because the particle size is larger and they have been allowed to dry, they form a more stable product and have a longer shelf life. The most common products manufactured as granules are antibiotics for suspensions, which are packaged in dispensing bottles designed for the addition of a prescribed amount of water at the time of dispensing.

Do not add the water to antibiotic granules for oral suspension until the day of dispensing because the formulation will expire 10–14 days after mixing.

CAUTION

Aerosols

Solid particles that are finely ground and suspended in a gas that is packaged under pressure will form an aerosol. These dosage forms may be intended for internal use as an inhalation for conditions such as asthma. They have the advantage of being delivered directly to the lungs for quick action with minimal systemic side effects. External aerosols are advantageous for topical administration to places that are difficult to reach. They can also be applied to irritated areas with little further irritation. Figure 8.17 shows a typical aerosol used for inhalation to treat asthma.

inhalation Administration route used to deliver medications to the lungs by breathing them in through the mouth.

Ointments, Creams, Pastes, and Gels

Ointments are dosage forms formulated to apply to the skin or mucous membranes. They utilize various bases depending on the purpose of the ointment. Oleaginous or

oleaginous A base in which the oil is the external phase, usually greasy and non-washable.

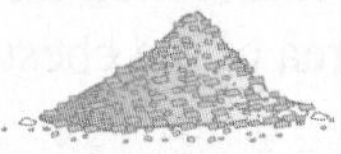

Figure 8.16 Powder granules are wetted and coarsely ground for a longer shelf life.

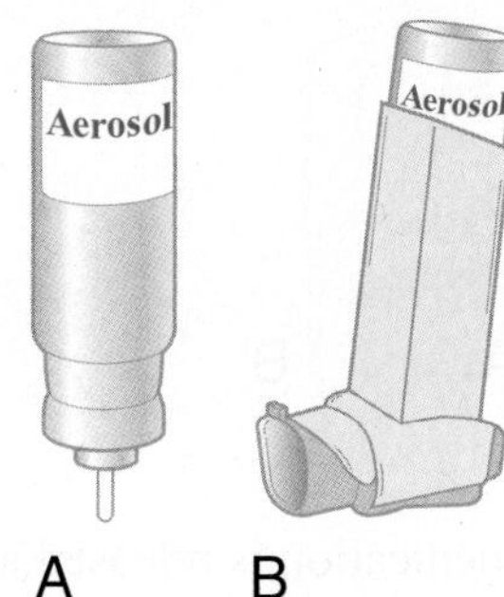

Figure 8.17 (**A**) Aerosol products are packaged in a small metal canister to be attached to an inhaler. (**B**) Plastic inhalers provide a mouthpiece for inhalation therapy with a metered-dose inhaler.

hydrocarbon bases Oil-based bases used to soothe and protect the skin.

occlusive Covered in a manner that does not allow penetration by air or moisture.

hydrophobic Bases that repel moisture.

anhydrous absorption bases Ointment bases that do not contain water but can absorb significant amounts of water and moderate amounts of alcoholic solutions.

hydrocarbon bases form emollients that soothe the area and are occlusive to protect the affected area from air. They also are hydrophobic, so they repel moisture, which is advantageous for diaper rash or other conditions in which moisture is a problem. An example of an oleaginous ointment base would be white petrolatum or Vaseline petroleum jelly. Anhydrous absorption bases are not water-washable but can absorb water. They also tend to be occlusive and greasy, so they make good emollients. Anhydrous lanolin is an example of this type of base. Absorption bases that contain water but can absorb only a limited amount of water and are not water-washable also have properties of being emollient, greasy, and occlusive. These are called water in oil (W/O) emulsions. Lanolin is an example of a W/O absorption base. In a W/O emulsion, the water is the internal phase and the oil is the external phase of the compound.

Creams are semisolid dosage forms that contain a drug dissolved or dispersed in a water-removable ointment base. A cream is insoluble in water, contains water, can absorb more water, and can be washed off the skin with water. These oil in water emulsions (O/W) are less protective, less emollient, and less occlusive than an ointment base. In an O/W emulsion the oil is the internal phase of the compound and the water is the external phase. The type of emulsion determines the properties of the compound.

Pastes are thicker and more absorptive than ointments because they contain higher amounts of dry ingredients. For example, in zinc oxide paste the amount of zinc oxide in the zinc oxide ointment is increased to form a thick paste that is more protective and stays on the skin longer.

Gels are semisolid preparations that are water-soluble and water-washable. They may be used topically or introduced into a body cavity (e.g., as nasal or vaginal gels) or they may be taken internally (e.g., as aluminum hydroxide gel).

TIP **It is important for the technician to understand the differences in these topical preparations because many active ingredients will be available in ointment, cream, or gel form, and dispensing an ointment instead of a gel or cream would be considered a medication error.**

Transdermal Patch

Transdermal patches are delivery systems in which the medication is enclosed in an adhesive patch designed to deliver the drug over a set time period by absorption through the skin. Nitroglycerin was one of the original medications formulated for transdermal delivery. It should be applied to a hair-free or shaven area of the chest or back for best results. Figure 8.18 shows a transdermal patch.

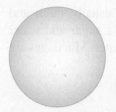

Figure 8.18 Transdermal patches are applied to a spot on the upper arm or torso to deliver medication contained in a reservoir on the patch.

CAUTION

The nitroglycerin patch should be removed at bedtime and a new patch applied in the morning to provide a drug-free period so that the patient does not build up a tolerance for the medication.

Scopolamine is available as a transdermal patch to be applied behind the ear for prevention of motion sickness. There are also transdermal forms of nicotine for smoking withdrawal, hormones for birth control, clonidine as an antihypertensive, and fentanyl as a narcotic painkiller. The technician should be familiar with the application methods and the duration of action of the various patches. Unless directed otherwise, the patient should always remove one patch before applying a new one.

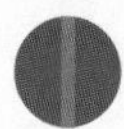

Liquid Dosage Forms

Liquid medication dosage forms use a fluid vehicle as a delivery system for the medication. The most common vehicles for liquid medications are water, alcohol, and mineral oil. Liquid dosage forms are advantageous because they are

- faster acting
- easier to swallow
- easier to adjust dose
- easier to administer to the eye or ear
- easier to administer to children or elderly patients

The disadvantages of liquid dosage forms are as follows:

- shorter expiration dates
- may need flavoring agents to mask bad taste
- inconvenient—may spill
- require a measuring device
- difficult to store—may require refrigeration

Solutions

A solution is an evenly distributed homogenous mixture of one or more medications dissolved in a liquid vehicle. Solutions are classified according to the type of vehicle used. Non-aqueous solutions can be alcoholic, hydroalcoholic, or glycerite. An alcoholic solution uses alcohol as the vehicle, and a common example is spirits of peppermint. Tinctures contain vegetable material in an alcoholic base. A hydroalcoholic solution uses a combination of alcohol and water as a vehicle. Elixirs are examples of hydroalcoholic solutions that are usually sweetened and flavored. Glycerites are medications dissolved in glycerin.

Aqueous solutions are medications that are dissolved with the use of water as a vehicle. Examples of aqueous solutions are douches, irrigating solutions, enemas,

vehicle A liquid, such as alcohol, mineral oil, or water, used to dissolve a drug for oral or topical administration.

glycerite A solution in which one of the vehicles is glycerin; such solutions are usually thick and oily in nature and sometimes used in the ear.

alcoholic solution A solution in which alcohol is used as the vehicle.

tincture An alcoholic solution of a drug that is much more potent than a fluid extract (do not substitute one for the other); alcoholic or hydroalcoholic solutions containing vegetable materials or chemicals made by percolation or maceration processes.

hydroalcoholic solution A solution in which both alcohol and water are used as vehicles; the ratio of alcohol to water may vary greatly.

elixirs Hydroalcoholic solutions that contain one or more dissolved drugs and are sweetened and flavored for oral use; liquids that are alcoholic or hydroalcoholic solutions.

viscous aqueous solutions Thick solutions that use water as a vehicle and contain high amounts of sugar.

gargles, washes, and sprays. Viscous aqueous solutions are usually thick and sticky. A syrup is a viscous aqueous solution that consists of a sugar and water mixture. Jellies are semisolid but have a high concentration of water. Mucilages are thick adhesive liquids.

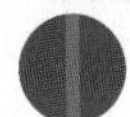

Routes of Administration

Oral

The most common route of administration for medications is the oral route, meaning that the drug is administered into the body through the mouth or through a G-tube. Dosage forms commonly administered orally are tablets, capsules, oral solutions, oral suspensions, and oral emulsions. The patient directions or Signa written on the prescription by the prescriber may indicate to take "po" or by mouth. These instructions should be included on the prescription label and communicated to the patient. The oral route of administration is advantageous because it is

- safe and convenient
- usually less expensive than other forms
- can be modified for extended release
- noninvasive

The disadvantages of oral administration are as follows:

- not appropriate for unconscious patients
- patient may be unable to swallow
- requires time for absorption and distribution
- absorption time is affected by food, drugs, stomach acid, and condition of patient

Sublingual and Buccal Tablets

Although a sublingual tablet is placed in the mouth, this is not considered an oral administration route because the absorption process is very different. The tablet is placed under the tongue and the drug is absorbed through the oral mucosa under the tongue into the bloodstream. The drug does not pass through the intestinal tract. This provides a much faster effect of the drug and eliminates many of the factors that might affect absorption rates. The most common drug available in a sublingual tablet is nitroglycerin. A rapid effect is very important with this drug because it is used to treat an attack of angina.

angina Chest pain caused by reduced blood flow in the coronary arteries.

A buccal tablet is placed inside the pouch of the cheek between the cheek and the gum. Similarly to a sublingual tablet, it is absorbed through the lining of the cheek and bypasses the intestinal tract. Metandren Linguets, a male sex hormone, is an example of a buccal tablet that is commercially available.

parenteral Medications given by injection that bypass the gastrointestinal tract.

Parenteral administration is the term used for medications given by injection that also bypass the gastrointestinal tract. This route of administration is used when the patient is not able to take oral medications (for example, if he or she is unconscious or has a health condition that prevents swallowing). In addition, some drugs are only available in the injectable form and this route provides for fast drug action. The disadvantages are that it is invasive because it penetrates the skin and may introduce bacteria into the system, causing infection, and it may be painful or frightening to the patient.

Intravenous Administration

Intravenous (IV) administration involves administering the drug through a needle placed directly into a vein. IV preparations are usually solutions that must be sterile and free of particulate matter. Methods of preparing IV medications using aseptic technique to ensure sterility will be discussed in a later chapter. Drugs administered by this route are immediately available to the body because they are introduced directly into the bloodstream. They have the advantage of being faster acting, but recovery is much more difficult if a medication error or an adverse reaction occurs. There are several methods of administering an IV medication that the technician should understand. Using the wrong method may result in serious injury or death of the patient. A bolus dose is a large dose injected over a short period of time. This method is also called IV push and usually involves a healthcare provider using a syringe with the medication and slowly injecting the drug over a predetermined time period. An example is using lidocaine by IV push to treat an abnormal heart rhythm. Another common method is continuous infusion, in which the drug is added to an IV bag and allowed to drip or infuse over a number of hours to supply a constant blood level of the drug. These IV bags are often mixed by the technician and may involve one or more drugs in a given amount of fluid to be administered over a prescribed amount of time. Technician accuracy is extremely important in performing IV admixture and will be discussed in detail in another chapter. Figure 8.19 is an example of an IV bag used for infusion.

intravenous (IV) administration An injection or infusion into a vein.

aseptic technique Procedure for mixing sterile compounded products with a complete absence of viable microorganisms.

bolus dose A large initial dose given to quickly bring the blood level of a drug up to a therapeutic level.

continuous infusion Administering a drug by placing it in solution in an IV bag and allowing the solution to slowly enter a vein over a prescribed period of time.

Intramuscular Administration

Intramuscular (IM) administration involves a direct injection into a large muscle mass. IM medications can be either solutions or suspensions, and some formulations can be given either IV or IM. It is important for the technician to be aware of the route of administration and the different reconstitution methods used for the different routes of administration. IM administration provides a faster rate of action than the oral route, but not as fast as an IV. IM suspensions can be formulated for extended release (sometimes lasting up to 3 months) by suspending the drug in a vegetable oil. The resulting preparation is called a "depot," so when the name of an injectable drug is followed by the word "depo" that indicates it is a long-acting preparation. Drug volumes up to 5 mL can be administered IM. Volumes greater than 5 mL can be divided into two doses. Drug absorption may be erratic depending on the site used, the muscle mass of the patient, and the amount of exercise performed by the patient. This is not a preferred route of administration for a patient with decreased muscle mass or bleeding problems, and it may cause considerable bruising. Although the medication is not absorbed directly into the bloodstream, it is difficult to reverse the drug action once it has been injected.

intramuscular (IM) administration An injection into a large muscle.

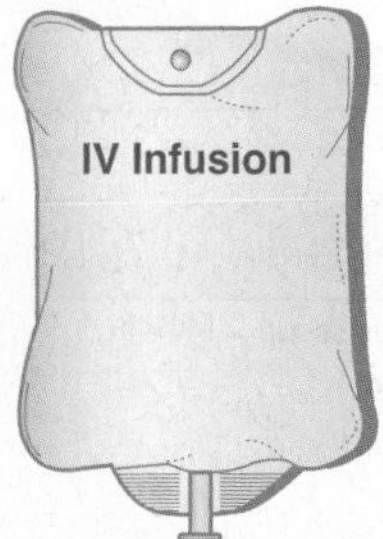

Figure 8.19 The IV bag provides a method for delivering medication directly into the veins for quick action.

Subcutaneous Administration

subcutaneous (SQ) administration Injection under the skin.

Subcutaneous (SQ) administration involves injecting a small amount of a solution or suspension immediately under the skin. Patients can be taught to self-administer SQ injections. The most common SQ medication is insulin, which is usually self-administered by diabetic patients to control their blood sugar. SQ injections are also used for emergency doses of epinephrine to counteract an allergic reaction, and for some ready-to-use treatments for migraines. There is a limit to the volume of medication that can be injected under the skin (usually 1.5 mL), and it may be difficult for patients with thin or frail skin. The rate of absorption is slower than the IV or IM routes.

Intradermal Administration

intradermal injection An injection between the layers of the skin.

An intradermal injection is inserted in the top layers of the skin and is not as deep as an SQ injection. The diagnostic test for tuberculosis involves placing the material in the tissue just beneath the epidermis. Allergen testing is also performed by injecting aliquots containing about 1 mL of various materials suspected of causing the allergic reaction intradermally in premarked areas on the back of the patient and checking for inflammation. See Figure 8.20 for an example of the above types of injections.

Intra-articular Administration

intra-articular administration An injection into a joint.

Intra-articular administration involves injecting a medication directly into a joint, such as the knee. This type of injection is often used to inject steroids into an inflamed joint to relieve pain and reduce inflammation.

Intra-arterial Administration

intra-arterial administration An injection into an artery.

Intra-arterial administration involves injecting the drug directly into an artery. This method delivers the drug directly to the desired location, so it decreases the side effects to other parts of the body. Cancer chemotherapy drugs are sometimes administered by this method, but extreme caution should be used because these drugs are toxic.

Intracardiac Administration

intracardiac administration An injection directly into the heart.

Intracardiac administration involves injection directly into the heart muscle. This method is used only in extreme life-threatening emergencies. Only healthcare per-

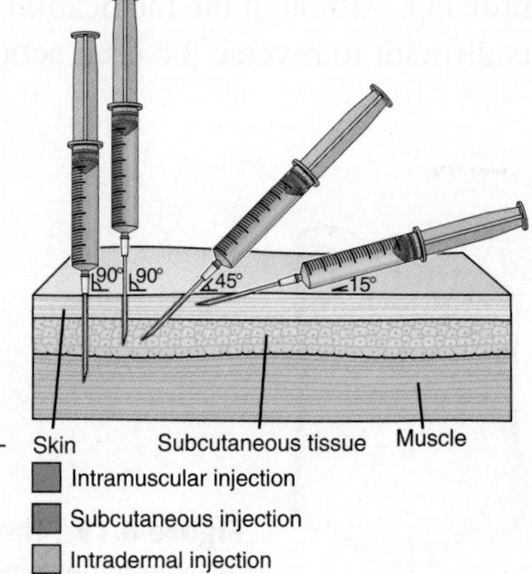

Figure 8.20 Injections: a comparison of the angles of insertion for intramuscular, subcutaneous, and intradermal injections. (Reprinted with permission from Stedman's Medical Dictionary for the Health Professions and Nursing. 5th ed. Baltimore, MD: Lippincott Williams & Wilkins, 2005.)

sonnel who are trained and experienced in performing this type of injection should attempt it because there is a risk of rupturing the heart.

Intraperitoneal Administration

Intraperitoneal administration involves injection into the peritoneal or abdominal cavity. This method of injection is often used to administer antibiotics needed to treat infections in the abdominal cavity, such as peritonitis resulting from a ruptured appendix. Peritoneal dialysis is sometimes used as a method to remove toxic substances that are normally excreted by the kidneys for patients suffering from end-stage renal disease.

intraperitoneal administration An injection into the abdominal cavity.

Intrapleural Administration

Injection of a drug into the pleura or the sac surrounding the lungs is called intrapleural administration. This may be done to eliminate or prevent excessive amounts of fluid from building up in the pleural sac surrounding the lungs.

intrapleural administration An injection into the pleural sac surrounding the lungs.

Implants

A medication pump, such as an insulin pump, or a medical device that is inserted into the body either permanently or for a prescribed amount of time and is designed to provide continuous administration of a drug over a predetermined amount of time is called an implant. Implants are used to treat long-term or chronic conditions, such as diabetes, or for cancer chemotherapy. There also is an implant system for long-term birth control lasting up to 5 years.

implant A drug or device temporarily placed under the skin to release a medication at a controlled rate.

Topical Application

Dosage forms used for topical treatment of skin conditions include ointments, creams, gels, and pastes, as well as solutions, lotions, and sprays. The drug should penetrate the skin to provide the therapeutic effect. The skin acts as a natural barrier that will affect the rate and amount of penetration. Usually the concentration needed to provide a therapeutic effect is difficult to determine. The condition of the patient's skin, the drug and delivery vehicle used, and whether an occlusive dressing is utilized all determine the final therapeutic effect of the product. Antibiotics, anesthetics, antiseptics, emollients, and corticosteroids are some of the medications delivered by topical application. In most cases, topical administration of a drug is intended for a local therapeutic effect where the product is applied. Some products are designed to produce a systemic effect by having the drug diffuse through the skin and into the bloodstream. Nitroglycerin ointment is an example of an ointment intended for its systemic effect. Topical corticosteroids should be applied sparingly and used for only the prescribed amount of time because they can be absorbed through the skin and produce unwanted side effects.

Inhalation

Use of the inhalation route of administration continues to increase as more drugs become available. Aerosol inhalers for the treatment of asthma are being replaced by dry-powder inhalers due to concerns about damage to the ozone layer. Asthma inhalation drugs include bronchodilators and corticosteroids. Other inhalation drugs for such things as nicotine replacement, insulin, and influenza vaccine are also being marketed.

Transdermal Route of Administration

transdermal route of administration Uses a patch formulated to release medication at a predetermined rate to be diffused through the skin.

The transdermal route of administration involves delivery of the drug across the top of the skin for percutaneous absorption to facilitate a systemic effect while bypassing the gastrointestinal tract. The drug is contained in an adhesive patch that slowly releases the medication at a predetermined rate. The skin assists in controlling the rate of absorption and delivery to the bloodstream. The patch may be applied to the skin every day, every 3 days, or every 7 days.

CAUTION **It is important for the technician to correlate the directions printed on the prescription label with the manufacturer's directions for use. Any discrepancy should be checked with the pharmacist and/or the prescriber.**

Professional Judgment Scenario 8.1

While preparing a fentanyl patch order for the medicine floor at the hospital, John noticed that the medication administration record (MAR) stated that a new fentanyl transdermal patch should be applied each morning. John felt sure that the fentanyl patch should be changed only every 3 days, but the administration record plainly stated "q am." The pharmacist who had verified the physician's orders was very experienced and did not like to be questioned. John wasn't 100% certain about the dosing time and thought he should just send the order as it was. Using your professional judgment, choose the course(s) of action you would take in this situation:

1. The patient may be in a lot of pain, so just send the order as is.
2. Check the package insert in the fentanyl for the manufacturer's dosing recommendations.
3. Confront the pharmacist to let him know he's made an error.
4. Approach the pharmacist as one professional to another and ask to discuss the dose indicated in the MAR.

If you approach the pharmacist and do not feel comfortable that the correct decision about the dose has been reached, what would be your next step? Remember the welfare of the patient always comes first!

Rectal Administration

percutaneous absorption Systemic diffusion through the lining of the skin as with a transdermal patch.

Rectal administration involves inserting a drug through the anus into the rectum. Rectal suppositories are solid dosage forms formulated in a base that is intended to dissolve and release the medication after it is inserted. The medication is absorbed through the rectal mucosa to provide a systemic effect, as in the case of antinausea and laxative drugs, or it may exert a topical effect, as in the case of hemorrhoid preparations. Rectally administered liquids are often in the form of enemas for bowel cleansing prior to diagnostic testing. Proctofoam is a foam packaged for rectal application to soothe inflamed tissue.

Vaginal Administration

Vaginal suppositories or tablets are intended for insertion into the vaginal canal and are designed to melt or dissolve and release the medication. Vaginal preparations also include creams, ointments, gels, solutions, and foams. They may contain a medication intended to be absorbed, or the effect may be topical and limited to the vaginal area. Preparations for treating vaginal yeast infections are available without a prescription and patients often need guidance in making this type of purchase. A vaginal infection should only be self-treated if the patient has previously experienced a yeast infection and is certain this is the problem, so that a more serious infection does not go untreated and cause complications.

Ocular, Otic, and Nasal Routes of Administration

Ophthalmic solutions, suspensions, and ointments must be sterile preparations free of any particulate matter that may irritate the eye. Solutions are instilled into the eye by tipping the head back and placing the required number of drops inside the lower lid of the eye while looking up. If several types of drops are being used, there should be a few minutes' wait time between the application of different medications. Ophthalmic ointments are applied by pulling down the lower lid and applying a thin ribbon of the ointment along the inside of the lid. There should be a 10-minute wait time between applications of two different ophthalmic ointments. In both cases, care should be taken to avoid touching the eye with the tip of the dropper or ointment tube. Ocular inserts are solid devices that are placed in the eye and release a drug at a constant rate, minimizing side effects due to rapid absorption. The disadvantage is that they are cumbersome to insert properly and the insert must be removed from the eye after the drug is released.

Otic preparations include solutions or suspensions that are administered into the ear canal and contain analgesics, antibiotics, and anti-inflammatory agents. The solvents traditionally used are glycerin or water. Glycerin helps the preparation remain in the ear for a longer period of time. Glycerin preparations are also used to soften earwax to facilitate removal of excess wax.

Nasal solutions are administered to the nasal passages in the form of drops or sprays and may be either suspensions or emulsions. Most nasal preparations are used to treat nasal congestion, but some products that use the nasal route for systemic effect are becoming available. Some asthma and allergy preparations are administered by nasal inhalation. A nasal spray to administer insulin for treatment of diabetes is in the testing phase.

Throat Sprays and Gargles

Throat sprays may contain antiseptics, anesthetics, deodorants, and flavorings. They are used to relieve minor sore throat pain or to improve bad breath. Chronic bad breath may be a sign of an underlying infection, so a trip to the dentist may solve the problem. Treating a sore throat with analgesics and anesthetics can cause a strep throat to be overlooked. An untreated strep throat can result in serious complications, including rheumatic fever. The technician should be alert for repeated purchases of sore-throat products and involve the pharmacist if patient counseling is indicated.

Drug Information Resources

Information about drugs, available strengths, dosage forms, and routes of administration is readily available in the manufacturer's package insert and a variety of reference books that may be available in the pharmacy. The technician should become familiar with the contents and layouts of the different reference books. (See the "Suggested Readings" section at the end of this chapter for full source information for these resources.)

- *Drug Facts and Comparisons*: Contains most comprehensive and current drug information, monthly updates, complete pharmacology, drug interactions, adverse effects, available doses, and administration; lists comparable brand and generic products together.
- *American Hospital Formulary Service Drug Information (AHFS)*: Comprehensive listing of available drugs, pharmacology, dosages, administration, and adverse effects; updated yearly with three supplements.
- *United States Pharmacopeia-National Formulary (USP-NF)*: Official compendium of all approved drugs and the required standards of purity and stability for each drug to be considered official.
- *United States Pharmacopeia-Drug Information (USP-DI)*: Volume I contains drug information for the healthcare professional, volume II contains advice for the patient in layman's terms, and volume III lists approved drug products and legal requirements.
- *Physician's Desk Reference (PDR)*: Book of package insert information for drugs chosen by manufacturers to be included; not a comprehensive reference; very few generics, color pictures of tablets, capsules, or packaging of included products.
- *Drug Interaction Facts*: Lists the drug interactions and ranks them according to severity of the interaction and the likelihood of its occurrence.
- *Redbook*: Lists all drugs and devices and the wholesale prices of the items; also contains many frequently-used tables, such as pregnancy categories, tablets that are not to be crushed, and addresses of drug companies.
- *Orange Book*: Lists generic drugs and rates their bioavailability in comparison with the brand-name product to determine whether they are legally substitutable.
- *American Drug Index*: A concise listing of available drugs, dosage forms, drug classes, "look-alike-sound-alike" drugs, pregnancy categories, discontinued drugs, and laboratory values.
- *Handbook on Injectable Drugs*: Complete information about injectable drugs, admixture procedures, compatibility, stability, and dilution.
- *Pediatric Dosage Handbook*: Lists drugs and doses appropriate for use in children.
- *Remington: The Science and Practice of Pharmacy*: Comprehensive information about all aspects of the practice of pharmacy in various practice settings.
- *Material Safety Data Sheets (MSDS)*: Information about the safe handling of chemicals and hazardous drugs in the workplace, including handling chemical spills and treating exposure to hazardous materials.
- *Micromedex*: A computerized reference system that contains comprehensive clinical information about drugs and toxicology, and a drug identification system.

Novel dosage forms and routes of administration are constantly being developed. Each dosage form has different advantages and disadvantages. As a professional technician, you should stay current with all new dosage forms released for sale so that you can provide up-to-date information to assist patients. Use your knowledge of available dosage forms and your ability to search available reference books for needed information as you perform prescription evaluations and choose the correct dosage form to enter into the computer. Be certain that the patient directions printed on the label are clear and accurate for the dosage form and route of administration of the product prescribed and dispensed.

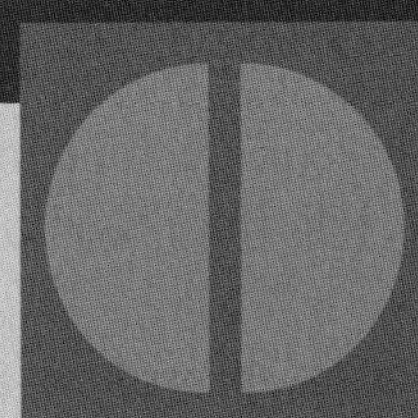

Case Study 8.1

Jim was assigned to the IV room during the afternoon when the total parenteral nutrition (TPN) orders were to be mixed for distribution to the patient floors. As he gathered the additives for the first preparation, he noticed he needed the following ingredients: calcium gluconate, sodium chloride, magnesium sulfate, potassium acetate, and potassium phosphate. Jim wondered whether all these ingredients were compatible in the same IV bag. He had a number of bags to compound that day and was trying to save time. "Surely," thought Jim, "if the doctor prescribed these ingredients to be added to the bag, they must be compatible." Jim didn't want to bother the pharmacist with a stupid question, so he asked another technician if the formula looked all right to her. She studied the formula for a few minutes and told Jim she thought she had read about a problem with one of the potassium additives but she couldn't remember what it was. Using the reference books, help Jim decide what he needs to do.

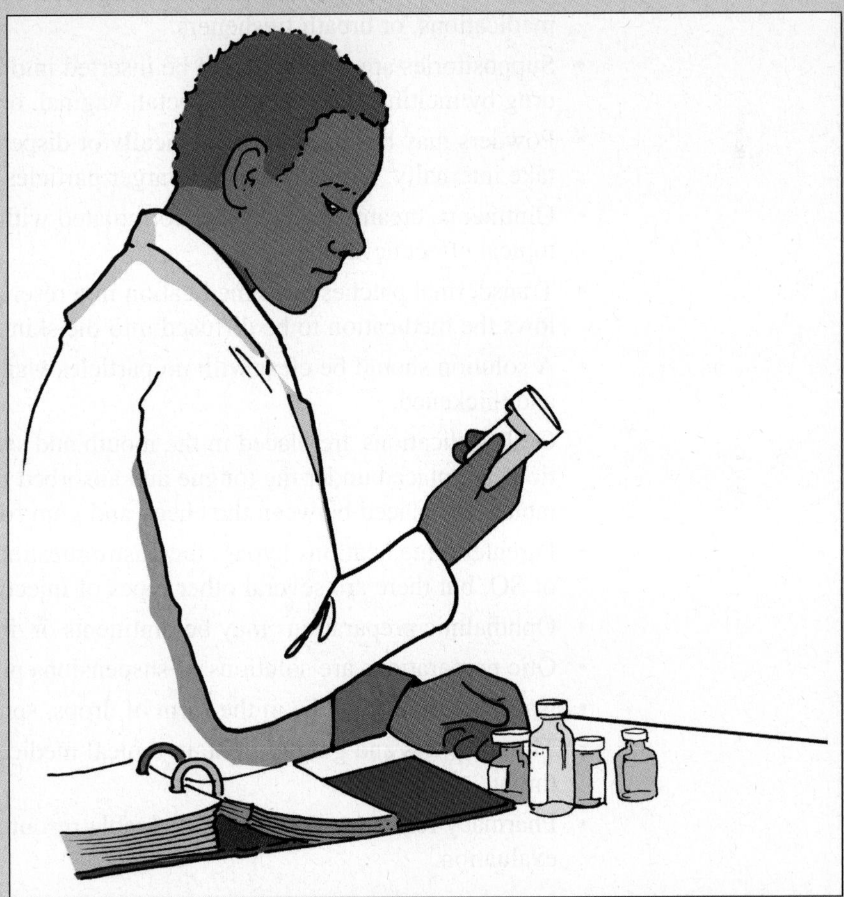

1. What reference book would provide the best information about IV compatibility issues?
2. After checking the desk copy of the reference book, did you discover any compatibility issues?
3. What important information did you learn about the order in which these electrolytes should be added to the mixture?
4. Discuss the possible consequences that might have occurred if Jim had not checked the reference book.

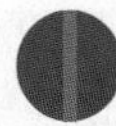

Chapter Summary

- Tablets are a common oral dosage form that contain an active ingredient and a number of excipients, such as diluents, binders, lubricants, coloring, flavoring, and disintegrates.
- Different tablet formulations produce variations in the release, absorption, and action of the medication.
- Capsules may contain drugs and diluents in the form of powders, liquids, or pellets that affect the rate of absorption of the drug.
- Lozenges, troches, and lollipops contain medication in a flavored base to provide a convenient dosage form for patients who are unable to swallow a tablet, and also produce a topical effect.
- Chewing gums are a portable and convenient dosage form.
- Medicated thin strips may contain analgesics, cough suppressants, anti-gas medications, or breath fresheners.
- Suppositories are formulated to be inserted into a body cavity and release the drug by melting. They may be rectal, vaginal, or urethral.
- Powders may be sprinkled on topically or dispensed in packets for solution to take internally. Granules contain larger particles that are more stable.
- Ointments, creams, and gels are formulated with different bases to produce the topical effect desired.
- Transdermal patches have medication in a reservoir enclosed in a patch that allows the medication to be diffused into the skin for absorption.
- A solution should be clear with no particles visible, although it may be colored and thickened.
- Oral medications are placed in the mouth and swallowed. Sublingual medications are placed under the tongue and absorbed through the mucosa. Buccal tablets are placed between the cheek and gum for absorption.
- Parenteral medications bypass the gastrointestinal tract and are usually IM, IV, or SQ, but there are several other types of injections.
- Ophthalmic preparations may be ointments or drops, but they must be sterile.
- Otic preparations are solutions or suspensions placed in the ear.
- Nasal solutions may be in the form of drops, sprays, or nasal inhalers.
- Throat sprays and gargles contain topical medications to treat conditions of the throat.
- Pharmacy reference books are a valuable resource to facilitate prescription evaluation.

Review Questions

Multiple Choice

Choose the best answer to the following questions:

1. When a rapid effect is needed to treat an asthma attack, the drug may be
   a. taken by mouth
   b. applied transdermally
   c. inhaled through the mouth
   d. sprayed on the chest

2. Ophthalmic drugs
   a. treat local conditions of the ear
   b. are delivered directly into the eye
   c. may be either an ointment or drops
   d. b and c

3. An elixir is an example of
   a. a hydroalcoholic solution
   b. an aqueous solution with no alcohol
   c. an emulsion
   d. none of the above

4. A semisolid medication dosage form that is applied to the skin or mucous membranes to lubricate and soften, or as a base for a drug, is a/an
   a. ointment
   b. cream
   c. gel
   d. all of the above

5. A parenteral route of administration is one that bypasses
   a. the kidneys
   b. the heart
   c. the stomach
   d. the lungs

Fill in the Blanks

Fill in the blank with the correct answer.

6. Powders that have been wetted, allowed to dry, and then ground into coarse pieces are called ________________________.

7. The most common vehicles for liquid medications are ______________, ________________________, and ________________________.

8. An evenly distributed, homogenous mixture of dissolved medication in a liquid vehicle is called a ______________________________.

9. ______________________________ tablets contain ingredients that bubble and release the active drug when placed in a liquid.

10. ______________________________ tablets have a coating that protects the tablet from stomach acid and protects the lining of the gastrointestinal tract from irritation by the drug.

Matching

Match the term with the route of administration.

11. ____ sublingual — A. Injection into the eye

12. ____ intra-articular — B. Injection into the sac surrounding the lungs

13. ____ intrapleural — C. Injection beneath the skin

14. ____ intravenous — D. Administration and absorption of a drug from under the tongue.

15. ____ intravitreous — E. Injection of a drug into a joint (e.g., the knee)

16. ____ subcutaneous — F. Injection directly into a vein

True/False

Mark the following statements True or False:

17. ____ Otic preparations are used to treat local conditions of the eye.

18. ____ Aerosols are suspensions of fine particles in a gas packaged under pressure.

19. ____ In an O/W emulsion the water is the internal phase.

20. ____ W/O emulsions are water-washable.

LEARNING ACTIVITIES

Use the most appropriate reference book to research the following problems:

1. Danny's mother presents the following prescription to the pharmacy from his dentist. Danny is 10 years old and weighs 110 pounds. He is going to have a dental procedure that requires conscious sedation, and the dentist has chosen Valium as the drug.

Joseph Drawer D.D.S. DEA#BDxxxxxxxxx
1806 South Maryvale, Wilmington, VT

Name: Danny Daylight, 6546 West Sunnyside, Wilmington, VT

12-06-09

RX: Diazepam 10 mg tablets

Disp: Dispense 2 tablets

Sig: Give two tablets (20 mg) 45 minutes before dental procedure

Refill: 0 void after 12-10-08

Dispense as written ______ May substitute Joseph Drawer D.D.S.

a. Would you question the appropriateness of this dose for this patient?

b. What reference book would give the best information about this issue?

c. What information did you find?

2. Mrs. Jones picked up her prescription for alprazolam today. After arriving home, she received a call from her gynecologist with the good news that her pregnancy test was positive. She called to share the good news with you. After congratulating her, you begin to think about the prescription she just picked up.

   a. What reference book would you check to see if there is cause for concern?

   b. What is the pregnancy category for alprazolam?

   c. What action would you take after reading this information?

3. Mrs. Sable brings in a prescription for her husband, who has just been diagnosed with terminal cancer. She tells you his liver is seriously impaired and he doesn't have long to live. He's been told not to take acetaminophen because of his hepatic impairment. She presents a prescription for Percocet.

   a. Using an appropriate reference book, list the ingredients in Percocet.

   b. Discuss any problem that might arise from Mr. Sable taking Percocet.

   c. Would Roxicet or Percodan be a reasonable alternative for Mr. Sable?

   d. List the strengths and ingredients of Roxicet, Percocet, and Percodan.

Suggested Readings

Allen L, Popovich N, Ansel H. Ansel's Pharmaceutical Dosage Forms and Drug Delivery Systems. 8th ed. Baltimore, MD: Lippincott Williams & Wilkins, 2005.

American Hospital Formulary Service Drug Information. Bethesda, Maryland: American Society of Health System Pharmacists, 2008.

Billups, Norman F., Shirley M., eds. American Drug Index, 50th ed. St. Louis, Missouri: Wolters Kluwer Health, 2006.

Drug Facts and Comparisons. 12th ed. St. Louis, Missouri: Wolters Kluwer Health, 2007.

Gennaro AR, ed. Remington: The Science and Practice of Pharmacy. Baltimore, MD: Lippincott Williams & Wilkins, 2006.

Medical Economics Staff. Drug Topics Redbook. Montvale, NJ: Thomson Healthcare 2006.

Orange Book-Approved Drug Products with Therapeutic Equivalence Evaluations. 28th ed. Rockville, MD US Department of Health and Human Services, 2007.

Physician's Desk Reference. 62nd ed Montvale, NJ: Thomson Healthcare, 2007.

Stedman's Medical Dictionary for the Health Professions and Nursing. 5th ed. Baltimore, MD: Lippincott Williams & Wilkins, 2005.

Taketomo, Carol K., Hodding, Jane H., Kraus, Donna M., Pediatric Dosage Handbook. 14th ed. Hudson, Ohio: Lexi-Comp, 2007.

Tatro, David. Drug Interaction Facts 2008 ed. St. Louis, Missouri: Wolters Kluwer Health, 2007.

Thompson J. A Practical Guide to Contemporary Pharmacy Practice. 3rd ed. Baltimore, MD: Lippincott Williams & Wilkins, 2004.

Trissel, Lawrence A. 14th ed. Handbook on Injectable Drugs, Bethesda, MD: American Society of Health System Pharmacists, 2007.

United States Pharmacopeia 43rd ed-National Formulary 39th ed. Rockville, MD: United States Pharmacopeial Convention, 2007.

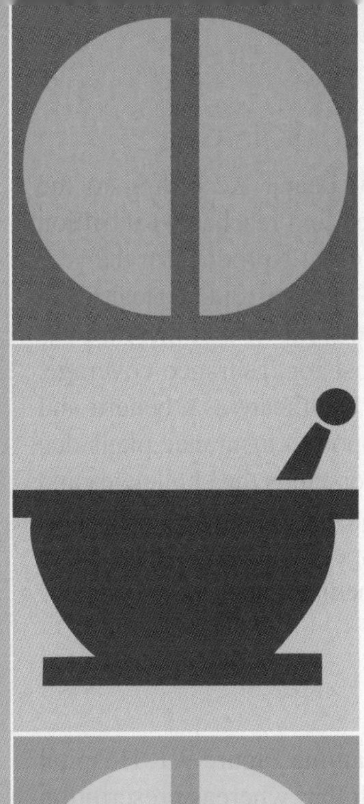

Chapter **9**

At the Right Price: Handling Payment

OBJECTIVES

After completing this chapter, the student will be able to:

- Describe factors that affect healthcare costs.
- Define the segment of healthcare costs related to pharmacy.
- Demonstrate a basic working knowledge of third-party insurance plans for prescriptions.
- Discuss patient insurance issues with physicians.
- Communicate with third-party insurers about billing issues.
- Assist patients to understand and optimize their prescription coverage.
- Assist patients in choosing a plan for Medicare Part D.
- Discuss pricing methods for patients who pay cash for prescriptions.

KEY TERMS

- Actual Acquisition Cost (AAC)
- Average Wholesale Price (AWP)
- co-pay
- deductible
- insurance formularies
- modem connection
- National Provider Identifier (NPI)
- network pharmacies
- noncovered drugs and devices
- on-line adjudication
- Pharmacy Benefit Manager (PBM)
- premiums
- prior authorization
- providers
- spend-down
- therapeutic drug class

The cost of healthcare has skyrocketed in the past 10 years. According to the National Coalition on Healthcare, in 2004 healthcare spending reached $1.9 trillion in the United States. That amounts to 16% of the gross domestic product for the year 2004. Predictions are that it will reach $2.9 trillion by the year 2009. Healthcare premiums paid by employers have risen by over 9%, and some of that increase has been passed on to employees who now pay a higher cost for insurance coverage. This has resulted in some employers no longer offering healthcare as a benefit and some employees opting not to sign up for employer-supported insurance plans due to high premiums. A knowledgeable technician who understands the challenges and choices patients face with their healthcare will be a great asset to the pharmacy. This chapter will discuss healthcare in general and, more specifically, the third-party insurance plans that provide coverage for prescription medications.

premiums Monthly fees paid by the patient to the insurance company for coverage of medical expenses.

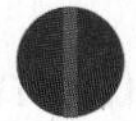

Healthcare Costs

To see how the nation's healthcare dollar is divided, examine Figure 9.1. Hospital care accounts for approximately 30% of the healthcare dollar, whereas prescription drugs account for approximately 10%. However, because most people are hospitalized infrequently, and insurance coverage for hospitalization is generally at a high level for insured patients, the expense incurred during a hospitalization is accepted as an expense that occurs rarely. Even though prescription drugs account for only 10% of the total healthcare dollar, this is a recurring expense that a patient deals with, and usually on a monthly basis. As medication costs increase and insurance companies pass more and more of the cost on to the consumer, patients who are on a fixed income often have to adjust their budget in a way that seriously changes their lifestyle. Sometimes patients can be better served by asking the physician to prescribe less expensive generic drugs even if it means they need to take the medication more often. The alert technician may be the first to notice that a patient is ordering refills less frequently than expected. The patient may share financial challenges with a technician more readily than with a pharmacist or a physician. Be sure to involve the pharmacist when this situation is noted.

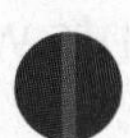

Types of Insurance Plans

There are hundreds of medical insurance companies and many types of insurance plans. Some plans offer prescription drug coverage and some do not. Although it is impossible to have knowledge of all the plans, it is helpful for technicians to

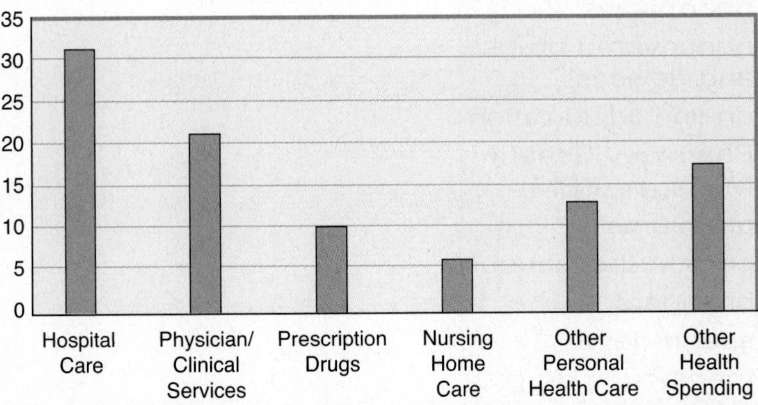

Figure 9.1 Healthcare dollar.

understand as much as possible about the plans available in the area in which they practice. An extensive discussion of individual plans is beyond the scope of this book, but some of the major types of plans will be discussed.

Private Insurance Plans

There are several different types of insurance plans available from private companies. Most of these companies include a prescription drug plan or offer it as an option for an additional cost. They vary in premiums, services covered, freedom to choose providers, and amounts of the co-pay and deductible.

- Preferred Provider Organization (PPO) plans (see Fig. 9.2):
  - Healthcare providers sign a contract with the insurance company.
  - Providers agree to accept the PPO fee schedule.
  - Members pay a co-pay at the time of service.
  - Members have a yearly deductible to meet before insurance coverage begins.
  - Insurance pays a percentage of the medical bills.
  - The percentage paid by the insurance is lower if the services are provided by an out-of-network provider.
  - The member can choose to see a provider of choice, but may pay more of the cost.
- Health Maintenance Organization (HMO) plans (see Fig. 9.3):
  - Healthcare providers work directly for the HMO.
  - The primary care physician (PCP) directs all medical care for the member.
  - Referrals can only be made by the PCP and usually to in-network providers.
  - Small co-pays.
  - Usually no deductible.
  - Little flexibility in choice of providers.
  - Low premiums.

providers Individuals or businesses that provide healthcare services to patients (e.g., a physician, laboratory, or pharmacy).

co-pay The amount of money that patients are required to pay at the pharmacy, which is determined by their insurance plan.

deductible The amount that patients are required to pay before their insurance begins to cover medical expenses.

Torch Insurance Company		PPO Green Plan
Member Name:	Office Visit	20%
Samuel E. Snively	Specialist	20%
Subscriber Name:	Emergency Room	20%
Susie Snively	Urgent Care	20%
	RX Tier 1/RX Tier2	10%/20%
Identification Number	RX Tier 3/RX Tier4	20%/20%
Y2k674S6512	Inpatient	20%
Group No.: 563	Other Outpatient	20%
Beginning Date: 01/01/20xx		

Figure 9.2 PPO insurance card

Group # 00000675 Member # 0005623789 Issued 12-22-20xx	EXCEL Plan	
Member: Sally Southern	Benefit Co-pays	
PCP: Herman Melville, MD	PCP	$20
PCP Phone # 543-784-6272	SPEC	$30
Network: Southland Medical Group	ER	$100
	UCC	$35
	MH	$30
XCEL Customer Center	DEDUCT	$200
6504 S. Hampton	RX	$20/$10
543-687-2302	Brand Non-Select $60	
www.excel.com		

Figure 9.3 HMO insurance card.

- Point of service (POS) plans:
  - The PCP directs the medical care.
  - The member may see out-of-network providers but must submit claims for reimbursement.
  - More freedom to see out-of-network providers.
  - Higher cost for out-of-network care.
  - Higher premiums.

Government-Funded Health Plans

- Medicaid
  - Government-funded program to provide healthcare services for the poorest of the poor.
  - Dually funded by the federal and individual state governments.
  - Each state administers the program for state recipients.
    - Sets policies for administration.
    - Sets eligibility standards.
    - Determines covered services.
    - Some states require a co-pay but the member is not obligated to pay it.
    - Federal government requires some basic services to be covered.
    - Eligibility is usually determined on a month-to-month basis.
      - Recipient must have a current Medicaid card to obtain services.
      - Some members must meet a monthly spend-down to be eligible for coverage.

spend-down The amount of money that a Medicaid recipient is required to pay each month for medications before coverage begins. The figure is based on the income and family circumstances of the recipient.

- Medicare
  - Federal program to provide healthcare for the elderly, persons with disabilities, and patients with end-stage renal disease (ESRD).
  - Largest healthcare program in the United States.
  - Divided into several parts:
    - Medicare Part A covers inpatient hospital care, skilled nursing facilities, hospice, and some home healthcare; no cost if the patient worked for 10 years in Medicare-covered employment.
    - Medicare Part B helps with doctor services, outpatient hospital care, and some physical and occupational therapy. Part B requires an extra monthly payment.
    - Medicare Advantage Plans: Participants in Medicare Parts A and B may choose to receive their care through an HMO or PPO for a managed care policy that covers more services for an extra cost.
    - Medigap or Medicare Supplement Policy: A policy sold by an insurance company to fill the gaps in the original Medicare plans.
    - Medicare Part D: A prescription drug plan that began in January 2006; provides coverage for prescription drugs, biologicals, insulin, vaccines, and medical supplies associated with the injection of insulin and not covered under Part A or Part B of Medicare. There are certain drug classes that are excluded from coverage, such as benzodiazepines, drugs for weight loss or gain, fertility drugs, cosmetic drugs, and over-the-counter (OTC) drugs.

The Technician's Role in Processing Insurance Claims

As pharmacists assume their role of providing excellent pharmaceutical care to patients through patient counseling and consultation with physicians and other healthcare professionals, a knowledgeable technician willing to become well versed in the parameters of the various third-party insurance plans will be an invaluable asset to the pharmacy team. Many patients do not understand the mechanics of their insurance plan, especially the guidelines for prescription drug coverage, and would benefit from a familiar person providing basic information about the insurance formularies, co-pays, deductibles, and noncovered drugs and devices.

insurance formularies Each insurance plan establishes a list of covered drugs and will not pay for any drug that is not on the list.

noncovered drugs and devices Any drug or device that is not listed on the formulary established by the insurance company.

Prescription Drug Plans

There are as many prescription drug plans as there are health insurance companies. Although there are similarities among the different plans, there are also many differences. It is unrealistic to attempt to memorize the guidelines for each plan, but understanding the basic components will facilitate data entry of insurance information and billing through on-line adjudication. The plans are usually a part of the patient's overall medical insurance package and the guidelines are dictated by the type of plan.

on-line adjudication Process of submitting an insurance claim for a prescription through a computer modem and receiving a response indicating the amount of coverage.

- PPO prescription drug plan: The member has a medical ID card listing prescription benefits. The patient sees a provider from the plans preferred list and takes the prescription to a member pharmacy that has a contract with the insurance plan. The insurance company has a preferred drug list (formulary) and prior authorization Required by insurance companies when a physician prescribes a drug that is not included in the formulary. The physician must call the insurance company or pharmacy benefit manager to request coverage.

modem connection Pharmacies under contract to an insurance company may establish a dial-up or wireless Internet connection through a modem to communicate via computer with an insurance provider to verify coverage of prescriptions.

pharmacy benefit manager (PBM) An individual or company that has contracted with an insurance company to manage formulary guidelines for the insurance company.

national provider identifier (NPI) A standard unique identifying number assigned to healthcare providers to facilitate transmission of health information in accordance with HIPAA regulations. Each pharmacy that is involved in providing Medicare and Medicaid services is required to apply for this number.

discourages use of nonpreferred drugs. Some nonpreferred drugs may require prior authorization. Brand-name drugs will have a higher co-pay than generic drugs. A 30-day supply of drugs may be purchased every 30 days unless a mail-order option is available to dispense a 90-day supply.

- HMO prescription drug plans: The patient's PCP directs the patient's medical care and must write all the prescriptions. Prescriptions written by another provider will be at the patient's expense unless they are ordered by a plan physician to whom the patient was referred by the PCP. Strict formulary guidelines are followed, with few exceptions. The use of available generics is often required and the co-pay is considerably higher for brand-name drugs. Mail-order opportunities exist for the patient to receive a 3-month supply of medication. At the retail pharmacy only a 30-day supply is allowed.
- Prescription discount plan: The insurance formulary may divide prescription drugs into classes or tiers that determine the percentage of cost paid by the patient. For example, RX Tier 1/RX Tier 2 10%/20% indicates that a drug classed as Tier 1 will be paid at 90% by the insurance and 10% by the patient, whereas a drug classed as Tier 2 will be paid at only 80% of cost by the insurance and 20% by the patient.

Most pharmacy software programs have an insurance screen to enter the data from the patient's insurance card(s). Some patients will have coverage from more than one plan (personal plan and spouse's plan). In this case both plans will need to be entered into the patient's profile, and they should be marked as the primary and secondary plans. The pharmacy signs a contract with each plan it is willing to accept. The contract contains specifics about how the cost of drugs is computed, the dispensing fee that will be paid to the pharmacy, and the co-pay to be paid by the patient. The pharmacy computer will have a modem connection to the insurance company or a pharmacy benefit manager (PBM) so that when the prescription is entered, the computer will connect to the insurance company and a quick response can be received detailing the insurance coverage and the co-pay to be collected from the patient. For this process to function, all the numbers from the patient's insurance card must be correctly entered into the computer. Figure 9.4 shows an example of an insurance screen that might be encountered in the pharmacy software. The technician needs to be familiar with the terminology so that the data will be entered in the proper locations.

Most insurance cards will have a member name and/or member code, which is different for each person covered on the policy whether it is a spouse or a dependent child. The subscriber name is the name of the person who has purchased the policy or has coverage because of their employment status. The subscriber ID number refers to the person who owns the policy and must be accurately entered for verification of coverage. The group number refers to the organization that has contracted with the insurance company to offer the insurance benefit to their employees. The plan number refers to the details of the coverage chosen by the organization for its employees. The insurance card may also indicate whether a PCP is required, and if so, the PCP's name may be listed on the card. The insurance card will also usually indicate whether the member has prescription benefits, and may list co-pays for brand and generic drugs. The back of the insurance card lists phone numbers to access insurance information and usually has a separate phone number for pharmacy inquiries, as well as a mailing address and often a Web address for further information.

Patient Name ____________ Sex ___ Medical Conditions ________

Patient Address ______________________ DOB ________

Patient Phone ____________________ Allergies ____________

Primary Insurance ____________

Plan ID ________ Plan Name ________ Person Code ________

Employer ID __________ Relationship to cardholder ________

Cardholder Name ________________ Cardholder ID ________

Pharmacy ID Number ____________ Plan Group Number ________

Secondary Insurance Plan Name ______________

Secondary Plan Group Number ________________ Plan ID ______

Employer ID ______________ Cardholder ID ______________

Cardholder ID ________________ Person Code ______________

Relationship to Cardholder ________________

Minimum Co-Pay Brand __________________

Minimum Co-Pay Generic ________________

Figure 9.4 Sample computer insurance screen.

The insurance card for Medicare Part D will look slightly different from cards for private insurance companies, although all Medicare Part D plans are administered by private insurance companies that have contracted with the Medicare organization to provide prescription services. Each pharmacy that participates in Medicare Part D insurance plans is required to obtain a National Provider Identifier (NPI) number to ensure secure, efficient transfers of health information between providers and health plans. See a sample Medicare Part D insurance card in Figure 9.5. As with other insurance plans, prescription coverage for Medicare Part D can only be obtained in network pharmacies. Patients must choose their Part D provider after carefully considering the provider's list of formulary-approved medications and comparing it with the medications that have been prescribed for them. The technician can be helpful in answering questions.

network pharmacies
Pharmacies that have contracted with an insurance company to accept its insurance.

AMERICAN INSURANCE COMPANY		
Medicare Rx Plan		
Effective Date: January 1, 20xx		
Rx Plan	63	
Rx PCN	02	Medicare Rx
Rx Group	09	Prescription Drug Coverage
ID 416-52-0035		
Ronald Tempe		

A

Medicare billing charges apply	
Submit Claims To:	
American Insurance Company 6403 W. Vermont Street Altoona WI 75306	Important Number
	Medicare Rx Plan 753-412-6906
	Member Services 753-412-6978

B

Figure 9.5 Sample Medicare Part D prescription drug insurance card, front **(A)** and back **(B)**.

Prescription Pricing

Prescription insurance plans have firm prescription pricing guidelines written in the contract agreement that must be signed by an agent for the pharmacy before the pharmacy can be listed as an approved provider. If the pharmacy is not willing to abide by the pricing guidelines, the insurance company will not reimburse the pharmacy for the cost of dispensing the prescription, and the pharmacy must tell patients that their insurance plan is not accepted at that pharmacy. The patients will then transfer their prescriptions to another pharmacy that will accept their insurance plan. Some insurance companies have exclusive agreements with a particular provider (such as a large chain) and other pharmacies are not allowed to enter into a contractual agreement with this insurance plan. Large chains or mail-order facilities may bid on the contract with an insurance company to be the exclusive provider.

There are published pricing guides that list average wholesale prices (AWP) of all prescription drugs on the market. These publications are updated monthly to reflect price increases, and the AWP is often used as the basis for pricing prescriptions. AWP is considered to be the average price that a wholesale establishment would charge a retail pharmacy for a certain package size of a given drug. The true wholesale price will vary in different locations because of quantity discounts and other factors that may affect costs. Most pharmacies have buying agreements with a primary wholesale drug company that offers a discount that has been negotiated by the pharmacy and the wholesaler. These buying agreements will be further discussed in a later chapter. The price the pharmacy actually pays for the drug (AWP minus any discounts) is called the actual acquisition cost (AAC). Because it is very difficult for the insurance company to determine the AAC for a particular drug in each pharmacy, most insurance plans base their reimbursement on the AWP. The insurance plan will then include in the contract agreement a percent deduction from the AWP to offset the difference between the AWP and AAC. For example, the contract may read that reimbursement will be at AWP minus 10% plus a dispensing fee. The insurance company dictates the amount of the dispensing fee it will pay. The pharmacy is also responsible for collecting the required co-pay from the patient at the time the prescription is dispensed.

average wholesale price (AWP) The calculated national average price that a retail pharmacy might pay for a given package size of a drug.

actual acquisition cost (AAC) The actual price that is paid for a drug after all discounts and shipping costs have been applied.

After the insurance software is entered into the computer system and the patient's insurance information is entered correctly into the patient profile, a prescription for that patient may be entered into the patient profile. The patient and prescription information is then transmitted via computer modem to the patient's insurance company or a PBM. The patient's eligibility will be verified and the prescription will be checked with the plan formulary and the days' supply. The computer terminal will then receive a message indicating the amount the plan will pay for the prescription and the amount of co-pay to be collected from the patient. If the drug is not on the plan formulary, there may be a message suggesting a similar drug that is on the plan formulary. Unless the suggested drug is an exact generic equivalent and generic substitution has been authorized, the physician will have to be called to authorize the change. This call may be initiated by the technician, but the pharmacist will need to take the information to make any change in the prescription order. The information may also be faxed on a secure fax line directly from the pharmacy to the physician's office, and the change may be received by return fax. The patient should be kept informed of any possible time delay necessitated by this process and the reason for the delay. The new prescription order should then be entered into the patient profile and resubmitted for insurance approval. The medication may then be prepared for a final check by the pharmacist and dispensing to the patient.

The pricing process for patients who pay cash for their prescriptions is determined by the pharmacy after careful consideration of the profit margin needed to meet expenses. Most pharmacies use the AWP as the basis for their pricing, but the AAC may also be used, especially for some of the more high-profile drugs that may be used in advertising. The pharmacy may use a percent markup on the cost of the drug, a markup plus a dispensing fee, or a sliding fee based on the cost of the prescription. See examples of each in the case study below.

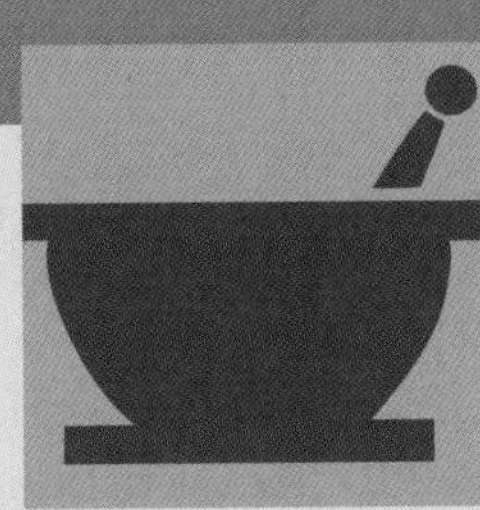

Professional Judgment Scenario 9.1

Marge receives a prescription for Lipitor from her physician to help lower her cholesterol. She is covered by her husband's insurance plan. Marge has been a regular customer at Nickelson's Pharmacy for years and is very trusting of the pharmacy staff. When she reaches the pharmacy counter, Jill greets her and checks her prescription for accuracy and completeness. Jill asks Marge if she has any additional medication allergies and Marge replies that she does not. Because Marge's insurance information is already in her profile, Jill begins to enter the prescription. When the information is transmitted to the insurance company, a response is returned that Lipitor is not on the formulary and the insurance plan recommends a change to simvastatin, which is the generic form of Zocor. Jill knows that Zocor is a different drug from Lipitor but is in the same therapeutic drug class. Both Lipitor and Zocor or simvastatin belong to the "statin" class of cholesterol-lowering drugs. This change will require authorization from the physician. Before proceeding, Jill discusses the options with Marge. Marge knows that her physician chose Lipitor for her because she believed it was the best drug for her condition. She asks Jill to give her a price on the Lipitor using the cash pricing system, and Jill is happy to do that for her.

therapeutic drug class Drugs are classified according to the use and means of action of the drug.

The AWP for a 30-day supply of Lipitor is $96.00. If the pharmacy uses a 30% markup to price cash prescriptions, the price for the Lipitor would be:

$96.00 × 0.3 = $28.80 markup

$96.00 + $28.80 = $124.80 prescription price for Lipitor.

If the pharmacy uses a 30% markup plus a $5.00 dispensing fee, the price would be:

$124.80 + $5.00 fee = $129.80 prescription price for Lipitor.

If the pharmacy uses the AWP plus a sliding fee scale, an example of a sliding fee schedule might be:

for AWP between	Fee
$1.00–$10.00	$4.00
$10.01–$25.00	$5.00
$25.01–$50.00	$8.00
$50.01 and above	$12.00

Using this sliding fee schedule, Marge's Lipitor prescription would be:

$96.00 + $12.00 = $108.00

Marge's prescription plan requires a $10.00 co-pay for generic medications. After comparing these costs, Marge requests that a call be placed to her doctor to see if she will authorize the change to simvastatin. Jill lets Marge know that it may be a few hours before the doctor's office returns the call, and offers to call Marge when the authorization is received and the prescription is ready. After consulting with the pharmacist, Jill receives approval to place the following call to the physician's office: "Hello, this is Jill, the pharmacy technician, calling from Nickelson's Pharmacy. One of Dr. Jones' patients, Marge Smithson, presented a prescription for Lipitor this morning. Lipitor is not on the formulary list of her insurance company and Marge requested that we ask if Dr. Jones would authorize a change to simvastatin, which is covered by her insurance." The medical assistant responds, "The doctor is with a patient, Jill, but I will place the request on her desk and return your call when she has had a chance to respond." Jill leaves the pharmacy phone number and continues with her work. Later, when the physician's office returns the call, Jill transfers the call to the pharmacist, who documents the change and returns the prescription to Jill for data entry and processing. When the prescription is complete, Jill calls Marge to let her know.

Discuss how Jill's professional knowledge of the pricing system and the insurance plan enabled her to deal with the situation effectively, allowing the pharmacist to concentrate on clinical issues and patient counseling.

Compare Jill's professional communication skills in the previous example with the following possible encounter in the same situation.

As Marge approaches the pharmacy counter, Jill greets her rather abruptly. "Hi, Marge. We're really busy today, but if you need to wait I'll try to get this ready for you." After entering the prescription and receiving a reply from the insurance company that the drug is not covered, Jill says, "Hey, Marge, doesn't your doctor know anything about your insurance formulary? This drug is not covered and the insurance says to switch to simvastatin. We can call your doctor and get it changed." When Marge requests a price comparison, Jill responds, "Lipitor will cost a fortune; we'll call the doctor and get it changed. You may as well go on home, it may be days before the doctor calls back." Which technician–patient encounter will you portray in your practice?

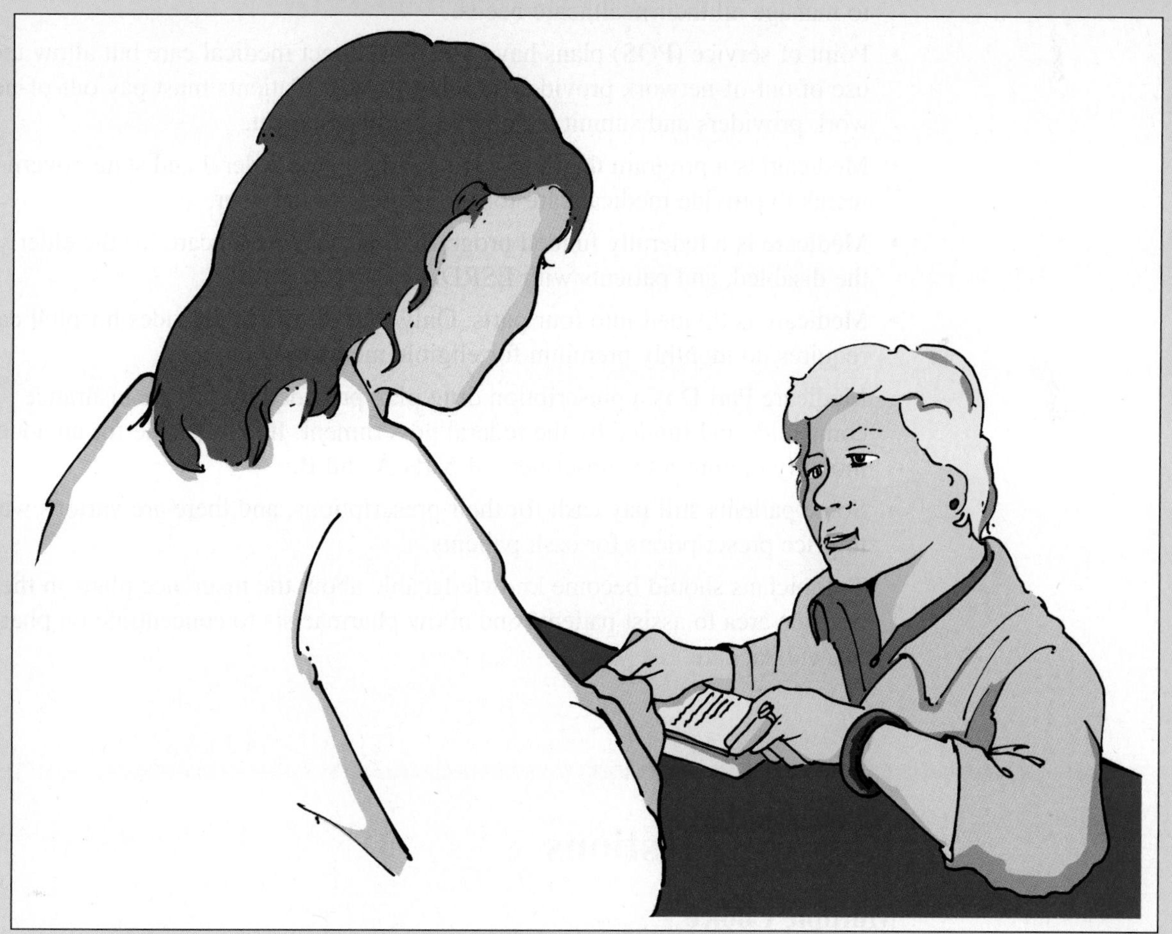

Prescription pricing is a very dynamic aspect of the practice of pharmacy. Formularies change daily as new drugs are introduced to the market, patents for brand-name products expire, and prescription drugs are transferred to OTC status. Insurance plans change their coverage guidelines and patients change insurance plans because of changes in employment status, disability or reaching retirement age, and coverage under Medicare. A knowledgeable technician will strive to be informed about these changes and assist patients by updating their insurance information when needed. This will enable the pharmacist to provide excellent pharmaceutical care to patients.

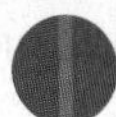

Chapter Summary

- Healthcare costs continue to rise, and insurance premiums have increased as the amount of coverage has decreased.
- Prescriptions account for about 10% of the healthcare dollar, but because this is a recurring monthly expense, it greatly affects the lifestyle of patients—especially those on a fixed income.
- A preferred provider plan (PPO) pays a higher percentage of healthcare costs when an in-network provider is used, but allows members to choose any provider.
- A health maintenance organization (HMO) requires members to choose a PCP to manage all their healthcare needs.
- Point of service (POS) plans have a PCP to direct medical care but allow the use of out-of-network providers at a higher cost. Patients must pay out-of-network providers and submit a claim for reimbursement.
- Medicaid is a program that is funded dually by the federal and state governments to provide medical care for the poorest of the poor.
- Medicare is a federally funded program to provide healthcare for the elderly, the disabled, and patients with ESRD.
- Medicare is divided into four parts. Only Part A, which provides hospital care, requires no monthly premium for eligible members.
- Medicare Part D is a prescription drug plan provided by private insurance companies and funded by the federal government. It is available for an added monthly premium to subscribers of parts A and B.
- Some patients still pay cash for their prescriptions, and there are various ways to price prescriptions for cash patients.
- Technicians should become knowledgeable about the insurance plans in their practice area to assist patients and allow pharmacists to concentrate on pharmaceutical care.

Review Questions

Multiple Choice

Choose the correct answer to each question below:

1. Prescription drugs account for what percentage of the annual healthcare dollar?
   a. 30%
   b. 20%
   c. 10%
   d. 40%

2. The price that a pharmacy pays for a drug after all discounts and shipping costs have been applied is called the
   a. average wholesale price
   b. premium
   c. actual acquisition cost
   d. discounted cost

3. The amount of money that a patient with prescription insurance coverage is required to pay at the pharmacy for their prescriptions is called the
   a. deductible
   b. co-pay
   c. discount price
   d. premium

4. A medication that is not listed in an insurance formulary may still be covered by the insurance plan if the physician
   a. signs on the "dispense as written" line
   b. writes "brand medically necessary" on the prescription
   c. calls the insurance company for prior authorization of the drug
   d. nonformulary drugs are never covered by insurance

5. The amount of medical expenses that a patient is required to pay before the insurance will begin to cover expenses is called the
   a. co-pay
   b. premium
   c. deductible
   d. acquisition cost

Fill in the Blank

Fill in the blank with the correct word or words.

6. A pharmacy that has contracted with an insurance company to accept its insurance plans is considered to be a ______________________ pharmacy.

7. The communication between a pharmacy computer and the insurance company to verify eligibility and prescription drug coverage is called ______________________.

8. An insurance plan in which all of the patient's medical care is managed by a PCP and prescriptions are covered only if written by the PCP is called a ______________________.

9. The government-funded program that was designed to provide healthcare to the poorest of the poor in this country is called ______________________.

10. The government-funded program that provides healthcare for the elderly and disabled is called ______________________.

Matching

Match the terms below with the correct definition:

11. _____ member code number
12. _____ subscriber ID number
13. _____ group number
14. _____ plan number
15. _____ co-pay

A. The number indicating the organization that has contracted with the insurance company to provide benefits to employees.
B. The number that indicates the details of the insurance coverage
C. The number indicating the person being covered by the insurance card.
D. The number indicating the person who owns the insurance policy.
E. The number indicating the amount the person must pay for the prescription.

True/False

Mark the following statements True or False.

16. _____ Most insurance pricing is based on the actual acquisition cost of drugs.

17. _____ Two drugs that are in the same therapeutic drug class can be substituted if the doctor authorizes the use of generics.

18. _____ A pharmacy benefit manager is an individual or company that has contracted with an insurance company to manage formulary guidelines.

19. _____ Medicare Part D covers prescription drugs for the elderly, who pay a monthly premium.

20. _____ Medicaid coverage is entirely managed and funded by the federal government to offer medical services to the poor.

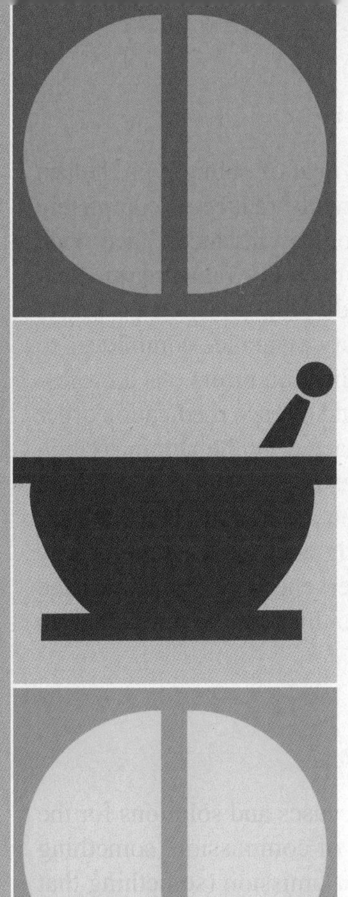

Chapter 10

Medication Error Prevention

OBJECTIVES

After completing this chapter, the student will be able to:

- Discuss the health consequences of medication errors.
- List the types of medication errors.
- Describe common causes of medication errors.
- Discuss the "systems approach" to medication errors.
- List the JCAHO National Patient Safety Goals pertaining to medication safety.
- Develop quality-assurance measures to assist in preventing medication errors.
- Categorize and track medication errors and their causes.

KEY TERMS

- Computerized Physician Order Entry (CPOE)
- E-prescribing
- errors of commission
- errors of omission
- quality assurance
- systems approach

The incidence of medication errors has received a great deal of publicity in the last few years, and a strong movement has developed to greatly reduce or completely eliminate errors from the healthcare setting. Technological advances have been implemented to improve patient safety. A systems approach to evaluating medication errors has directed the focus away from blaming individual healthcare workers for errors and has encouraged the establishment of quality assurance committees to examine procedures for lessening the likelihood of medication errors. As a professional pharmacy technician, you understand that at the end of each medication order there is a patient whose health may be profoundly impacted by the administration of medications. Your responsibility to your patients does not end with the accurate performance of your responsibilities as a technician. You are morally and ethically obligated to use your professional knowledge and judgment to be alert for any potential problems in the medication process, and intervene if necessary for the good of the patient. If you are unable or unwilling to do this, you do not belong in healthcare.

systems approach Examining the processes and procedures in the pharmacy to determine the cause of medication errors rather than placing blame on an individual.

quality assurance A set formula to analyze and improve pharmacy procedures to provide excellent pharmaceutical care to patients.

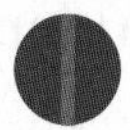

Types of Medication Errors

Categorizing medication errors helps to determine the causes and solutions for the different types of errors. The two basic types are errors of commission (something was done that should not have been done) and errors of omission (something that should have been done was omitted). Each type of error can cause great harm to the patient. Even if the patient discovers the error before a dose of medication is taken, the trust relationship between the patient and the pharmacy staff may be impaired. Concerns about medication safety may prevent patients from being compliant with life-saving medications. The following sections detail the most common medication errors.

errors of commission Errors resulting from something that was done that should not have been done.

errors of omission Errors that occur as the result of something that should have been done but was not done.

Incorrect Label Instructions on the Prescription Vial

Description: The physician writes the instructions for the patient's medication on the prescription blank. Often Latin abbreviations are used and the physician's handwriting may not be ideal. The technician translates the abbreviated instructions to the prescription label in a form that the patient can understand.

Quality Assurance Solutions:

- Screen the prescription for accuracy. Before entering the data, the technician must read the entire prescription and translate all abbreviations. Any discrepancy concerning legibility must be verified with the pharmacist and/or physician.
- Evaluate the prescription information. After verifying the legibility, the technician must evaluate the prescription and instructions to the patient to ascertain that the directions are reasonable for the medication ordered. The dosage form prescribed must also be correct for the instructions to the patient.
- The technician is often the person who makes the offer of patient counseling by the pharmacist. The technician should be certain that the patient understands how to take the medication.
- Computerized physician order entry (CPOE) is a technological approach to eliminating issues involving poor handwriting. The physician must be adequately trained in entering orders, and the technician and pharmacist must still screen the prescriptions for accuracy.

computerized physician order entry (CPOE) A plan to use technology to eliminate handwriting errors by having physicians enter orders directly into the computer.

Incorrect Drug Name on Label

Description: The name, strength, and form of the drug must be accurate on the prescription label to prevent dosing errors. If the wrong drug, strength, or dose has been entered into the patient profile, the next time the prescription will be filled with the wrong drug.

Quality Assurance Solutions:

- The technician should verify after data entry that the prescription label correctly indicates the drug, strength, and dosage form as written on the prescription.

Incorrect Drug Quantity in the Vial

Description: The correct quantity of the medication and the correct number of refills must be entered into the computer so the patient can receive the proper therapy regimen.

Quality Assurance Solutions:

- The technician should verify that the label indicates the correct quantity of drug and number of refills.
- The technician should exercise caution in counting the number of doses placed in the prescription container.
- Automated dispensing machines should be properly maintained to ensure delivery of correct amounts of medication.

Incorrect Drug Dispensed

Description: The many distractions in the practice of pharmacy, and the number of look-alike/sound-alike drugs may cause the technician to choose the wrong drug to dispense.

Quality Assurance Solutions:

- The technician should check the label of the medication bottle three times before completing the prescription. The label should be checked when the bottle is removed from the shelf, again when the drug is poured onto the counting tray or into the dispensing bottle, and a third time after the prescription is completed and placed for the final check by the pharmacist.
- The technician should exercise caution when placing drugs back on the shelf after use and when placing newly ordered drugs on the shelf. Many manufacturers use labels on medications that look very similar. If two products with similar labels are switched on the shelf, an error is likely to occur.
- The technician must double-check the medication label before refilling automated dispensing machines to prevent errors resulting from the wrong medication being dispensed by the machine.

Medication Dispensed to the Wrong Patient

Description: In a community pharmacy, when a new prescription is entered into the computer system for a patient, that patient's name will appear on the screen for the next new prescription. In a hospital setting, the nursing staff may administer the medication to the wrong patient.

Quality Assurance Solutions:

- The technician should always check to be sure the correct patient name is on the computer screen before beginning data entry of the prescription. If several family members are entered into the computer system, be certain that the correct name is chosen.
- When prescriptions are being prepared for multiple patients, be sure to separate the orders for each patient to avoid putting someone else's medication in the patient's prescription bag.
- Label inpatient medications according to protocol to prevent the nursing staff from administering them to the wrong patient.
- If medication administration records (MAR) are prepared in the pharmacy, check them carefully for accuracy.

Wrong Dose

Description: The physician may prescribe an incorrect dose based on the age, weight, or disease state of the patient. The medication may not be commercially available in the dose prescribed. A prescription for a compounded medication may have a miscalculation, resulting in a wrong dose. The wrong dose of the medication may be chosen by the technician.

Quality Assurance Solutions:

- The technician should check the patient's date of birth during the screening of patient information to note whether the patient is a child or an adult. If a parent and child have the same name, be certain the correct person is chosen from the data screen.
- The technician should be careful to enter all allergies and diagnoses (if known) in the patient profile so the pharmacy software can indicate any problems with the medication being entered. Any interaction should be brought to the attention of the pharmacist.
- Calculations for a compounded prescription or an IV admixture should be double-checked. A leading zero before a decimal should always be used (e.g., 0.3 mg), but a trailing zero after a whole number (e.g., 1.0 mg) should never be used. Be certain that the units (e.g., milligrams, grams, or ounces) are correctly labeled.
- The technician should read the label three times. The pharmacist should also check the medication label, the drug inside the container, and the hard copy of the prescription to ensure that all are correct.
- In an institutional setting where automated dispensing machines are used, the person removing the medication from the shelf in the warehouse should have it checked by another technician or a pharmacist before placing it in the machine. When removing a medication from an automated machine, the nurse or health-care professional should double-check the drug and strength, and do so again before administering it to the patient. Automation helps to prevent medication errors, but it does not replace careful attention to detail by health professionals.

Wrong Administration Time Error

Description: The patient may not understand the directions. For example, he or she may think that 1 tid means that the medication can be taken at any time during the day as long as three doses are taken. A hospitalized patient may not receive his or her medication at the correct time, or might receive the dose twice due to an error in documentation on the medication administration record.

Quality Assurance Solutions:

- Encourage patients to accept counseling from the pharmacist. If the patient refuses counseling, ask the patient if they understand the directions.
- Hospitals have established medication administration times. It is considered an administration error if the patient does not receive medication before it is time for the next dose to be administered. If the patient is away from the room for a laboratory test, the missed dose is not classified as an error. The nursing staff must be diligent about documenting medication administration to avoid giving a second dose.

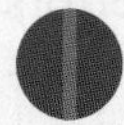

The Technician's Professional Approach to Medication Errors

Too often, the procedure observed on the discovery of a medication error is to correct it as quickly as possible and pretend it never happened. This approach developed as a result of the punitive manner in which blame and often punishment were meted out to the person held "responsible" for the error. It is now understood that medication errors are failures of the system and the underlying causes of the error must be analyzed to develop a plan to prevent the error from recurring. The first step in this process is to put in place a formal procedure for reporting medication errors. A number of organizations have developed organized plans and specific reporting forms to facilitate this process.

Often the technician is the first person to receive the report of an error. A patient, nurse, or another healthcare professional may call the pharmacy to report a discrepancy. The professional technician should discuss the pharmacy's protocol for handling medication errors early in the training process to be aware of proper handling of any incidents before they occur. The technician should use excellent communication skills and follow pharmacy protocol when speaking with the patient or healthcare professional. Pay close attention to any details given and the demeanor of the reporting person, and politely refer the phone call to the attention of a pharmacist. Assist the pharmacist in locating the paper work for the order in question and offer any pertinent information you may have about the order.

CAUTION

If the patient reports that a medication looks different from the last time and you are pretty sure that a different generic was given, take the time to double-check the prescription and the patient's description of the tablet or capsule received, and check with the pharmacist to be certain before telling the patient the medication is correct.

If the pharmacist determines that a medication error has occurred, the first steps to resolving the error depend on a number of factors. If the patient has ingested one or more doses of the incorrect medication, the physician should be notified and any corrective procedures should be instituted immediately. If the patient is at home and discovered the error before taking the medication, he or she may be willing to return the medication to the pharmacy so the error can be corrected, or the pharmacist may send someone from the pharmacy to pick up the medication so the correction can be made. The health and safety of the patient are the primary concerns. If the incorrect medication is administered in a hospital or other healthcare facility, the patient and/or the patient's family should be informed of the error. They should be advised of any known reasons for the error, possible adverse effects, and the steps being taken to rectify the situation. After the patient has been adequately served and any concerns have been addressed by the pharmacist, nurses, and physicians, the process of determining the causes of the error can begin.

The first step in this process is to report the error through the proper channels in the organization and to one of the national error-reporting organizations. The Institute for Safe Medication Practices (ISMP) provides an online error-reporting system that will assist in disseminating information nationally to prevent the same error from being repeated in other pharmacies.

TIP **Go to http://www.ismp.org to view this form and get more information on safe medication practices.**

This is especially important with look-alike/sound-alike medications or errors that are the result of similar or confusing package labeling. The ISMP also compiles a list of drugs that have a high error rate or have especially serious consequences when involved in errors. See Appendix A of this text for an abbreviation watch list, and Appendix B for a list of high-risk medications. This information can assist in alerting health professionals to situations that cause repeated medication errors due to a system that is faulty.

In a large organization, there should be a quality assurance committee to examine all medication errors on a regular basis, categorize them, and list possible causes and solutions to prevent repetition of the same error. The committee should be comprised of pharmacists, physicians, nurses, and technicians. Technicians are very involved in the handling processes in the pharmacy and often can see a potential problem situation before an error occurs.

Improving processes in the pharmacy to prevent medication errors should be the constant concern of every technician. Even in a small pharmacy with only a few employees, quality assurance should be constantly evaluated. Often a medication misadventure that is discovered before it reaches the patient is not considered an error, but these incidents should be included in the analysis. In addition to using the reporting form of the ISMP or the MedWatch form of the FDA, each pharmacy should create an internal form to document and categorize all medication errors, including those that never reach the patient. The form should include the date and time the prescription was filled, information about the working conditions at that time, any comments about distractions that may have contributed to the error, how the error was discovered, and an analysis of possible causes and possible solutions. This form should be discussed at staff meetings or, if no staff meetings take place, all pharmacy personnel should read the report and offer comments. Awareness of medication misadventures will increase the alertness of the staff in preventing repeated errors.

Several of the 2006 JCAHO National Patient Safety Goals are directly related to pharmacy and medication dispensing. One of the goals is to improve the accuracy of patient identification. This is important not only in an institutional setting where medications are administered to the patient, but also in outpatient pharmacy settings. Many patient names are similar or may sound similar when the patient is called to the pharmacy, and many patients have the same name. When a patient comes to the pharmacy counter to pick up a medication, the name and address of the patient should always be verified to prevent dispensing the medication to the wrong patient.

The effectiveness of communication among caregivers is vitally important in the pharmacy setting. Verbal or telephone orders should be reduced to writing immediately and read back to the person phoning the order for verification. They should also be dated and the name or initials of the person phoning the order in as well as the person accepting the order should be documented in case there is a question later. The JCAHO also provides a standard list of abbreviations that may not be used, to prevent confusion between words with dual meanings.

A standardized approach to "handing off" communications at the change of a shift will assist in continuity of care. Other medication safety goals, especially in a large institution, include standardizing and limiting the number of drug concentrations available. Institutions may compile a list of "high-alert medications" that are known to cause serious consequences when an error occurs, and require a second person to double-check the medication and dose before it leaves the pharmacy. Periodic reviews of a list of look-alike/sound-alike drugs and development of a plan to differentiate these drugs will assist in error prevention. The JCAHO also requires that all medications and medication containers be labeled. An open container must be labeled with the date opened, the expiration date, storage conditions, and drug name. Medication reconciliation (communicating a complete list of all patient medications when the patient arrives at a facility and each time the patient is moved to another area) is a recent addition to the requirements for patient safety.

Prescription evaluation will become more exact as more physicians begin to perform electronic prescribing (E-prescribing), and many of the evaluation issues will be resolved online at the point of prescribing. This will eliminate many of the phone calls to physician offices involving formulary concerns and dose, and dosage form errors can be corrected electronically at the point of prescribing. Bar coding of unit of use medications has been shown to improve dispensing accuracy, as does the use of automated dispensing machines.

E-prescribing Using an electronic health record system that checks formulary compliance of the patient's health plan and performs a drug utilization review (DUR) at the point of prescribing, with computer messages that allow the physician to correct issues before the prescription is transmitted to the pharmacy.

Not all of these goals are the responsibility of a technician, but it is the technician's responsibility to be constantly alert for any patient safety initiative that has been neglected. Regardless of the level of technology available in an institution, conscientious observations by every healthcare worker are imperative for preventing medication errors. The five "rights" of medication administration—right patient, right drug, right dose, right route of administration, and right time—should become a mantra that is constantly in the minds of all healthcare workers. With the constant diligence of all healthcare providers, the number of medication errors can be diminished or eliminated.

Case Study 10.1

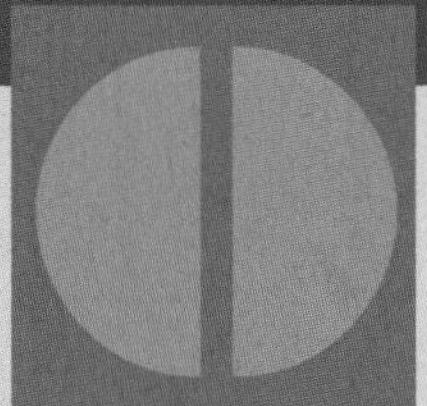

As Jim began taking some of the introductory courses in his pharmacy technician program, he requested a transfer from his job in the hospital to the hospital pharmacy department. There was so much to learn, and Jim was a very enthusiastic learner. The experienced technicians were happy to answer his questions and participate in his training. He frequently accompanied experienced technicians as they delivered medications to the floors and restocked the Pyxis machines. After he completed his Pyxis training, Jim received his own code for the Pyxis machines. He was proud of the fact that he could now restock the machines without supervision. He understood that his code was to be kept private because it would document any functions he performed in the automated dispensing cabinets.

Jim liked working weekends so that he could attend classes during the week. One Saturday afternoon, Jim was working with a technician who had been hired a few weeks after him. Jim and Bob had become friends as they went through some of their training together. Jim knew that Bob had been trained on the Pyxis machines but had not yet received his code. Two technicians had called in sick that day and the pharmacy was quite busy. Even though Jim was still fairly new to the position, he was the most experienced technician that day and he was anxious to prove that he and Bob could handle all the technician tasks. The pharmacy received a printout saying that several of the Pyxis machines were out of stock for a number of items. Jim felt that he needed to stay in the pharmacy to complete IV admixtures and answer the phone. He asked Bob if he would feel comfortable gathering the out-of-stock medications and taking them to the floors to fill the dispensing machines. Bob was anxious to help and agreed to this, so he gathered the medications and placed them on a cart. Jim gave him a card with his Pyxis code so that Bob could access the machine. Jim admonished Bob to proceed slowly and carefully as he followed the protocol for restocking the Pyxis, because the procedures would be documented with Jim's code. Bob returned to the pharmacy after completing the process and reported to Jim that there were no problems. Bob and Jim left the pharmacy at the end of their shift feeling proud that they were able to keep things running smoothly. Later that night as Jim was watching the evening news, he was horrified to see a report that a child had died at the hospital where he worked. The cause of death was an overdose of heparin. Heparin is a blood thinner that prevents blood clots from forming and is used in patients receiving IV therapy to keep the IV lines open. It comes in several different strengths, and it is critical to use the correct strength. The different strengths of heparin are packaged in vials that look the same

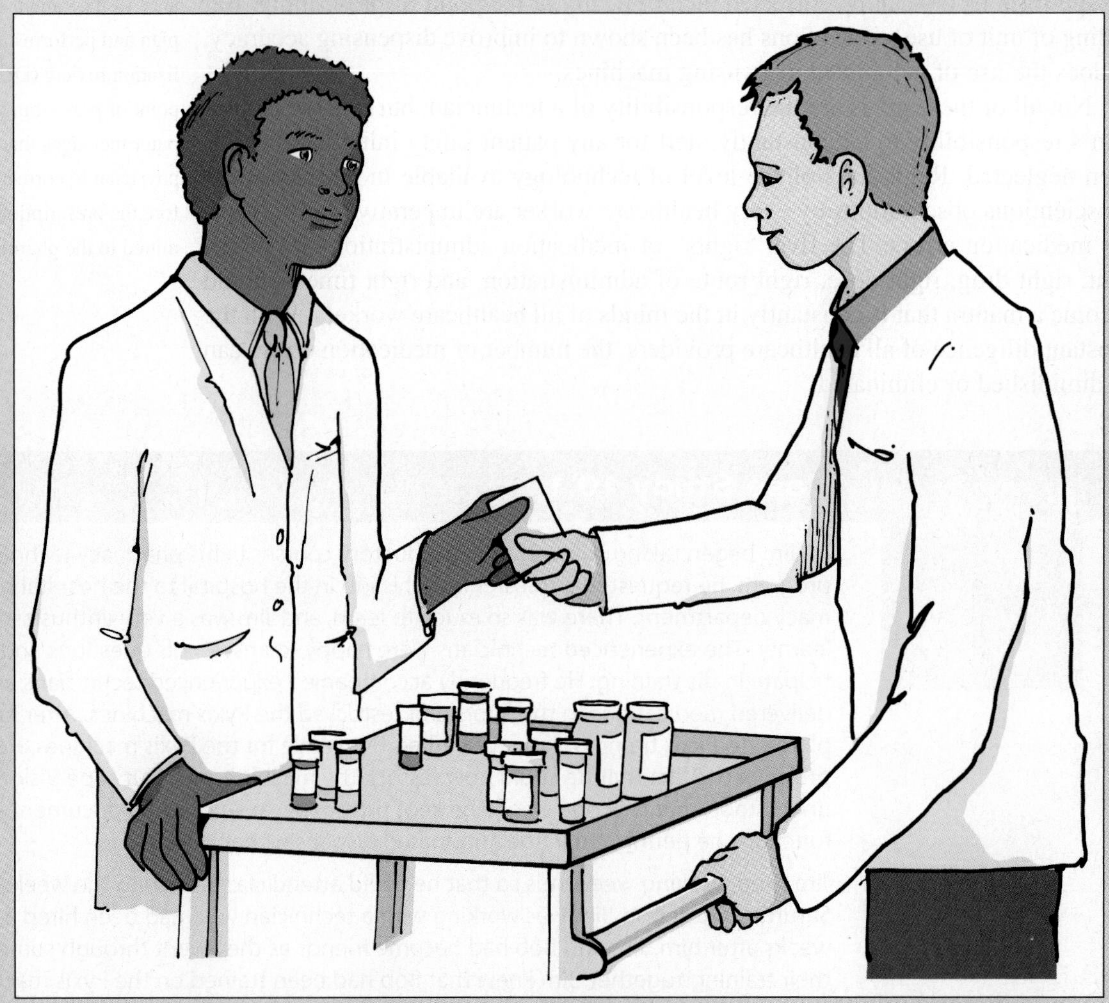

except for the strength listed on the vial. The news report stated that a nurse removed a vial of heparin from the Pyxis machine and administered it to a child. Several hours later the child began to show signs of hemorrhaging. When the vial was rechecked, it was discovered that the incorrect strength of heparin had been placed in the Pyxis machine and subsequently administered to the child.

1. Name the person or persons responsible for this tragic error.
2. Discuss the breaks in protocol that allowed this tragedy to occur.
3. List other circumstances that contributed to this situation.

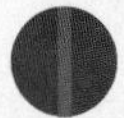

Chapter Summary

- Medication errors can profoundly impact the health of patients.
- Every healthcare professional must be actively involved in error prevention.
- Categorizing medication errors will improve awareness of problem situations that may result in an error.
- Medication errors should be considered a system problem rather than the fault of an individual.
- Quality assurance committees should analyze all medication errors to determine causes and possible solutions.
- Quality assurance committees should meet with all pharmacy personnel regularly to report medication errors and preventive measures to be instituted.
- Technicians should be constantly alert for potential sources of medication errors in the pharmacy and make suggestions for process improvement.
- All pharmacy staff must be familiar with the JCAHO "do not use" abbreviation list, and each institution should add problem abbreviations to the list.
- Look-alike/sound-alike drugs should be reviewed periodically to alert pharmacy staff to the danger of an error.
- High-alert medications should require a double-check by a second staff member.

Review Questions

Multiple Choice

Circle the best answer in the questions below.

1. Choose the statement that best describes the proper approach to medication errors:
   a. Medication errors are rare and cause little impact on the healthcare system.
   b. The healthcare worker involved in a medication error should be severely reprimanded.
   c. A systems approach to medication errors directs focus away from the individual and assesses processes for quality improvement.
   d. A medication error that is caught before it reaches the patient should not be reported.

2. Incorrect patient instructions on the prescription vial can be prevented by
   a. carefully counting the number of doses placed in the container
   b. accurate screening and evaluation of the prescription by the technician
   c. checking the manufacturer label of the drug three times
   d. none of the above

3. Manufacturers can assist in preventing medication errors by
   a. choosing drug names that do not look or sound like other drug names.
   b. using labels that accent differences in drugs
   c. highlighting drug strengths of multiple strength drugs
   d. all of the above

4. The systems approach to medication error
   a. holds the individual(s) involved in a medication error responsible for the error
   b. reprimands the entire pharmacy department when an error is discovered
   c. resolves the error as quietly as possible
   d. involves categorizing and evaluating errors to establish safe procedures

5. Quality assurance committees
   a. have all pharmacy staff as members
   b. are established after medication errors become a problem
   c. should be in place in all pharmacy departments to establish medication safety protocols
   d. do not include technicians as members

Fill in the Blank

Fill in the blanks with the correct term.

6. Having physicians enter medication orders directly into a computer to eliminate handwriting errors is called ______________________.

7. An error that occurred as a result of something that should have been done but was not done is called an error of ______________________.

8. A ____________________ zero should always be used before a decimal, but a ____________________ zero should never be used after a whole number.

9. If a patient in the hospital does not receive a scheduled medication dose before the next dose is due, the error is called a ____________________ error.

10. The JCAHO has a standard list of medical ____________________ that should not be used in prescription writing to eliminate confusion.

True/False

Mark the following statements True or False:

11. ________ All medication containers in the pharmacy must be labeled with the drug name and expiration date.

12. ________ An error of commission is an error resulting from something that should have been done and was not done.

13. ________ When an incorrect medication is dispensed to a patient, there is no harm done if the patient discovers the error before taking a dose.

14. ________ Automated dispensing machines will eliminate medication errors involving the drugs included in the machine.

15. ________ Neglecting to affix an auxiliary label to a medication that may cause drowsiness is an example of an error of omission.

Matching

Match the correct term with the statements below.

16. ____ wrong administration time error
17. ____ quality assurance
18. ____ wrong dose error
19. ____ wrong patient directions error
20. ____ incorrect drug dispensed

A. The process of categorizing and analyzing medication errors to improve safety procedures.
B. The directions printed on the prescription label are incorrect.
C. The medication in the prescription vial is not the medication ordered.
D. The medication dosing schedule is not followed according to directions.
E. The strength of the drug dispensed is different from the strength ordered.

LEARNING ACTIVITY

After completing the quality assurance analysis in the previous case study, devise a formal plan to ensure that this type of medication error will never occur again in this hospital. Include protocols that were already in place but were not followed and additional steps to prevent a recurrence. What action by the manufacturer might provide an additional safety feature?

UNIT IV

Mechanics of Medication Dispensing and Inventory Control

Chapter **11**

Over-the-Counter Medications, Herbal Products, and Diagnostic Aids

OBJECTIVES

After completing this chapter, the student will be able to:

- List the classes of over-the-counter medications
- Describe several drugs in each class
- List products that are sugar- and alcohol-free
- Demonstrate initiative in the sale of over-the-counter medications
- Describe procedures for the sale of the growing list of drugs that are kept behind the prescription counter but do not require a prescription

KEY TERMS

- adsorbent
- analgesic
- anti-inflammatory
- antipruritic
- antipyretic
- antitussive
- decongestant
- electrolyte imbalance
- expectorant
- hypercalcemia
- prodrugs
- rebound congestion
- Reye's syndrome
- rhinitis
- salicylates
- stimulant laxative
- tineas

Managing the over-the-counter (OTC) drug department often becomes the responsibility of a technician. Although this may seem to be an overwhelming responsibility, with a little experience and some organizational skills it can become a rewarding task. The technician should acquire a working knowledge of the nonprescription products and their drug classifications. The technician must be confident in knowing which types of patient questions may be answered by a technician and which must be referred to a pharmacist. The technician should be alert to signs of confusion as a patient attempts to choose an OTC product. Offer to assist patients who seem unsure about their purchase. With a few questions, you can discern whether you can guide them in their choice or they should be directed to the pharmacist for counseling. Once you take ownership of this department, you will be better able to assist customers as they search for medications to manage their symptoms at home. This chapter will discuss OTC medications, including vitamins and herbal preparations and the many new at-home test kits available. A complete listing of all nonprescription medications is beyond the scope of this book, but the basic categories and examples from each category will be listed. Chapter 11 will address the purchasing and inventory functions for this department.

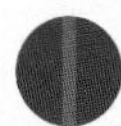

Categorizing Nonprescription Drugs

Analgesics and Antipyretics

salicylates Aspirin-containing products or products that contain compounds from the same class as aspirin.

Reye's syndrome A serious condition that can occur in children as a result of taking a product containing a salicylate.

analgesic A substance that provides pain relief.

antipyretic A substance that lowers fever.

anti-inflammatory A substance that reduces inflammation caused by allergic reaction, irritation, or disorders such as arthritis.

OTC pain medications consist of three basic types of oral medications. The first group is the salicylates, which consist of aspirin and aspirin-related drugs and combinations. Aspirin is available in many strengths, including an 81-mg tablet that in some cases may still be called children's aspirin. However, because of its association with a serious condition called Reye's syndrome, aspirin is no longer used in children. The 81-mg dose is primarily used as a daily dose for preventing blood clots in adults, especially those who have already had a heart attack. Regular-strength aspirin contains 325 mg or 5 grains, but there are higher strengths available that can be used for more severe pain and the pain of osteoarthritis. In addition to their analgesic properties, salicylates also have antipyretic and anti-inflammatory effects. A disadvantage of salicylates is their potential to cause gastrointestinal bleeding; however, there are enteric-coated formulations to help guard against that effect. Aspirin use is also contraindicated for patients who are taking a blood thinner, such as Coumadin (warfarin), unless prescribed by a physician. Aspirin may also be combined with sodium bicarbonate to create an effervescent tablet, and is formulated in a long-acting tablet.

The nonsteroidal anti-inflammatory drugs (NSAIDs) include ibuprofen, naproxen, and many others. These drugs are also analgesic and antipyretic, and are available in several formulations. Strengths of ibuprofen above 200 mg and naproxen over 220 mg require a prescription. Ibuprofen is also available in a liquid suspension (100 mg/5 mL) and drops (50 mg/1.25 mL) for convenient pediatric dosing. Both of these products are alcohol-free. In addition to acute pain, the NSAIDs are also useful for treating chronic pain conditions such as arthritis. The chronic use of NSAIDs has been implicated in the development of heart problems and should be supervised by a physician.

The third class of OTC analgesics is acetaminophen. It is available in tablets, capsules, and liquid formulations. Acetaminophen is analgesic and antipyretic, but it has no anti-inflammatory properties and does not cause gastrointestinal bleeding. Acetaminophen, however, can be extremely toxic and can cause liver failure if consumed in too high a dose or taken with alcohol. The maximum dose for acetaminophen is 4 grams and it can be toxic in lower doses when combined with alcohol. Acetaminophen is combined with many other drugs, both prescription and nonprescription, so it is important to check the labels of compound products to prevent overdosing. Children's formulations include both a liquid (80 mg/half teaspoonful) and infant drops (80 mg/0.8 mL). Both products are alcohol-free. It is also imperative for the caregiver to administer the correct dose according to the weight of the child, because a child may easily be overdosed.

Antacid Preparations

Antacid products are designed to reduce the symptoms of sour stomach, heartburn, and indigestion that are caused by overeating or eating problem foods. They are safe to use for self-treatment if no other serious symptoms, such as serious vomiting, vomiting of blood, excessive diarrhea, or blood in the stool or vomitus, are present. Indigestion should be self-treated with OTC preparations for no longer than 2 weeks without the advice of a physician to ensure that a more serious condition is not overlooked. Antacid products should not be given to a child under 2 years of age.

Most antacid preparations are available in both liquid and tablet formulations. They contain various amounts of aluminum hydroxide and magnesium hydroxide or calcium carbonate and magnesium hydroxide to help neutralize the acid in the stomach. Some preparations also contain simethicone, which helps to relieve gas and the bloated feeling that accompanies it, and some have calcium carbonate alone.

Tums has several formulations that consist of calcium carbonate alone. This is the most potent and fast-acting antacid, but excessive use can cause a rebound effect due to hypercalcemia. An excess of calcium can also increase the risk of kidney stones and constipation. Because of their high levels of calcium carbonate, Tums and other products of the same potency are often used as calcium supplements.

hypercalcemia A condition of excess calcium in the bloodstream, possibly from overconsumption of chewable antacid tablets containing calcium.

The most common combination products are Maalox, which contains magnesium hydroxide and aluminum hydroxide, and Mylanta, which has simethicone added to the combination.

Both are available in various formulations, and some formulations of Mylanta contain calcium carbonate with magnesium hydroxide. Mylanta is sugar- and alcohol-free. Magnesium hydroxide may cause a laxative effect, which is balanced by the constipating effects of calcium carbonate.

Bismuth subsalicylate is advertised for heartburn and upset stomach as an agent that provides a protective coating for the gastrointestinal mucosa. It is not a true antacid and there are some concerns regarding its use for an upset stomach. It is a salicylate similar to aspirin and therefore can cause irritation to the gastric mucosa and lead to stomach bleeding. It also carries the risk of Reye's syndrome and should not be used in children. Bismuth subsalicylate is sugar- and alcohol-free.

Antacids will neutralize acid better if taken after meals. If the antacid is in a tablet form, it is important to chew the tablet very well. Suspensions are usually quicker acting and more effective because they cover a larger area. All OTC antacids carry a label warning that they may interfere with certain prescription medications. Lower levels of stomach acid may increase the absorption of some medications. Many drugs may have reduced or slowed absorption that will result in decreased effectiveness when combined with antacid use.

H-2 Antagonists

H-2 blockers were originally introduced as prescription products, but as the patents began to expire on these medications the manufacturers sought FDA approval to market them OTC. They differ from antacids in that they actually block the production of acid. The nonprescription formula is half the strength of the prescription products, and it is recommended that such products be used for only 2 weeks without the advice of a physician.

Tagamet HB, or cimetidine, was the first H-2 antagonist to achieve nonprescription status, but it is the only one in the category to require drug interaction warnings on the label. The dose is one tablet up to 30 minutes before a meal, up to twice daily. Pepcid AC (famotidine 10 mg) is taken 60 minutes before a meal up to twice a day, and Axid AR (Nizatidine 75 mg) can be taken just before eating or up to 60 minutes before a meal, up to twice a day. All of these products are effective for treating existing symptoms, but Zantac (ranitidine) cannot be labeled to be taken just before a meal to prevent symptoms.

Proton Pump Inhibitors

The first proton pump inhibitor (PPI) to be introduced to the market as a prescription-only product was omeprazole (Prilosec). In 2003, Prilosec was granted OTC status by the FDA. PPIs act by inhibiting up to 90% of the secretion of gastric acid. They are much more effective at lowering the acid content of the stomach, but because they are prodrugs, the acid suppression does not begin for several hours. These drugs are most effective when taken 30 to 60 minutes before the first meal of the day. They are not effective for reducing the acid that is already present in the stomach, so they will not offer immediate help once heartburn has begun. As with other OTC gastrointestinal drugs, continued use should be monitored by a health professional to ensure that serious conditions are not overlooked.

prodrugs Drugs that need to be metabolized to the active form in the body.

Anti-Gas Medication

Bloating and flatulence are among the most common complaints of patients today. This may be the result of a diet high in foods that produce large amounts of intestinal gas, swallowing of excess air by patients, or more serious physical problems. Simethicone (Mylanta) is the only OTC anti-gas agent recognized by the FDA. Simethicone is available as a liquid, chewable tablets, or a drop preparation to be used for infant colic. It relieves the feelings of pressure and fullness caused by excess gas and allows it to be more easily eliminated by the patient. Because it is not absorbed from the GI tract, there are no adverse effects and it is considered safe for all ages. Patients for whom this is a continuing problem may benefit from a consultation with the pharmacist about lifestyle modifications.

Antidiarrheals

Diarrhea is characterized by an increased frequency of loose, watery stools, and is experienced by most individuals at some time in their life. Generally, it is an acute condition that subsides in a few days with or without treatment, but it can be extremely dangerous and is, in fact, the second leading cause of death in most developing nations. Excessive fluid loss can result in dehydration and electrolyte imbalance, which can result in death. Chronic diarrhea should always be managed by a physician and any acute attack that lasts longer than 2 days should be

electrolyte imbalance A debilitating condition that occurs due to a loss of electrolytes resulting from diarrhea or poor nutrition.

checked by a physician. Acute attacks are usually caused by an infection (either viral or bacterial) or ingesting foods with large amounts of fiber or lactose (for patients who are lactose-intolerant). Diarrhea can also be caused by many types of drugs, including antibiotics, antihypertensives, NSAIDs, and others.

Adsorbent types of antidiarrheals include Pepto-Bismol (bismuth subsalicylate) and several formulations containing attapulgite. Loperamide is an antidiarrheal that should only be administered to patients over the age of 6. It is a very effective product and often stops diarrhea after only one or two doses. Adverse reactions are rare and usually mild.

adsorbent An anti-diarrheal product that promotes fluid and electrolyte absorption by the intestine to prevent dehydration and electrolyte imbalance.

Laxatives

Constipation is a common occurrence among patients and is usually described as having less than three bowel movements per week. Although constipation can affect people of all ages, it is much more prevalent among the elderly. Chronic constipation can often be managed by lifestyle changes, such as increasing the amount of fiber ingested, increasing fluid intake, and increasing exercise.

Fiber or Bulk Laxatives

Patients with chronic constipation may benefit from maintenance use of a fiber laxative such as Metamucil or Perdiem (psyllium) or Citrucel (methylcellulose). It is imperative that these bulk-forming laxatives be taken with adequate amounts of fluid to prevent the formation of a blockage in the gastrointestinal tract. Fiber or bulk laxatives may also interact with several medications, but when used correctly they are safe and effective.

Stool Softeners

Stool softeners act by using a surface-active agent to increase fluid in the fecal matter, making it softer and easier to pass through the colon. Colace (docusate sodium) and Surfak (docusate calcium) are two common stool softeners. They are useful in the elderly and in children over the age of 2 because they are relatively safe and cause few adverse reactions. Stool softeners may increase the absorption of some medications, so medical advice is needed for patients taking other medications.

Stimulant Laxatives

Stimulant laxatives should be used for no more than 7 days for cases of acute constipation or for bowel cleansing prior to diagnostic testing. Habitual use of stimulant laxatives will lead to damage of bowel tissues. Dulcolax, Correctol, and Fleet laxative tablets, all of which contain bisacodyl 5 mg, are common examples of stimulant laxatives.

stimulant laxative A laxative that acts by directly stimulating the nerves in the intestine.

TIP

A technician should be alert for repeated purchases of laxatives by patients and report this to a pharmacist for counseling.

Hemorrhoid Preparations

Hemorrhoids are enlarged blood vessels in the anorectal area that may cause symptoms of pain, itching, and sometimes bleeding. Treatment choices are Preparation H cream or ointment containing phenylephrine, Anusol ointment, and Proctofoam containing pramoxine and Anusol HC, with the addition of hydrocortisone to the Anusol formula. Another choice would be Nupercainal anesthetic ointment with Dibucaine.

If the problem persists after 7 to 10 days of self-treatment with nonprescription medications, a physician should be consulted.

Vaginal Antifungals

Vaginal fungal infections are the only vaginal infections that may be self-treated with nonprescription medications. Such infections are generally caused by an overgrowth of *Candida albicans*, a normal resident of the genital tract. Symptoms of candidal fungal infections include itching, vaginal discharge, burning, and pain. Patients who have previously had a candidal infection diagnosed by a physician are candidates for self-treatment with OTC medications. If the condition is not cleared up after a 7-day course of therapy, a physician should be consulted to ensure that a more serious condition is not being overlooked. Monistat (miconazole), Gyne-Lotrimin, and Mycelex (clotrimazole) are all available in various treatment forms using both 3- and 7-day therapies, as well as creams, suppositories, and prefilled disposable applicators.

Topical Antifungals

tineas Fungal skin infections.

Fungal skin infections, also known as tineas, are some of the most common infections found in patients because the organisms that cause them are found in so many places. Athlete's foot (tinea pedis) is often contracted at swimming pools, gyms, or summer camps, and thrives in warm, moist places such as sneakers. Jock itch (tinea cruris) is often contracted in the summer months when warm, moist areas of the body are in contact with each other for long periods of time. Ringworm of the scalp (tinea capitis) is spread by contact with infected hairbrushes, toys, telephones, or blankets. Topical antifungals are available in lotions, powders, sprays, and solutions to facilitate treatment in the required area of the body. Some OTC antifungals are Lamisil AT (terbinafine), Lotrimin AF (clotrimazole), and Tinactin (tolnaftate).

Topical Wound Care

Superficial wounds are a common occurrence among patients and generally respond well to self-treatment with OTC products. The technician should be alert for signs of an infection, such as swelling, redness, or pain. Any puncture wound, extensive wound that may need stitches for proper healing, wound from an animal bite, or wound suffered in a contaminated environment should be referred to the pharmacist for counseling and possible referral to a physician.

Topical Antiseptics

Antiseptics may be applied to a superficial wound to prevent infection. Common first-aid antiseptics include alcohol and hydrogen peroxide, which should be applied after washing the skin with plenty of water. Hydrogen peroxide has a cleansing effect and will assist in cleansing the wound through its effervescent action, but should only be used in early treatment of the wound because it will continue to debride the tissue and prevent healing. Other OTC antiseptics are Bactine, Betadine solution and ointment, and Campho-phenique. Merthiolate and Mercurochrome were widely used in the 20th century, but are now considered unapproved for use by the FDA.

Topical Antibiotics

Commonly used first-aid antibiotics include Bacitracin ointment, Polysporin ointment (in which polymixin B is added to bacitracin), and Neosporin, which includes bacitracin, polymyxin B, and neomycin. There are a number of other brands and combinations of these three ingredients that are packaged for OTC use. A combination of the three antibiotics has been shown to be more effective against different organisms. All are safe for short-term use on small areas to reduce the risk of infection. They should not be used for more than 1 week and should not be used in the eye or ear. Long-term use or use over large portions of the body may result in systemic absorption and side effects.

Anesthetic Ointments

Topical ointments for relief of pain usually contain benzocaine or lidocaine, both of which are topical anesthetics. They are sometimes combined with menthol or another antipruritic product to relieve itching. These products can help with the pain and itching of insect stings or bites, the minor pain of wounds, and the pain and itching of sunburn. They can also be used for temporary relief of the pain from superficial first-degree or less severe second-degree burns that are not caused by electrical or chemical contact. Americaine, Dermoplast, Lanacane, and Nupercainal are examples of frequently used anesthetic formulations.

antipruritic A drug or chemical that reduces itching.

Topical Corticosteroids

Nonprescription corticosteroid formulations all contain hydrocortisone at either a 0.5% or a 1% concentration. Creams, ointments, and sprays are available to accommodate the expected uses of the product. Hydrocortisone is antipruritic and anti-inflammatory, so it may be used for a minor skin rash or insect bite, or to aid in comfort and healing of minor sunburn. It should not be used for long periods of time or over large areas of the body, to reduce the risk of systemic absorption that may result in side effects. Common brand names for hydrocortisone formulations are Cortaid, Cortizone, and Lanacort.

Cough, Cold, and Allergy Preparations

The common cold occurs so frequently that it is estimated that each person suffers from 3 to 12 episodes each year. Because colds are caused by a number of different viruses, they cannot be cured, and it is impossible to develop a vaccine that will prevent them. There are many products on the market to treat the various symptoms of the common cold. The nonprescription cough and cold section is constantly changing as new products are switched from prescription to nonprescription status, and new research indicates that some previously used drugs are not safe for general use or that a nonprescription product is widely used for the illegal formulation of a drug of abuse.

Adult Antitussives

Nonprescription antitussives contain various amounts of dextromethorphan (DM) and are intended to silence a nonproductive cough by suppressing the cough center. They are safe for use in patients above the age of 6 years, but do have some drug interactions, especially with MAOI inhibitors. Products containing DM are sometimes abused and the sale of these products may soon be regulated. Single-entity preparations that contain DM include Robitussin Cough Gels, Benylin, and Hold DM Lozenges.

antitussive A substance that inhibits or reduces the cough reflex.

Many states also allow the nonprescription sale of cough products containing 10 mg of codeine per 5 mL. These products are schedule V narcotic nonprescription products and there are special requirements for their sale. They must always be stored behind the pharmacy counter where the sale can be monitored and recorded by the pharmacist. Some brand names for codeine-containing products are Cheracol, Robitussin AC, and Novahistine DH.

Expectorants

expectorant A substance that helps to thin mucus so it can be coughed up.

Guaifenesin is a nonprescription expectorant that is available in many cough preparations. It helps thin the mucus and make the cough more productive. Guaifenesin is the main ingredient in all the Robitussin products, and when combined with DM (as in Robitussin DM), it is one of the most recommended cough and cold products on the market. A newer, extended-release formulation of guaifenesin is available as Mucinex.

Antihistamines

rhinitis An inflammation of the nasal passages.

Nasal discharge associated with the common cold is often treated with antihistamines to dry up the watery mucuos secretions. Antihistamines are also used for allergic rhinitis and hay fever. The older sedating antihistamines are Benadryl (diphenhydramine), Chlor-Trimeton (chlorpheniramine), and Tavist (clemastine). They may cause considerable drowsiness, which may add to the discomfort of the cold. One of the newer nonsedating antihistamines, loratidine (brand names: Claritin and Alavert), has been approved for nonprescription use.

Oral Decongestants

decongestant A drug that reduces swelling in the nasal passages and sinus cavity.

Twice in the last decade, nonprescription cough and cold preparations have been reformulated due to FDA restrictions on decongestants. Phenylpropanolamine, a common ingredient in many cold preparations, was found to cause serious health problems in healthy adults and removed from the market, necessitating the reformulation of many products. Most manufacturers replaced the phenylpropanolamine with pseudoephedrine as the decongestant in cough and cold products. Pseudoephedrine is a safe and effective decongestant, but it is a primary ingredient in methamphetamine and became a drug of abuse as large quantities of it were purchased for that purpose. In 2006, the FDA required pseudoephedrine and all nonprescription products containing pseudoephedrine to be stored behind the counter where each sale can be documented and monitored. Most manufacturers of multisymptom products reformulated the products again, using phenylephrine as the decongestant. In 2007, all cough and cold preparations marketed for children under 2 years of age were removed from the shelves as pediatricians expressed agreement that they were ineffective for children this young and children were often overdosed with these medications, putting them at risk for side effects. All children's cough and cold formulations are to be relabeled with the warning to consult a physician before administering to a child under 2 years of age.

Topical Decongestants

Topical decongestants include Afrin (oxymetazoline), Vicks and Neo-Synephrine (phenylephrine) nasal sprays, Vicks VapoRub, and Vicks Inhaler. The nasal sprays and drops should not be used in children under the age of 2 and carry a warning not to use for more than 3 days to prevent rebound nasal congestion. They are also contraindicated in patients with heart disease, high blood pressure, thyroid disease, diabetes, or enlarged prostrate. Benzedrex inhalers contain propylhexedrine, a central nervous system stimulant that is abused in several ways and should be kept behind the prescription counter so its sale can be monitored. Patients who use oral or topical decongestants should read the labels carefully and request counseling from the pharmacist if they are unsure about their safe use.

Technicians should be alert for repeated sales of topical decongestants to the same patient and alert the pharmacist about the possibility of rebound congestion and the need for pharmacist counseling. TIP

Multisymptom Cough and Cold Products

Combination products for cough and cold are abundant. Patients like the idea of taking only one medication to alleviate all their symptoms. Because the different cold symptoms tend to come and go during the course of a cold, these multiple-drug preparations will result in the patient being overmedicated during most of the days the cold is treated with such a product. Examples of these products include Dayquil, Nyquil, and TheraFlu Severe Cold and Congestion. These products typically contain an antihistamine, a decongestant, an analgesic, and an expectorant and/or antitussive. The possibility of a drug or disease interaction resulting from one or more of these ingredients is high.

Cold Sore Products

Cold sores, also called fever blisters, are viral lesions that usually occur on the outer surface of the lips, causing considerable discomfort and embarrassment to the patient. Technically these blisters are called herpes simplex labialis and are caused by herpes simplex type 1 virus. This virus is extremely contagious and can be passed to others by direct touch or by touching objects that an infected person has touched. Once infected, the person may have recurrent events throughout life, followed by periods when the virus is dormant. Attacks usually last 10 to 14 days and result in complete healing and no resultant scarring. Therapy consists of a combination of external analgesics, anesthetics, and protectants. Some nonprescription products for cold sores are Abreva (Docosanol), Zilactin gels (with either lidocaine or benzocaine), Blistex Lip Medex (menthol, camphor, and phenol), and Carmex (menthol, camphor, and phenol; also contain salicylic acid and alum, which have not been proved safe or effective and could be harmful).

Artificial Tears

Dry eye is a common condition that affects many people. There are a number of factors that could cause this condition, including tear deficiency due to aging, exposure to dry air, wearing soft contact lenses, and a number of drugs, such as antihistamines, anticholinergics, and diuretics. Tears are made up of three layers: mucin (coats and wets the surface), aqueous (intermediate layer), and lipid (inhibits evaporation and helps prevent dry eye). Artificial tear products contain compounds similar to mucin that coat and protect the surface and prevent drying and irritation. Examples of these products are Tears Plus, Refresh Plus, and Murine Tears. Ophthalmic ointments contain emollients to help lubricate the eye and protect against irritation. Examples of emollient ophthalmic ointments are Hypo Tears lubricant eye ointment and Lacri-Lube S.O.P.

Ophthalmic Vasoconstrictors

Redness of the eye caused by minor irritations can be treated with ophthalmic vasoconstrictors that will help to constrict swollen blood vessels. Glaucoma patients should be advised to check with a physician before using these products. These products should be used only for short time periods to prevent rebound congestion and redness. Common vasoconstrictor products are Clear Eyes (naphazoline), Visine (Tetrahydrozoline), and OcuClear (oxymetazoline).

rebound congestion
Congestion caused by use of a decongestant for more than 3 days.

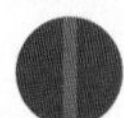

Herbal Remedies

Although herbal medicines were once found only in health food stores, they are gaining popularity due to widespread advertising campaigns that play on the belief that herbal medicines are safe and natural and produce therapeutic effects with no side effects.

Certainly, many of the drug products on the market originate from plants and other natural sources, so plants can and do have therapeutic effects. The dangerous misconception is the thinking that because plants are natural they cannot be toxic. The herbal industry is not well regulated, and in many cases it is impossible to ascertain whether a product actually has an active ingredient, how much is present, and if it is in a form that is bioavailable to the body. Recently, some of the more reputable herbal companies have allowed the USP to evaluate their products so that at least the quantity of active ingredient can be documented. The label will indicate this, but all herbal remedies must carry the warning "This statement has not been evaluated by the Food and Drug Administration. This product is not intended to diagnose, treat, cure, or prevent any disease." Following are a few of the most common herbal products that have found a place in many pharmacies, and their advertised uses:

1. Echinacea comes from the sunflower plant and has been touted to stimulate the immune system and reduce the severity of cold and flu symptoms. It has moved from the strictly herbal section into some throat lozenges in the regular cough and cold section. Its effectiveness has not been proved and it carries the added risk of severe allergic reactions in individuals with sensitivity to sunflowers and related plants.
2. Garlic is considered to have many therapeutic effects, most of which have not been documented with valid research. It is marketed to lower cholesterol and help with cardiovascular health, and to assist with viral, fungal, and bacterial infections. As a food product it is safe, and as an oral herbal supplement it has a low toxicity; however, as a topical agent it is not safe and may result in serious burns. Kwai and Kyolic are common garlic extract products.
3. Gingko biloba (Ginkoba) has been purported to improve memory, concentration, vertigo, and circulation. Some studies have shown some improvement in memory and peripheral circulation, but there is a lack of amply documented trials proving its efficacy and safety.
4. St. John's wort (Kira) has been widely marketed to assist in mild depression and anxiety. Some studies have shown some benefit in mild depression, but these studies failed to meet the standards required by the FDA. This product has many side effects, including stomach irritation, tiredness, dizziness photosensitivity, and even fatal liver failure. St. John's wort is also a factor in many serious drug interactions. In addition, depression is an extremely serious condition that should not be self-treated with a questionable product.

There are many unanswered questions about whether untested herbal products should be stocked on the shelves of a pharmacy. Health food stores are not staffed by health professionals and do not have the risk of liability that a pharmacist may incur just by selling a product of questionable efficacy and safety.

Vitamins and Minerals

Most people who eat a normal, well-rounded diet receive an adequate amount of the vitamins essential for good health. Advertising claims have convinced many people that taking vitamin supplements will result in more energy and better health. There is no evidence to support this fact or the belief that more expensive organic or natural vitamins are superior to other supplements. Vitamins are divided into two general categories: fat-soluble and water-soluble.

Fat-Soluble Vitamins

The fat-soluble vitamins are vitamins A, D, E, and K.

- Vitamin A (retinol) affects the bones, teeth, skin, eyes, and urinary system.
- Vitamin D (ergocalciferol) is important to facilitate the absorption of calcium and affects the bones and joints.
- Vitamin E (alpha tocopherol) has been advertised as an antioxidant to improve cardiovascular health and is often used topically to promote healing of scars from wounds. These uses have not been approved by the FDA.
- Vitamin K (menadiol/phytonadione) is a factor in clotting of the blood, and a deficiency can result in coagulation defects.

Fat-soluble vitamins can be stored in the body for long periods of time, and this increases the risk of toxicity if supplements are taken.

Water-Soluble Vitamins

Water-soluble vitamins are the various B vitamins and vitamin C.

- Vitamin B_1 (thiamine) aids in the metabolism of carbohydrates.
- Vitamin B_2 (riboflavin) is vital for eye and skin health.
- Vitamin B_6 (pyridoxine) aids in the utilization of amino acids.
- Vitamin B_{12} (cyanocobalamin) aids in DNA synthesis and red blood cell formation.
- Niacin (nicotinic acid) helps the body use carbohydrates as energy and maintains healthy tissue.
- Folic acid (folate) helps prevent anemia and reduces the risk of spina bifida in infants if taken during pregnancy.
- Vitamin C (ascorbic acid) helps maintain healthy bones, blood vessels, and teeth.

Minerals

There are several minerals that are essential to good health.

Calcium

Calcium is essential for normal growth and bone health. Adequate amounts of calcium are essential to prevent osteoporosis in older men and women, and most people should take 500 to 1200 mg a day as a supplement.

Iron

Iron is essential for preventing anemia. It is extremely toxic to children in large doses and is a major cause of poisonings. It is important to understand the various forms of iron available:

- Ferrous sulfate 325 mg (Ferro-Sequels) contains 65 mg of elemental iron.
- Ferrous sulfate elixir 220 mg/5 mL contains 44 mg of elemental iron.
- Fer-In-Sol drops 75 mg/0.6 mL contains 15 mg of elemental iron/0.6 mL.

Home Testing Kits

As more home testing kits become available and people become more knowledgeable about their health, it is important for technicians to have a working knowledge of the various products sold in the pharmacy. Although the technician must not enter into counseling the patient about his or her test results, it is within their scope of practice to demonstrate the use of the various test kits and complete the sale while reminding the patient to discuss their results with their physician. One of the earliest testing kits on the market was the blood-glucose monitoring machine. Over the past several decades this machine has evolved from a large cumbersome box to a small hand-held meter that can fit in the pocket and produce accurate test results in a matter of seconds. Each machine has unique features and specific directions for use. The technician should read the directions and become familiar with the function of each machine, and be able to explain the directions to the patient.

Another important home diagnostic testing kit (e.g., ColoCare and EZ Detect) is used to detect fecal occult blood that is indicative of possible colon cancer. Colon cancer awareness has increased greatly in recent years as it became known that early detection usually results in a cure, whereas a late diagnosis is often fatal. Patients are often reluctant to submit to a colonoscopy as a routine screening because it is an invasive and uncomfortable procedure, but they may be willing to perform these simple tests in the privacy of their bathroom.

The CholesTrak Kit is a testing device that uses several enzymes that react with a blood sample from the patient to indicate total cholesterol by a color change on a measuring device included with the kit. Many things can affect a single cholesterol reading, but if the test shows a high reading, a physician should be consulted.

Home pregnancy tests detect the presence of human chorionic gonadotropin (HCG) in the urine of pregnant patients, allowing for early detection of pregnancy so that precautions such as eliminating alcohol and caffeine use can be instituted promptly. Examples of home pregnancy tests are Clearblue Easy, 1 Step E.P.T., and Precise. Ovulation predictor kits are helpful for couples who are having difficulty conceiving, because they can help predict the exact day of ovulation. The kits come with sufficient materials to test the urine for 5, 6, or 9 days. The older tests require many specific steps to obtain accurate results, but the newer tests only require the absorbent tip to be held in the urine stream for 5 seconds. Examples of newer tests are First Response 1-Step Ovulation Predictor Test, One-Step Clear Plan Easy, and OvuQuick 1 Step.

New diagnostic testing kits are being developed at a rapid rate. There are also several kits on the market to test for various drugs. As new products are released to the market, the professional technician should make an effort to study the instructions in each kit and become knowledgeable to provide expert customer service to patients.

Nonprescription Drugs Restricted to Behind-the-Counter Sales

There has been some discussion in the past few years about establishing a third class of drugs that would not require a prescription but could be prescribed and dispensed only by a pharmacist. Although this concept has not met with widespread acceptance, the number of products that are now kept behind the counter is increasing. The requirements for sale of these products vary from state to state and are established by the state boards of pharmacy. Some schedule V exempt narcotics, generally cough syrups with small amounts of codeine may be sold without a prescription. A pharmacist is required to complete the sale of these products by recording the quantity, date, and name of the product; the name and address of the purchaser; and the pharmacist's initials. As illegal drug users began purchasing insulin syringes to administer the drugs, many pharmacies began to document purchases of syringes in much the same manner as for exempt narcotics. Recently all products containing ephedrine or pseudoephedrine have been restricted to sales behind the counter. They do not require a pharmacist and are sold in grocery stores and gas stations, but the new regulations require written documentation of each sale and mandatory training for anyone involved in selling these products. There is now an age restriction for OTC sales of the controversial birth control product Plan B, and purchasers under the age of 18 are required to have a prescription.

There is serious discussion about the possibility of establishing a new class of drugs that would be kept in the pharmacy to be dispensed by the pharmacist without a prescription from a physician. There is also a continuing trend to transfer prescription drugs to OTC status, and the technician must stay current on the different strengths of drugs that are available in lower strengths as OTC drugs but still require a prescription at higher strengths. It is important for the technician to be cognizant of the regulations and the scope of practice in his or her state.

Case Study 11.1

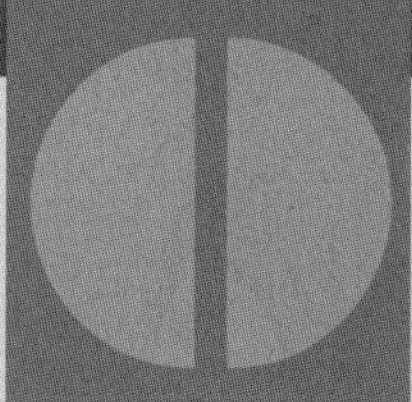

As Jill progressed in her pharmacy technician program and her level of experience working at Nickelson's Pharmacy, she felt ready to accept more challenges. She began to extend her knowledge to the OTC drug section near the pharmacy counter. She soon realized that many patients were confused by the vast array of products and often turned to her for answers to their questions. Jill developed an understanding of the types of questions she could answer for patients and those that needed input from the pharmacist. Let's listen to how Jill responded to questions she received in a typical day at the pharmacy and decide whether her answers were appropriate.

A lady approached the counter with a piece of paper in her hand. She stated, "My doctor told me to get this from the drugstore. I can't pronounce it but I wrote it down the way he spelled it to me." She handed the paper to Jill and it read "diphenhydramine." Jill asked, "Is this for you or another family member?" The lady replied, "It's for my 9-year-old son, so I hope it comes in a liquid." Jill replied, "I can show you where the liquid is, but did your doctor tell you how much to give your son?" The lady said, "Yes, he told me to follow the directions on the package for his age and weight." Jill took the lady to the section where the diphenhydramine was stored and showed her the name "diphenhydramine" on the label. She then showed her the panel on the back where the dosing directions were located and asked if she understood the directions or had any questions for the pharmacist. When the lady assured Jill that she understood the directions, Jill completed the purchase.

As Jill returned to the pharmacy counter, she saw Mr. Jackson, a regular customer approaching the counter. "Hi, Mr. Jackson," she said, "how can I assist you today?" "Well Jill," he replied, "I just came from the doctor's office and was told that I have diabetes. I spent an hour with a diabetes educator learning about the diet I should follow. They didn't start me on any medicine but I need to monitor my blood sugar to keep it in the range they set for me. They told me to purchase an AccuChek Advantage machine and they taught me how to use it. I think I understand everything they want me to do, but could you go through the testing process with this machine before I purchase it?" Jill had carefully read the directions for each of the testing devices stocked in the pharmacy, so she was able to take him through the process step by step. After demonstrating the machine, Jill asked Mr. Jackson if he had any questions for the pharmacist and he assured her that all his questions had been answered at the doctor's office. She completed the purchase and told him to be sure to call the pharmacy if any questions arose after he returned home.

Mrs. Champion approached the counter waving a bottle of a children's multisymptom cold preparation and asked, "Is it okay to give this to my 6-year-old daughter? She has a terrible cold and the label says it is for children 6 years and older." "Just a moment, Mrs. Champion," Jill responded, "I'll get the pharmacist to answer your question." If the cold preparation was intended for children the age of her daughter, why did Jill feel that she needed the pharmacist to answer the question?

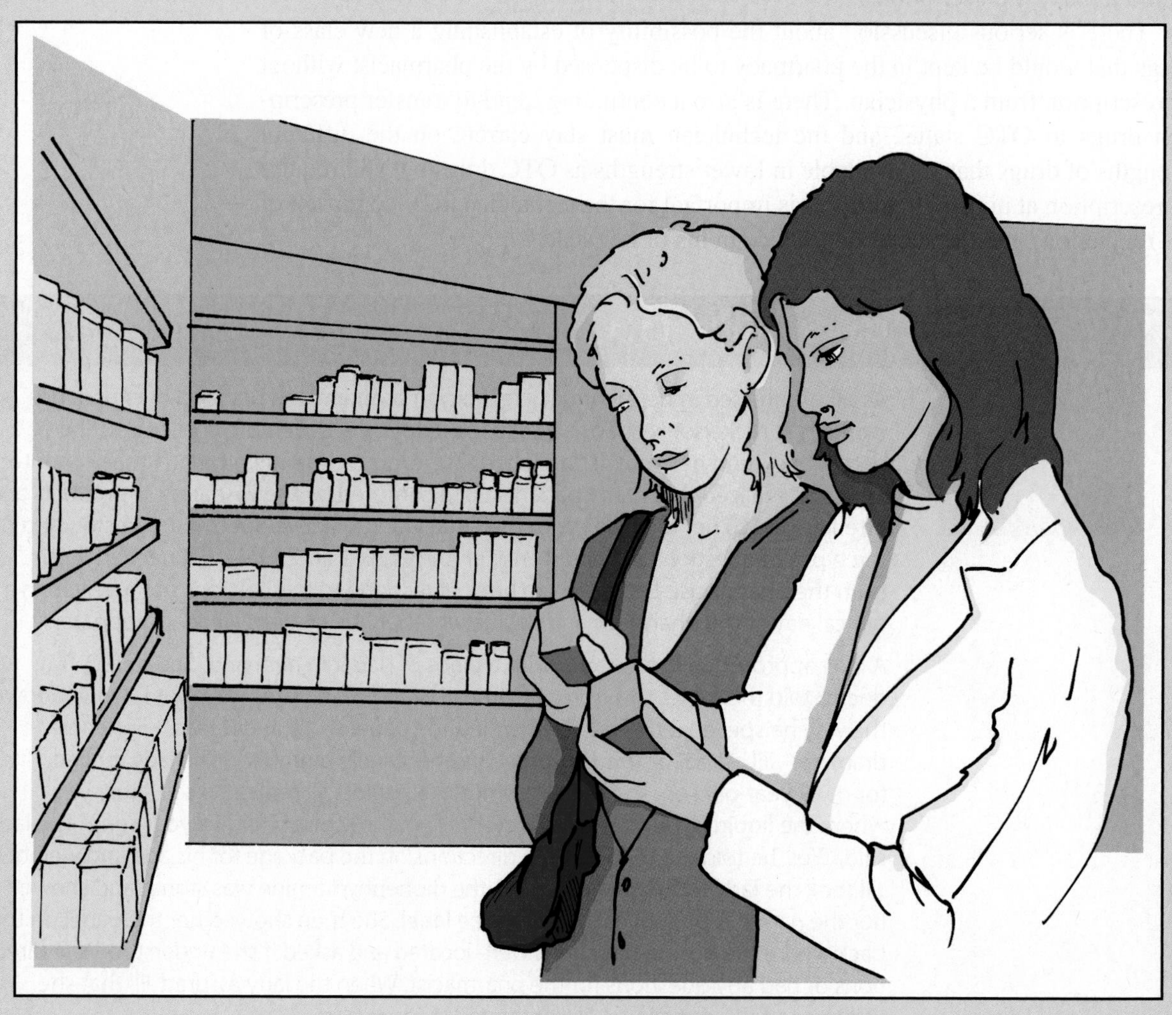

Mr. Gray arrived at the pharmacy counter to pick up a refill of his prescription for Vicodin. He had called the refill line earlier, so his prescription was ready. Jill asked if he had any questions for the pharmacist and he stated that his questions had been answered when he filled the original prescription. As Jill entered the amount into the cash register, Mr. Gray handed her a bottle of Tylenol that he wished to purchase. He stated that sometimes the Vicodin doesn't totally relieve the pain, so he just takes a few Tylenol along with it. Jill remembered that Vicodin contains hydrocodone and acetaminophen, and that Tylenol is a brand name for acetaminophen. She knows that too much Tylenol can cause liver toxicity. Jill said, "Excuse me a minute, Mr. Gray." She discreetly explained the situation to the pharmacist, who then came to the counter to counsel Mr. Gray.

As Marie, the pharmacist, was counseling Mr. Gray, the phone rang. Jill picked it up promptly and said, "Good afternoon, Nickelson's Pharmacy, this is Jill the technician speaking. How can I assist you?" "Hi Jill, this is Dr. Moore. I have a patient who needs a home cholesterol screening kit. I wanted to be certain that you have one in stock and that someone in the pharmacy can explain how to use it. I have instructed him on his target cholesterol level and that he is to report the results to me." Jill quickly checked the shelf and saw the CholesTrak. She had read the instructions and watched a demonstration by the salesman. "Yes, Dr. Moore," she said, "we have one in stock and can explain its use to him. Thank you for calling to let us know." "Thanks, Jill. I'll send the patient right over and tell him to ask for you." Marie was able to continue with her important work as a pharmacist while offering minimal supervision of Jill. She had developed a trust relationship with Jill based on her observance of Jill's skills, and a sense of confidence that Jill would use her professional judgment and her understanding of the scope and standards of a technician's practice to determine which questions she could answer and which required a pharmacist's intervention. Jill left the pharmacy that day with a feeling of professional satisfaction knowing that she had made a difference in the health of patients and had provided competent assistance to Marie, the pharmacist, so that she could perform the functions that required the professional judgment of a pharmacist.

Chapter Summary

- Nonprescription oral analgesic drugs can be classified as salicylates, NSAIDs, and products containing acetaminophen.
- Salicylates and NSAIDs exhibit analgesic, antipyretic, and anti-inflammatory properties.
- Acetaminophen has analgesic and antipyretic properties, but no anti-inflammatory action.
- Antacid preparations are designed to help neutralize acid in the stomach and work better if taken with a meal.
- H-2 antagonists help block the production of acid and should be taken before a meal.
- PPIs should be taken 30 to 60 minutes before the first meal of the day.
- Simethicone is often added to antacid products and is the only anti-gas agent approved by the FDA.
- Diarrhea lasting more than 2 days can cause serious dehydration and requires consultation with a physician.

- Fiber laxatives require adequate fluid intake to prevent a blockage from forming.
- Stool softeners increase fluid in the fecal matter, helping it pass through the colon.
- Stimulant laxatives should be used only for acute constipation or bowel cleansing prior to diagnostic tests.
- Hemorrhoid preparations help with pain and itching because they contain topical anti-inflammatories and anesthetics.
- Topical antifungals are available to treat various infections. It is important to use the correct formulation for the type of infection being treated.
- Superficial skin wounds can be treated with antiseptic, anesthetic, and/or antibiotic ointments. Rashes, sunburns, and insect bites are treated with hydrocortisone ointments or creams.
- The common cold is treated by treating the symptoms the patient is experiencing.
- Multisymptom cold preparations may contain an antitussive, an antihistamine, a decongestant, and an analgesic/antipyretic.
- Oral and topical decongestants may cause rebound congestion if used for more than 3 days.
- Artificial-tears products help to relieve dry-eye conditions, whereas ophthalmic vasoconstrictors help clear redness of the eye and carry a warning against use by glaucoma patients.
- Some herbal products have demonstrated therapeutic effects, but these products have not been approved by the FDA and should be used with caution. Herbal product use should be included in the patient profile to screen for drug interactions.
- Fat-soluble vitamins can be stored in the body, causing toxic levels to build up over time.
- Adequate amounts of vitamins and minerals are essential to good health, but eating a well-balanced diet supplies the essential vitamins and minerals.
- Home diagnostic test kits require the consumer to strictly follow step-by-step directions to obtain accurate results. A knowledgeable technician can help instruct patients in the proper use and care of such products.
- The number and type of nonprescription products restricted to behind-the-counter sales are increasing. It is vital for the technician to understand the regulation of these products in the state in which he or she practices.

Review Questions

Multiple Choice

Choose the best answer for the questions below.

1. Nonprescription products that have analgesic, antipyretic, and anti-inflammatory properties include:
   a. aspirin
   b. acetaminophen
   c. ibuprofen
   d. a and c

2. The OTC product that is not given to young children because of the risk of Reye's syndrome is:
   a. ibuprofen
   b. naproxen
   c. aspirin
   c. acetaminophen

3. PPIs, such as omeprazole, work best when taken:
   a. after a meal to treat an attack of heartburn
   b. 30 minutes before each meal to prevent heartburn
   c. 30 minutes before the first meal of the day to inhibit secretion of gastric acid
   d. at bedtime if needed for nighttime heartburn

4. Skin infections known as tineas can be treated with:
   a. hydrocortisone cream
   b. topical antifungals
   c. topical antibiotics
   d. topical antiseptics

5. The common cold is best treated with
   a. antibiotics
   b. single-entity products to treat symptoms
   c. multisymptom products to treat all symptoms that may arise
   d. all of the above

Fill in the Blank

Fill in the blanks below with the correct word or words.

6. Oral and topical decongestants can cause ____________________________ if used for more than 3 days.

7. Vitamins A, D, E, and K are ____________ __________________ vitamins and can build up in the body to toxic levels.

8. Topical ointments that contain lidocaine or benzocaine and are used for pain relief are called ____________________ ointments.

9. Guaifenesin is a nonprescription __________________________ that helps to thin mucus and create a more productive cough.

10. Artificial-tear products provide relief for a common condition called ______________________.

True/False

Mark the following statements True or False.

11. ________ All people should take vitamin supplements to maintain good health.

12. ________Calcium is essential for normal growth and bone health.

13. ________ OTC herbal products have been tested and approved by the FDA.

14. ________ Cold sores or fever blisters are caused by a virus.

15. ________ Antitussives silence a nonproductive cough by suppressing the cough center.

Matching

Match the descriptions in column B with the correct home testing kits in column A.

Column A	Column B
16. _____ EZ Detect Test Kit	A. Home pregnancy test
17. _____ CholesTrak Test Kit	B. Blood glucose monitoring
18. _____ Clearblue Easy	C. Fecal blood test
19. _____ One-Step Clear Plan Easy	D. Cholesterol screening
20. _____ AccuChek Advantage	E. Ovulation predictor

LEARNING ACTIVITY

Design an OTC medication section in a small professional pharmacy. Decide how much space can be allocated to OTCs and which products should be carried. Develop a rationale for placement of the items in relation to the prescription counter. Are some products more likely to require consultation with a pharmacist? Where should the home monitoring test kits be located? Discuss your plan with the class.

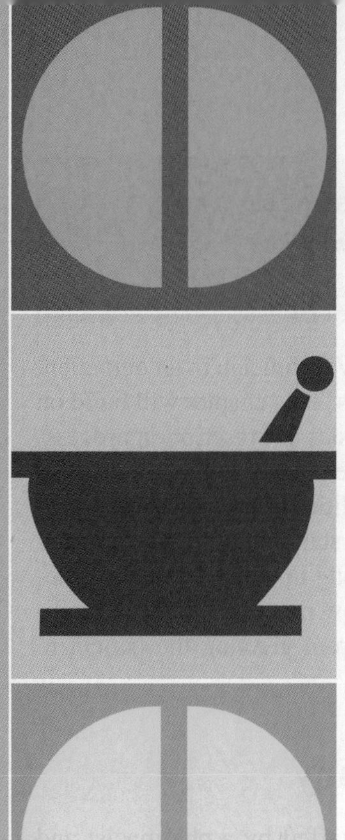

Chapter **12**

Outpatient Prescriptions

OBJECTIVES

After completing this chapter, the student will be able to:

- Recognize the required parts of an outpatient prescription.
- Discuss pharmacy software alerts and technician responses to alerts.
- Demonstrate accurate evaluation of outpatient prescriptions.
- Demonstrate how to choose the correct drug from the drug file.
- Establish procedures for accurate prescription processing.
- Design an efficient workflow process for an outpatient pharmacy setting.
- Evaluate and process outpatient prescriptions.

KEY TERMS

- absorption
- chain pharmacy
- clinic pharmacy
- compliance
- cross-sensitivity
- drug–disease interaction
- drug–drug interaction
- duplicate therapy interaction
- eutectic mixture
- extemporaneous compound
- independent retail pharmacy
- interaction override
- invoice

- lead technician
- merchandise facing
- order verification sheet
- prioritizing prescriptions
- rotating the stock
- spatulate
- workflow

One of the most important responsibilities of a pharmacy technician in an outpatient setting is to accurately evaluate and process prescriptions. This chapter will build on the knowledge established in Chapter 2, in which the basics of prescription processing were introduced. A busy outpatient pharmacy can be chaotic without a plan for an efficient workflow process to organize the responsibilities of each pharmacy professional. A competent technician will have a firm understanding of the process and the standards and scope of practice in the particular setting in which he or she practices. This chapter will discuss several different workflow processes that can facilitate the efficient delivery of outpatient prescriptions from greeting the patient to completing the sale.

workflow An established procedure for organizing the daily work in a given practice setting.

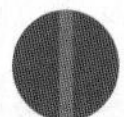

Independent Retail Pharmacy

independent retail pharmacy A pharmacy owned by one or more individuals who make all the management and buying decisions.

Pharmacy A is a small independent retail pharmacy staffed by a pharmacist and one technician. See Figure 12.1 for the layout of the pharmacy as we discuss the workflow process.

The technician, Jill, and the pharmacist, Marie, have just opened the pharmacy for the day when the first patient arrives at the counter. Jill greets the patient and accepts the prescription. She quickly searches the prescription for any missing information, checks the spelling of the patient's name, and verifies the address. As she enters the patient information into the computer, Jill discovers that he has not had prescriptions filled in their pharmacy before.

"Mr. Campbell," she says, "I'd like to set up a patient profile for you to aid the pharmacist in preparing your prescriptions. Are your prescriptions covered by insurance or do you pay cash?"

"Oh, I do have an insurance card. Thanks for asking," says Mr. Campbell.

"Could I have your date of birth, Mr. Campbell, so I can enter the insurance information into the computer?"

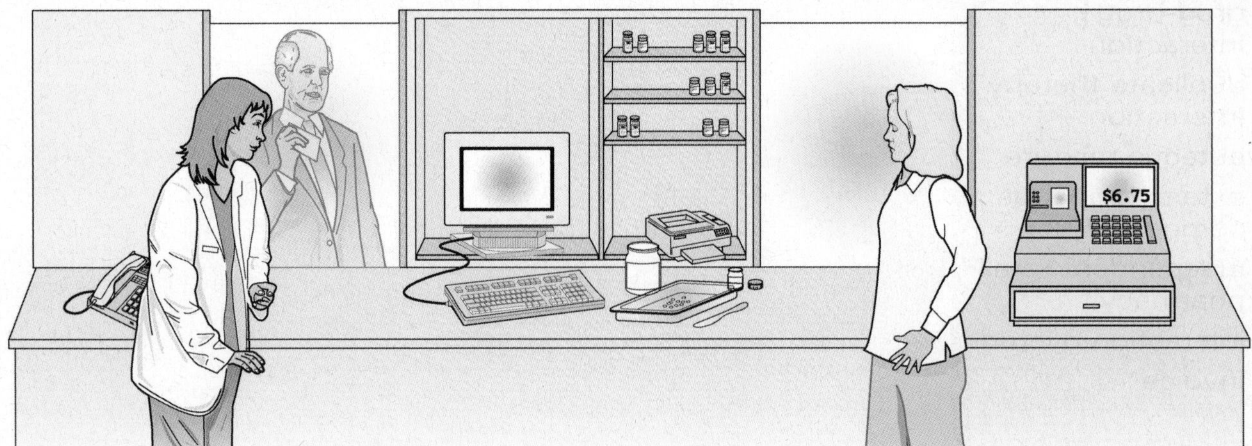

Figure 12.1 Technician gathering patient information and performing data entry in a small independent retail pharmacy.

"My date of birth is 12-22-39," he replies.

"Do you have any drug allergies that you are aware of, Mr. Campbell?"

"Penicillin is the only drug I'm allergic to as far as I know," says Mr. Campbell.

"I'll make a note of that in your profile. Are you taking any other medications?"

"No, I'm not taking anything else, except some chewable antacid tablets at bedtime," he remarks.

"Thanks, Mr. Campbell, we'll have your prescriptions ready in a few minutes."

Jill made a note of the antacid tablets in the patient profile.

After completing the data entry for the patient profile, Jill begins to enter the prescriptions. The first prescription is for amoxicillin and the computer indicates a drug allergy alert because amoxicillin has a cross-sensitivity with penicillin. Jill knows that only the pharmacist can authorize an interaction override, so she asks the pharmacist to check the alert. The pharmacist asks Mr. Campbell if he has ever taken amoxicillin before and if the doctor knows he is allergic to penicillin. Mr. Campbell replies that he has not taken amoxicillin before, and the clinic where he received the prescription had not asked about drug allergies. The pharmacist calls the clinic and alerts them to the penicillin allergy, and the physician changes the prescription to cephalexin. He asks the pharmacist to counsel the patient about the possible cross-sensitivity with cephalexin and give him instructions to be alert for any signs of an allergic reaction.

cross-sensitivity Some medications have similar structures to another medication and may cause an allergic reaction in a patient who is allergic to either medication.

interaction override An interaction indicated by the pharmacy software during the prescription-filling process that requires the pharmacist's judgment to override or ignore the interaction and continue filling the prescription.

Jill begins to enter the second prescription for Vicodin 5/500 as the pharmacist consults with the physician. She types "vic" in the drug field of the pharmacy prescription-filling software. Figure 12.2 shows the drug file screen as it appears on the computer, showing the drug choices beginning with "vic." Jill chooses the Vicodin 5/500 tablet and enters "no" in the DAW field of the prescription screen. This changes the drug name to hydrocodone 5 mg with acetaminophen 500 mg. Jill enters the directions and refill status, and prints the label. She retrieves the bottle of hydrocodone-acetaminophen 5/500 from the shelf, counts the tablets, and applies the label and auxiliary labels.

The pharmacist then hands her the cephalexin 500 mg prescription with the corrected documentation and she enters "ceph" into the computer. See Figure 12.3 for the drug file screen. Jill chooses cephalexin 500 mg capsules, completes the data entry, retrieves the medication from the shelf, counts the tablets, applies the labels, and leaves the medications in the appropriate checking area for the pharmacist to perform the final check. She mentions to the pharmacist that Mr. Campbell takes antacid tablets every night, because she remembers that they might interfere with absorption if taken at the same time as an antibiotic.

absorption The process by which a drug enters the bloodstream.

	NDC number	Generic for	NDC number
Hydrocodone/APAP 5 mg/500	00044-0727-02	Vicodin	00406-0357-05
Hydrocodone/APAP 7.5/750 ES	00044-0728-02	Vicodin ES	00406-0360-01
Hydrocodone/APAP 7.5/500 elixir	00406-0375-16	Lortab Elixir	00406-0375-16

Figure 12.2 Choosing the correct entry from the drug file screen for generic Vicodin 5/500 tablets.

Cephalexin 250 mg capsules 000777-0869-02 Keflex 63304-0657-01
Cephalexin 500 mg capsules 000777-0870-02 Keflex 63304-0657-01
Cephalexin susp 125 mg 00003-2201-03 Keflex
Cephalexin susp 250/5 00093-4177-74 Keflex

Figure 12.3 Choosing the correct entry from the drug file screen for cephalexin 500 mg capsules.

After the pharmacist completes the counseling session, Jill takes the prescriptions to the checkout counter to complete the sale. Mr. Campbell has picked up a bottle of Tylenol Extra Strength to purchase along with the prescriptions "in case the pain medicine isn't enough to take care of the pain." Jill remembers that generic Vicodin contains acetaminophen and that an overdose can have serious consequences. She discreetly mentions to the pharmacist that Mr. Campbell is purchasing Extra Strength Tylenol, and the pharmacist comes to discuss the maximum safe dose of Tylenol with Mr. Campbell before he leaves the pharmacy.

Jill then answers the phone to accept refill orders from patients. If the refills have all been used, Jill will either call or fax the physician's office to request refill authorization. When the physician's office returns the fax or call with refill authorizations, Jill documents the information, fills the prescriptions, and leaves them in the appropriate area for the pharmacist to check. When the daily order arrives, Jill carefully checks the items against the invoice, placing them in the correct spot on the shelf and rotating the stock. Jill enjoys being proficient in performing all of her responsibilities, but she realizes the customer is the most important part of her work day, so she is always attentive to any customers who approach the prescription counter, as well as customers in the over-the-counter (OTC) medication aisles who might need her assistance. In this way she is able to provide assistance to the pharmacist so that she can perform the clinical requirements of her profession with the knowledge that Jill understands the scope of her practice as a professional technician and will consult her on all matters that require the professional judgment of a pharmacist.

invoice Document that accompanies each order and lists the items sent, the quantity, the cost of each item, the total invoice cost, and the terms of payment.

rotating the stock When stocking merchandise, the newer items should be placed behind the stock already on the shelf to keep expired merchandise to a minimum.

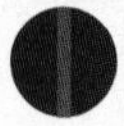

Clinic Pharmacy

clinic pharmacy A pharmacy in an outpatient clinic building to serve the patients of physicians located in the clinic.

Pharmacy B is a high-volume clinic pharmacy that employs two pharmacists and four pharmacy technicians. The prescription volume and the workflow are very different from those experienced in a small community pharmacy, but many of the tasks remain the same. An educated and well-trained technician could function efficiently in any of these practice settings with a brief orientation to the procedures of each facility. Refer to Figure 12.4 as the technician responsibilities in this practice setting are described. Meet the two pharmacists: Kevin and Samantha. Assisting them in this clinical practice setting are four pharmacy technicians: Sasha, Amber, Scott, and Chris. The pharmacy is located in a busy clinic in which six physicians and two dentists practice. The patients come directly from their appointment to have their prescriptions filled, so many of the patients are quite ill or have just had dental procedures performed, and it is vital that they receive prompt and efficient care.

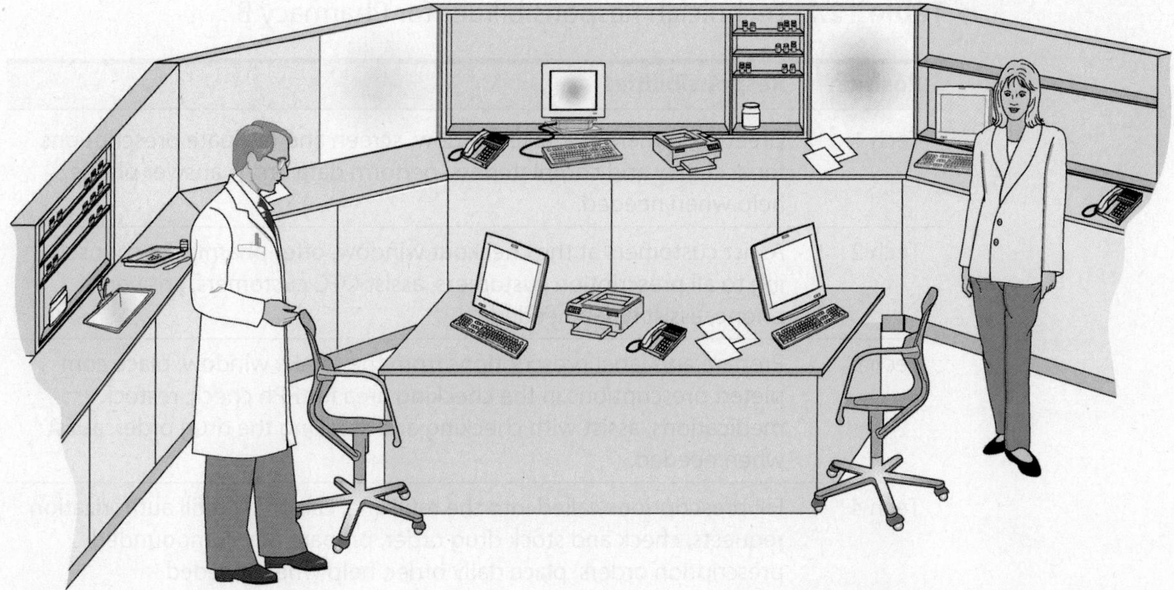

Figure 12.4 Workflow process for four technicians working in a high-volume clinic pharmacy.

Prioritizing prescriptions is sometimes necessary to accommodate the needs of very ill patients. The pharmacy has an intake window where prescriptions may be dropped off, a pick-up window, a pharmacist consultation window, and a work table where prescriptions are prepared for the pharmacist to check. There are four computers, two label printers, and three telephones. One of the phones is a doctor line to ensure that physicians or their nurses have immediate access to the pharmacy to call in prescriptions or ask questions. This line is answered by one of the pharmacists unless they are both busy, in which case a technician will answer and refer the call to a pharmacist if necessary.

prioritizing prescriptions Establishing the order of processing prescriptions based on special needs of patients.

Scott is the lead technician who does the weekly scheduling. Although each technician is assigned to certain duties each day, the technicians understand that it is imperative that they work together and assist where the work load is heaviest at any one time. Table 12.1 shows an example of the weekly schedule for the four technicians, and Table 12.2 lists the responsibilities for each technician position. Referring to Figure 12.4 and Tables 12.1 and 12.2, follow the workflow on a Monday morning in Pharmacy B. Amber greets Mrs. Aloe at the intake window and accepts her insurance card and her three prescriptions. (See Figures 12.5, 12.6, and 12.7 for the written prescriptions, which are for Lasix 40 mg #30 1 daily am, digoxin 0.125 #60 1 daily am ad, and menthol 200 mg-thymol 200 mg-Dermabase 60 gm 1 jar apply to knee PRN arthritis pain.)

lead technician The technician assigned to establish technician schedules, track attendance, and assist with technician concerns as a liaison between the management and the technicians.

Table 12.1 Weekly Technician Schedule for Pharmacy B

	Monday	Tuesday	Wednesday	Thursday	Friday
Tech 1	Amber	Sasha	Scott	Chris	Amber
Tech 2	Sasha	Scott	Chris	Amber	Sasha
Tech 3	Scott	Chris	Amber	Sasha	Scott
Tech 4	Chris	Amber	Sasha	Scott	Chris

Table 12.2 Technician Responsibilities for Pharmacy B

Position	Responsibilities
Tech 1	Greet customers at intake window, screen and evaluate prescriptions for accuracy and completeness, perform data entry, answer phone, help when needed.
Tech 2	Assist customers at the checkout window, offer pharmacist counseling to all prescription customers, assist OTC customers, answer phone, assist when needed.
Tech 3	Prepare and label prescriptions from the intake window, place completed prescriptions in the checking area for RPh check, restock medications, assist with checking and stocking the drug order, assist when needed.
Tech 4	Fill prescriptions called into the refill line, call or fax refill authorization requests, check and stock drug order, prepare any compounded prescription orders, place daily order, help where needed.

Amber asks, "Mrs. Aloe do you have any drug allergies?"

"No, I'm not aware of any," she responds.

Amber enters the patient information into the computer and finds that her patient profile is complete. She checks the prescriptions for any missing information and realizes that one of the prescriptions is a compound.

"Mrs. Aloe, one of these prescriptions will need to be mixed and may take a little more time, so would you like to pick them up later?"

"Well, I have some errands to run and I'll return after lunch," says Mrs. Aloe.

"Thanks, Mrs. Aloe. We'll have them ready for you."

extemporaneous compound A medication compounded in the pharmacy pursuant to a prescriber's order for a given patient.

drug–drug interaction An adverse event that may occur as the result of two incompatible drugs being used together.

Amber enters the prescriptions into the computer and lets Chris know that there is an extemporaneous compound promised for early afternoon.

After Amber enters the Lasix prescription, she begins the entry of the digoxin and the computer indicates a drug–drug interaction. Amber lets the pharmacist, Kevin, know there is an interaction. He reads the reaction warning and performs an override because he knows that the two drugs are often used together and the adverse reaction is rare. Amber continues the data entry of the two prescriptions and places

Dr. Barry Weiss
901 Sheridan St., Austin, TX 90902
874-555-1300

Name: Katherine Smith 498 E 11th St.

RX: Lasix 40 mg

Disp: #30

Sig i – q am

Dispense as written

Dr. Barry Weiss
May substitute

Figure 12.5 Handwritten prescription for Lasix ready for data entry by the technician. (Reprinted with permission from Mohr ME. Lab Experiences for the Pharmacy Technician. Philadelphia: Lippincott, Williams & Wilkins, 2006.)

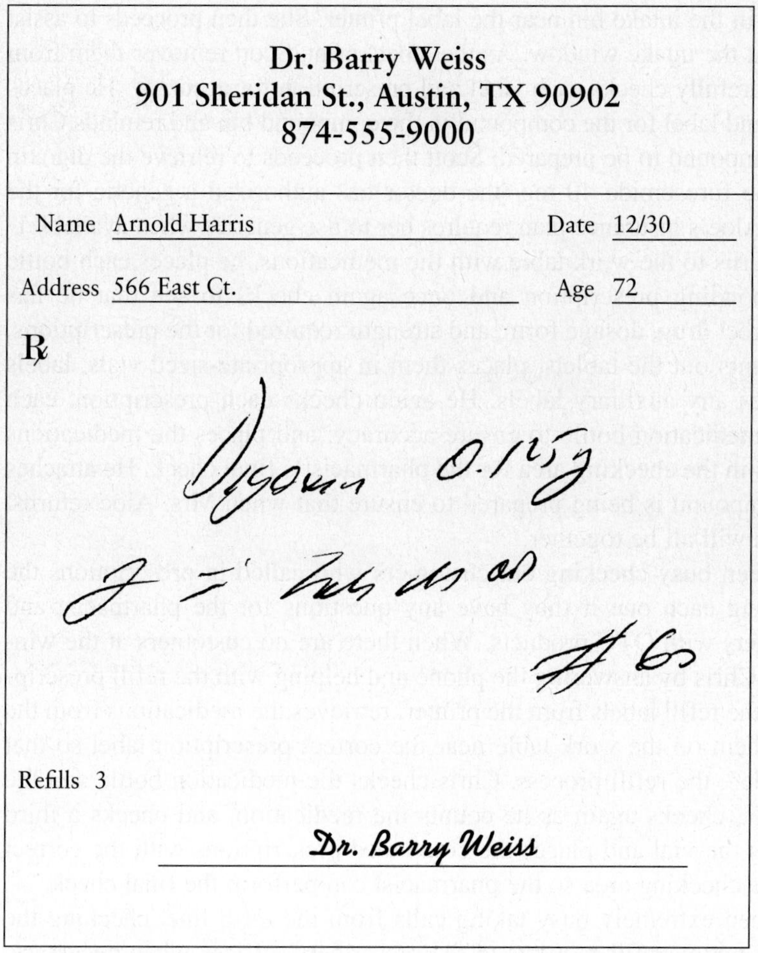

Dr. Barry Weiss
901 Sheridan St., Austin, TX 90902
874-555-9000

Name Arnold Harris Date 12/30

Address 566 East Ct. Age 72

℞

Digoxin 0.125 g

1 tab po qd

#60

Refills 3

Dr. Barry Weiss

Figure 12.6 Handwritten prescription for digoxin ready for data entry by the technician. (Reprinted with permission from Finkel R. Patient Care Management Lab, 2nd ed. Philadelphia: Lippincott, Williams & Wilkins, 2008.)

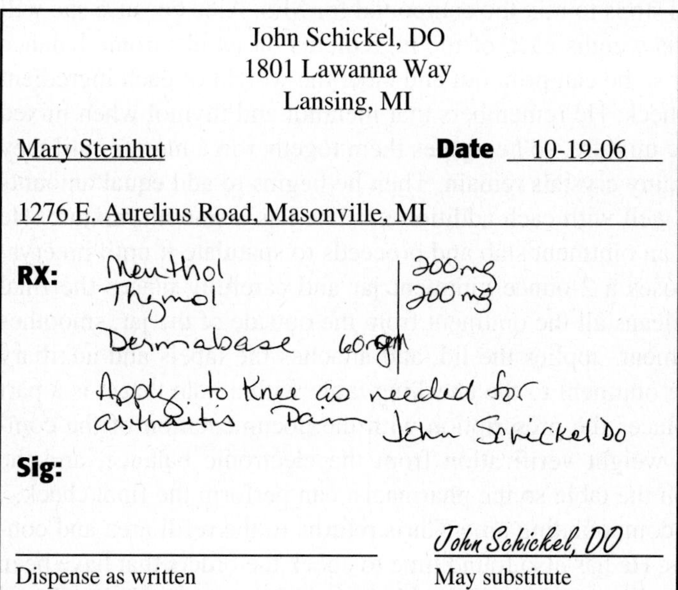

John Schickel, DO
1801 Lawanna Way
Lansing, MI

Mary Steinhut **Date** 10-19-06

1276 E. Aurelius Road, Masonville, MI

RX: Menthol 200 mg
Thymol 200 mg
Dermabase 60 gm
Apply to knee as needed for arthritis pain John Schickel DO

Sig:

Dispense as written

John Schickel, DO
May substitute

Figure 12.7 Prescription formula for an extemporaneous compound to be prepared by the compounding technician. (Reprinted with permission from Mohr ME. Lab Experiences for the Pharmacy Technician. Philadelphia: Lippincott, Williams & Wilkins, 2006.)

the prescriptions in the intake bin near the label printer. She then proceeds to assist the next patient at the intake window. As the labels print, Scott removes them from the printer and carefully checks each label and prescription for accuracy. He places the prescription and label for the compound in the compound bin and reminds Chris that there is a compound to be prepared. Scott then proceeds to retrieve the digoxin 0.125 mg and the furosemide 40 mg (the doctor has authorized a generic for the Lasix, and Mrs. Aloe's insurance plan requires her to use generics when available).

As Scott returns to the work table with the medications, he places each bottle near the corresponding prescription and once again checks to see that he has retrieved the correct drug, dosage form, and strength required for the prescriptions. He carefully counts out the tablets, places them in appropriate-sized vials, labels them, and applies any auxiliary labels. He again checks each prescription, each label, and each medication bottle to ensure accuracy, and places the medications and stock bottles in the checking area for the pharmacist's final check. He attaches a note that a compound is being prepared to ensure that when Mrs. Aloe returns, her prescriptions will all be together.

Sasha has been busy checking out customers who called in prescriptions the day before, asking each one if they have any questions for the pharmacist and assisting customers with OTC products. When there are no customers at the window, she assists Chris by answering the phone and helping with the refill prescriptions. She takes the refill labels from the printer, retrieves the medications from the shelf, and sets them on the work table near the correct prescription label so that Chris can complete the refill process. Chris checks the medication bottle and the prescription label, checks again as he counts the medication, and checks a third time as he labels the vial and places the completed prescriptions with the correct paperwork in the checking area so the pharmacist can perform the final check.

Chris has been extremely busy taking calls from the refill line, checking the refill status, and faxing refill requests to the prescribers' offices when necessary. He accepts the daily drug order from the wholesaler, signs for the order, and takes the controlled-drug tote to the pharmacist to be checked and the order verification sheet signed. He prints labels for the called-in refills that do not need authorization from the physician, and stops to mix the compound for Mrs. Aloe because she will be returning soon. Chris weighs each of the ingredients on an electronic balance equipped with a printer so he can print out and label the weight of each ingredient for the pharmacist to check. He remembers that menthol and thymol when mixed together form a eutectic mixture, so he titrates them together in a mortar until they are liquefied and no grainy crystals remain. Then he begins to add equal amounts of Dermabase, mixing well with each addition until he has a smooth mixture. He places the ointment on an ointment slab and proceeds to spatulate it until no crystals remain. Chris chooses a 2-ounce ointment jar and carefully places the final product in the jar. He cleans all the ointment from the outside of the jar, smoothes the surface of the ointment, applies the lid, and attaches the labels and auxiliary labels. Chris moves the ointment to the checking table with a note that it is a part of another order. He places the prescription with the documentation of the compounding method, the weight verification from the electronic balance, and the ingredient containers on the table so the pharmacist can perform the final check.

order verification sheet An order container with controlled drugs will be secured and have a form requiring the signature of the pharmacist to verify that the correct drugs were delivered.

eutectic mixture Two or more chemicals that change from a solid form to a liquid when mixed together.

spatulate The process of using a spatula to evenly mix an ointment and eliminate graininess in the final product.

After cleaning the compounding area, Chris returns to the refill area and continues processing refills. He has also found time to check the orders that have been received and to stock the items on the shelves, being careful to rotate the stock and check expiration dates. Scott assists him with the orders when he can. By mid-afternoon the intake and checkout windows are very busy with walk-in customers and Chris is able to assist by answering phones and filling prescriptions from the intake window to keep the pharmacy wait times at a reasonable level (usually no more than 15–20 minutes).

The technicians for the evening shift begin to arrive and assist through the rush hour so that Chris can place the orders for the next day. The technicians consult with each arriving technician in their same position to ensure a smooth transition as the morning shift leaves for the day and the evening shift begins. Amber, Sasha, Scott, and Chris hang up their technician jackets, knowing they have made a difference in the lives of patients and worked efficiently as a team, and that their teamwork has allowed the pharmacist to perform the cognitive and consultative responsibilities that are essential for providing excellent pharmaceutical care to patients. Each walks out the door with the same thought: "I am a professional pharmacy technician. I understand the scope and standards of practice for my profession and I am living them. I made a difference today."

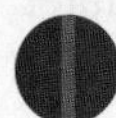

Chain Pharmacy

Pharmacy C (shown in Fig. 12.8) is a high-volume chain pharmacy in a large metropolitan area. One pharmacist and two technicians on each of the two shifts staff the pharmacy. The primary responsibility of both technicians is to assist the patients in the pharmacy to maintain reasonable wait times. Karen and Teresa work the day

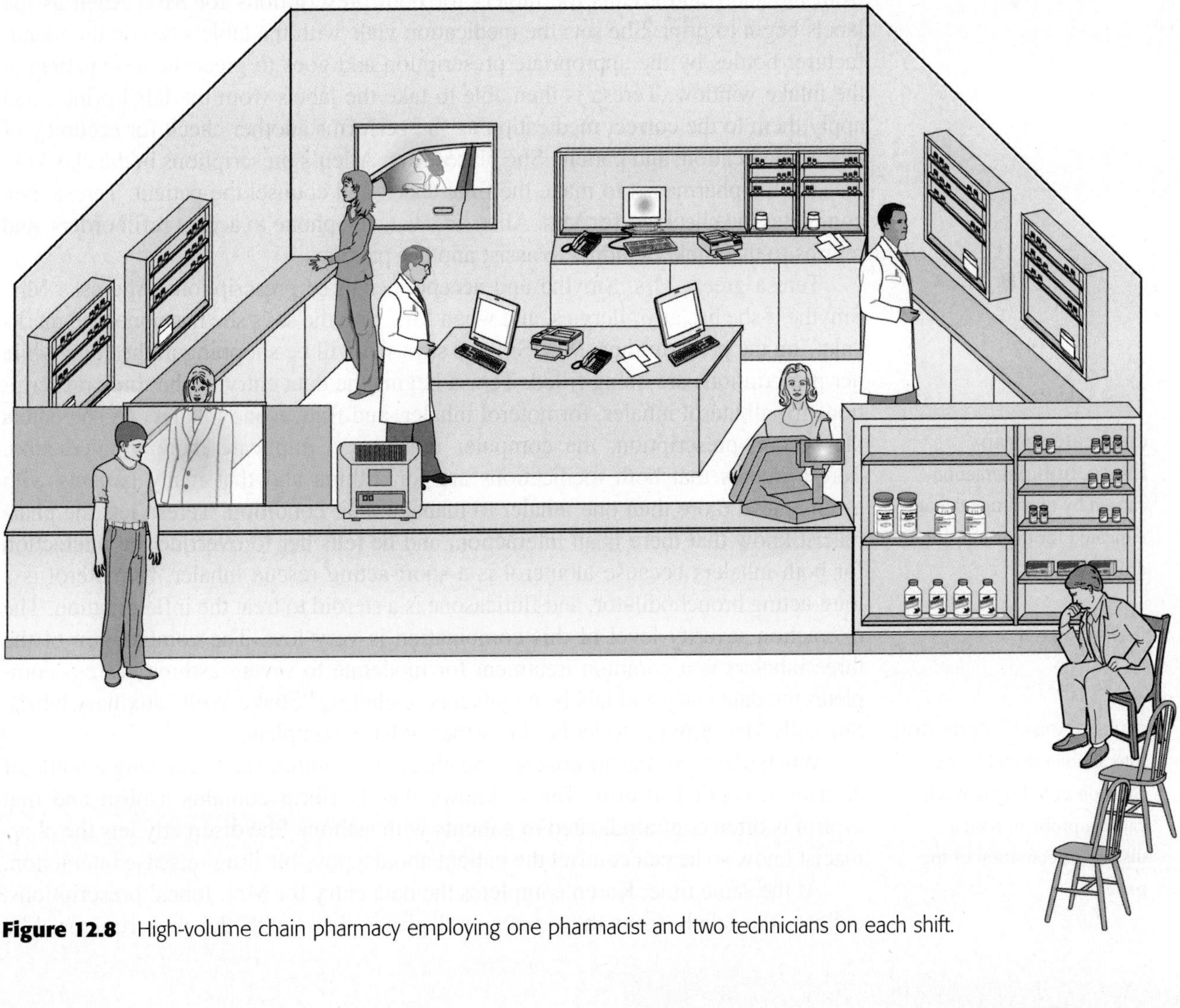

chain pharmacy One of a group of pharmacies owned by an individual or a corporate group that makes all management and policy decisions.

Figure 12.8 High-volume chain pharmacy employing one pharmacist and two technicians on each shift.

shift and have established a pattern of teamwork to facilitate the workflow. Both technicians are very attentive to the intake window and greet each patient promptly as they arrive at the window.

As Mrs. Jones walks up to the window, Karen greets her and accepts her prescriptions. She knows Mrs. Jones is a regular customer and that her profile is up to date. As she examines the prescriptions, she asks Mrs. Jones if she has experienced any new allergies since her last visit. Mrs. Jones says she will return in an hour for her prescriptions, and Karen begins to enter them into the computer.

As she is performing the data entry, another patient arrives at the window. Teresa immediately greets the new patient and begins the prescription evaluation.

"Mrs. Allen, do you have any drug allergies?"

"I'm only allergic to codeine."

Teresa notes the allergy on the prescription and checks to see that neither prescription has codeine as an ingredient.

"Would you like to wait for the prescriptions or will you pick them up later, Mrs. Allen?"

"I'd like to wait for them because I need to take them right away."

"We'll have them ready for you in a few minutes. Please have a seat and we'll call you when they are ready."

Karen finishes the data entry on Mrs. Jones' prescriptions. She sets Mrs. Jones' prescription aside and reads the drug names on Mrs. Allen's prescriptions. As Teresa enters Mrs. Allen's prescriptions into the computer, Karen retrieves the medication from the shelf and counts the tablets for both prescriptions for Mrs. Allen as the labels begin to print. She sets the medication vials with the tablets beside the manufacturer bottles by the appropriate prescription and goes to greet the next patient at the intake window. Teresa is then able to take the labels from the label printer and apply them to the correct medication as she performs another check for accuracy of labels, medication, and patient. She places Mrs. Allen's prescriptions in the checking area for the pharmacist to make the final check and counsel the patient. Teresa then completes the checkout for Mrs. Allen, answers the phone to accept refill orders, and returns to the intake window to assist another patient.

Teresa greets Mrs. Smythe and accepts her three prescriptions. She asks Mrs. Smythe if she has any allergies, and when Mrs. Smythe says she has none, she marks "nka" on the prescriptions. Mrs. Smythe says she will be shopping in the store while her prescriptions are being filled. Teresa begins the data entry of the three prescriptions for albuterol inhaler, formoterol inhaler, and fluticasone inhaler. As she enters the second prescription, the computer indicates a duplicate therapy interaction. Teresa knows that both medications are for asthma and that many patients with asthma need more than one inhaler to manage their condition. Teresa lets the pharmacist know that there is an interaction, and he tells her to override the interaction for both inhalers because albuterol is a short-acting rescue inhaler, formoterol is a long-acting bronchodilator, and fluticasone is a steroid to treat the inflammation. The interaction severity level of this combination is very low. The combination of the three inhalers is a common treatment for moderate to severe asthma. Teresa completes the data entry and labels the inhalers, including "Shake Well" auxiliary labels. She calls Mrs. Smythe to let her know her order is complete.

duplicate therapy interaction Interaction caused by two drugs that are indicated for the same condition.

When Mrs. Smythe approaches the checkout counter, she is carrying a bottle of arthritis-strength Bufferin. Teresa knows that Bufferin contains aspirin and that aspirin is often contraindicated in patients with asthma. She discreetly lets the pharmacist know so he can counsel the patient about a possible drug–disease interaction.

drug–disease interaction Interaction created by the addition of a drug that will cause a problem with a disease or condition of the patient.

At the same time, Karen completes the data entry for Mrs. Jones' prescriptions, collects the labels from the printer, and places them with the prescriptions. She checks the labels with the prescriptions to be certain that she has entered everything correctly. Karen retrieves the medication bottles from the shelf and double-checks each bottle to be certain it has the correct drug, strength, and dosage form required for each prescription. Karen carefully counts out the correct number of dosage forms for each prescription, places them in appropriate-sized vials, and applies the correct labels and auxiliary labels. The pharmacist checks Mrs. Jones' prescriptions and places them alphabetically in the pick-up area while Karen answers the phone and takes another refill order.

The refill is for atenolol and the patient received 30 tablets 2 months ago with directions to take one tablet daily for blood pressure. As Karen processes the refill, she makes a note for the pharmacist to discuss medication compliance with the patient when she arrives because she knows that it is important to take blood pressure medication exactly as directed.

compliance Medication compliance requires that the patient take their medication exactly as directed.

Karen and Teresa continue to work as a team to ensure excellent customer service and assist the pharmacist. They are attentive to customers in the OTC drug aisle and offer to assist customers who seem unsure about which product to buy. Both technicians understand their scope of practice and are able to direct questions to the pharmacist that require consultation. Often the customers only need assistance in finding a product or getting information about brand or generic products that is easily provided by the technicians. Karen is responsible for ordering and stocking the OTC section, and she takes every opportunity to perform "merchandise facing" to keep it looking neat. Teresa takes responsibility for ordering and stocking the inventory behind the prescription counter. Each technician is responsible for checking expiration dates on prescription medications monthly to ensure that all expired medications are removed from stock. Recall notices are promptly checked and the results documented. Karen and Teresa have familiarized themselves with the third-party plans prevalent in their practice setting and are able to troubleshoot insurance problems. With their professional assistance, the pharmacist is able to perform the consultative and cognitive functions that ensure excellent pharmaceutical care can be extended to the patients.

merchandise facing The process of bringing all merchandise on a shelf to the front edge of the shelf in an orderly manner.

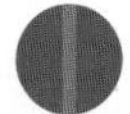

Chapter Summary

- A technician's role will vary according to the practice setting.
- Many technician responsibilities are the same in every practice setting.
- It is important to establish an efficient workflow process for each practice setting and the pharmacy professionals.
- Basic technician knowledge is important for prescription evaluation in every practice setting.
- Proper handling of computer interaction alerts that require a pharmacist's intervention is critical.
- Teamwork is essential to ensure an effective workflow process in a large pharmacy.
- Merchandising responsibilities are an important aspect of the technician's work in an outpatient setting.
- A knowledgeable and alert technician can prevent drug interactions by alerting the pharmacist to problems that require consultation.
- Prescriptions may need to be prioritized to accommodate patients who are very ill or in pain.

Review Questions

Multiple Choice

Choose the best answer for each of the following:

1. When an asthmatic patient takes a medication that is contraindicated in patients with asthma, the resulting interaction will be a
   a. drug–drug interaction
   b. drug–food interaction
   c. drug–disease interaction
   d. duplicate therapy

2. The probability that an adverse drug interaction will occur and the degree of harm it may cause is indicated in *Drug Interaction Facts* by categorizing it according to
   a. probable cause
   b. severity level
   c. alphabetical listing
   d. bioavailability

3. The process by which a drug enters the bloodstream is
   a. metabolism
   b. administration
   c. elimination
   d. absorption

4. Medication compliance can be improved by
   a. patient counseling
   b. extended-release products to be taken less often
   c. refill reminders
   d. all of the above

5. A procedure for organizing the daily tasks in a practice setting is called a
   a. timeline
   b. workflow process
   c. job list
   d. none of the above

Fill in the Blank

Fill in the blank(s) with the correct term.

6. A small pharmacy owned and managed by one or two pharmacists and designed to serve the pharmacy needs of walk-in customers is called a(n) ______________________________.

7. The document that lists the quantity and price of items included in the order is called the ____________________.

8. To keep the OTC section looking neat, the technician can ____________ the merchandise during slow times in the work day.

9. When checking the order and stocking the shelves, it is important for the technician to ____________________ the stock.

10. When the manufacturer discovers a problem with a drug, it will issue a ____________________ to alert the pharmacies.

True/False

Mark the following statements True or False.

11. _____ A eutectic mixture results from a solid being dissolved in a gas to form an aerosol.

12. _____ Extemporaneous compounding can only be done by a pharmacist.

13. _____ A technician should always consult the pharmacist before overriding a drug interaction.

14. _____ A duplicate therapy interaction alert indicates that two drugs are being prescribed for the same indication.

15. _____ Questions about nonprescription drugs do not require consultation with the pharmacist.

Matching

Match the items in column A with the statements in column B.

Column A	Column B
16. _____ lead technician	A. A pharmacy owned and managed by a large company.
17. _____ clinic pharmacy	B. Placing new merchandise behind the items with earlier expiration dates
18. _____ chain pharmacy	C. Responsible for scheduling and serving as a liaison with management
19. _____ rotate the stock	D. A pharmacy located in a building with physician offices to serve the patients
20. _____ merchandise facing	E. Straightening the merchandise and bringing it to the front of the shelf.

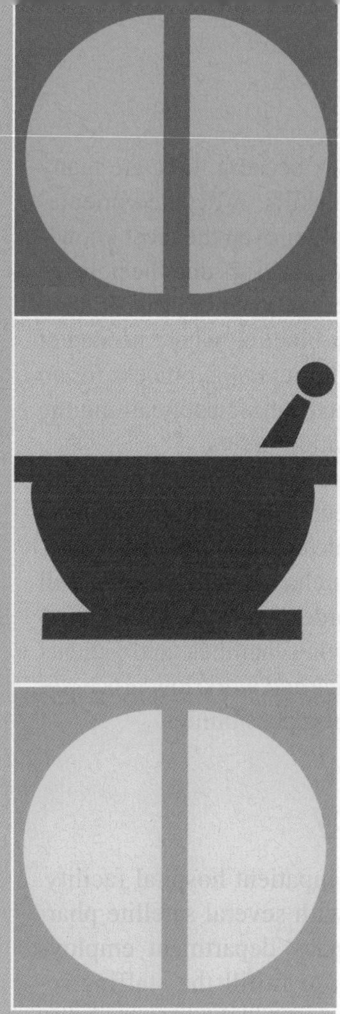

Chapter **13**

Inpatient Hospital and Homecare Prescription Processing

OBJECTIVES

After completing this chapter, the student will be able to:

- Process inpatient medication orders.
- Discuss delivery systems for inpatient medication orders.
- Diagram a technician workflow process for an inpatient hospital setting.
- Discuss the importance of technicians being cross-trained to perform in all areas of the inpatient setting.
- Process inpatient medication orders in a homecare setting.
- Discuss delivery systems in a homecare setting.
- Plan a workflow process for a homecare setting.

KEY TERMS

- barrier isolator
- bingo card
- biological safety cabinet
- cleanroom
- laminar flow hood
- log book
- pneumatic tube system
- Pyxis
- robot room
- Total Parenteral Nutrition (TPN)
- TPN compounder
- unit dose packaging machine

The technician's role in an inpatient pharmacy is complex because there are many different areas and each involves special knowledge and skills. A detailed orientation to each particular inpatient hospital setting is essential for even the most knowledgeable technician to become proficient in the workflow processes and the policies and procedures of each institution. A professional technician should be cross-trained in every area of the practice setting so that he or she can function where needed at any given time. The first part of this chapter simulates an orientation process for an educated technician who is beginning to work in a hospital setting and learning the hospital procedures for processing and delivering medication orders.

There are numerous specialty pharmacies that require specific skills and training. Having a position in a specialty pharmacy gives a technician an opportunity to become an expert in a field of interest and make a valuable contribution to the practice setting. Some specialties were discussed in an earlier chapter. This chapter will also discuss evaluation and processing of medication orders in a homecare pharmacy that serves a number of nursing homes, assisted-living facilities, and patients receiving medication therapy at home. The practice settings and workflow processes described here are just basic examples of the many existing possibilities.

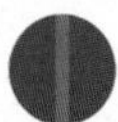

Inpatient Hospital Pharmacy

Falls City General Hospital is a 300-bed, full-service, inpatient hospital facility. The main pharmacy is an around-the-clock operation with several satellite pharmacies staffed during the daytime hours. The pharmacy department employs 20 pharmacists and 30 certified pharmacy technicians to fulfill the staffing requirements for the three shifts. The scheduling of technicians is the responsibility of Pam, the technician supervisor who also serves as a liaison between the technicians and management. The training and orientation of new technicians are accomplished through a well-organized plan implemented by Marcia, the technician educator. Today Pam and Marcia will begin the training of a newly hired technician, Susie. Susie recently graduated from a formal pharmacy technician program. She has learned the standards of practice for her profession and completed experiential time in several different practice settings. Today Susie is excited to begin her first position as a professional pharmacy technician in a hospital setting. After checking in with Pam to complete the paperwork, sign the confidentiality statement, receive her employee handbook, and discuss scheduling, she is introduced to Marcia, who will facilitate her training. This chapter will follow Susie as she learns to process medication orders and fulfill the responsibilities of each area of the hospital pharmacy.

Front Window

The area of the front window of the pharmacy provides a place where health professionals can visit the pharmacy to seek information or pick up medications. Pam introduced Susie to the technician who was assigned to that area and left her to begin her training. Susie learned how to check emergency drug kits (EDKs) in when returned, and the proper procedure for checking them out to a department when a request was received. She remembered from her experiential time in a hospital setting the procedure for checking returned EDKs for missing and expired drugs. When a drug is missing there will be a billing record with the name of the patient who received the drug. Susie learned the procedure for entering the billing into the patient's record. She then replaced the missing item(s) and rechecked the expiration dates of all the drugs in the box, being sure to follow the hospital protocol of pulling any drug with less than 6 weeks left before it expires. As she sealed the box with a safety lock, she applied an expiration sticker for the box listing the earliest expiration date of any item in the box. The hospital also used a pneumatic tube system to send drugs to various units in the system. Susie learned how to operate the system and was able to send "stat" drugs to the floors without leaving the pharmacy. She also learned that some items, such as glass containers, controlled drugs, and hazardous materials, could not be "tubed." She was careful to request assistance from a pharmacist when asked a question that was beyond the scope of practice of a technician.

pneumatic tube system A system of tubes connecting the units of a hospital with the pharmacy so that certain medications can be sent immediately from the pharmacy department.

In a teaching hospital, interns, medical residents, nursing students, and other allied health students often stop at the pharmacy window with questions. Be certain that your answers are accurate and within the scope of your practice because they will accept your answers as fact.

CAUTION

Delivering Medications to the Floor

As Susie developed a proficiency working at the front window, it was time to expand her training to other areas of the pharmacy. The hospital used Pyxis automated dispensing cabinets. Susie had received her password for the Pyxis machines and was anxious to learn another aspect of her position as a technician. She was paired with an experienced technician to begin making the runs to the floors delivering IV medications and stat items that could not be tubed, and loading needed medications into the Pyxis machines. This task required a great deal of organization and stamina. Susie learned to check the printout of items that needed to be replaced in the Pyxis machines. She began to gather these items on a cart and then gathered the IV bags and any other medications that were ready to be distributed to the units. She organized the items according to their destination and began the trip through the hospital. Susie was glad to have an experienced technician with her because she wasn't familiar with all the units yet.

Pyxis Automated dispensing machine to provide easy access to patient medications for the nursing staff.

As they arrived at each unit, Susie learned where the medications were stored and was careful to check the auxiliary labels to see whether they needed refrigeration and to procure a signature from the nurse when needed. After delivering the medications, Susie picked up any returns, again noting whether they required refrigeration and whether they had been properly stored and could be reissued from the pharmacy. She then entered her code into the Pyxis machine and began the reloading process for the medications ordered for that dispensing cabinet. See Figure 13.1 for a picture of a technician beginning the reloading process on a Pyxis machine. She was careful to log out when her task was completed.

Susie repeated this process at each of the units, delivering medications, picking up returns, and restocking the Pyxis machines until she had completed her rounds. She and her supervising technician returned to the pharmacy, and Susie was shown how to return useable medications to stock and how to dispose of medications that were no longer useable. Between runs to the floors, Susie worked in the unit dose area. She learned to operate the unit dose packaging machine for medications that are not commercially available in unit dose form. Susie learned to enter the drug name and strength, NDC number, lot number, and expiration date in the software program for the machine, load the labeling strips, and place the number of tablets or capsules needed in the proper area of the machine. She then recorded the information in the unit dose log book with her initials and

unit dose packaging machine A machine capable of packaging medications in individual dose containers with proper labels.

log book A book used to document compounding ingredients and techniques, or the repackaging of bulk products into single-dose packaging.

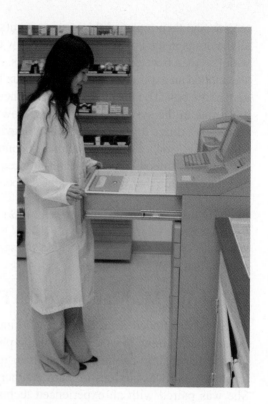

Figure 13.1 Pyxis machine.

placed the packaged medication with the manufacturer's bottle and the log book in the checking area for the pharmacist to check. After the medications were checked by the pharmacist, Susie placed then in the appropriate bin on the shelf, being careful to double-check that it was the correctly labeled bin to prevent a medication error in the future. Susie then checked the IV area and the Pyxis central printer and discovered that it was time for another run to the floors to deliver medications. She was able to load the cart and perform all the necessary functions without assistance this time, although another technician accompanied her on the rounds. After returning all the items to their proper place in the pharmacy, Susie learned the procedure for filling and labeling unit dose oral syringes. She quickly developed a routine to fulfill the responsibilities and establish an efficient workflow process for this area of the hospital pharmacy. Her confidence as a professional pharmacy technician continued to increase as she attained competence in each position in the pharmacy.

IV Admixture

The next morning Susie checked her training schedule and was excited to see that she would be working in the IV room. She reviewed the USP 797 regulations she had learned in school as she waited to meet the technician who would facilitate her training and explain the hospital protocols for IV admixture. Because she understood the theory behind aseptic technique, her trainer began to walk her through the hospital procedures beginning with removing jewelry, hand washing, gowning, and gloving. See Figure 13.2 for a diagram of a cleanroom. They entered the cleanroom through a small anteroom with sticky paper on the floor. The cleanroom was equipped with a positive air pressure system and two horizontal flow laminar hoods.

cleanroom An enclosed room with smooth walls, floors, and ceilings that are resistant to damage from sanitizing agents; the air quality meets ISO Class 8 standards.

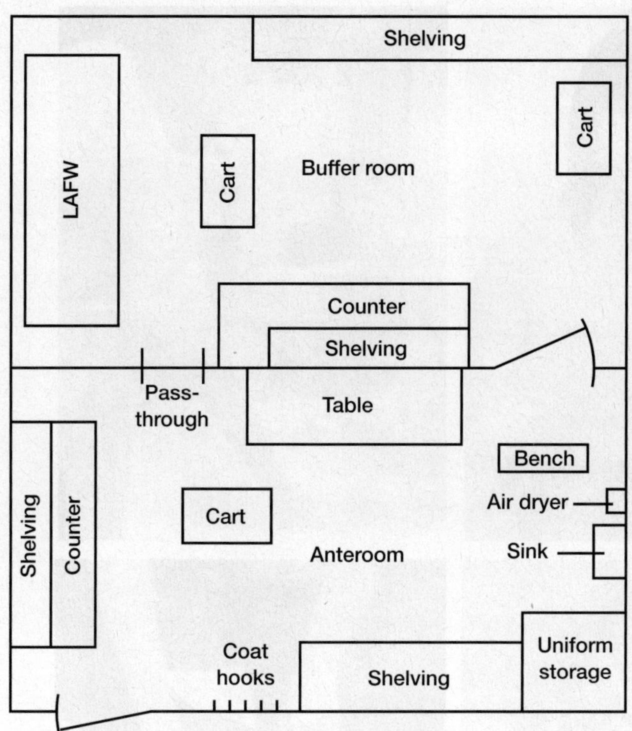

Figure 13.2 Cleanroom layout. (Reprinted with permission from Thompson JE. A Practical Guide to Contemporary Pharmacy Practice, 2nd ed. Baltimore, MD: Lippincott, Williams & Wilkins, 2004.)

There was an anteroom to facilitate bringing materials into the area and returning the finished product to the pharmacy area. The hoods were never turned off because this was a 24-hour operation. Susie gathered the IV orders from the printer and began to retrieve the needed materials to prepare the admixtures. She calculated the number of vials of each ingredient that would be needed to fill each order and carefully noted each calculation on the paperwork. She placed the materials on a cart in the anteroom, cleaned them with alcohol, and began the gowning and gloving procedure in preparation to enter the cleanroom. (See Preparation Method 13.1 for gowning and gloving procedures.)

Preparation Method 13.1
Gowning and Gloving

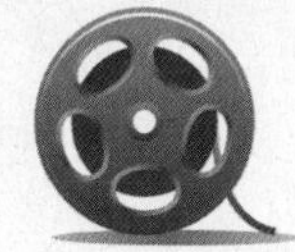

See the student CD and website for a video of this procedure.

1. Remove outer lab jacket (see Fig. 13.3A).
2. Remove all jewelry (see Fig. 13.3B).
3. Scrub hands and arms to elbows with soap or special sponge, and dry (see Fig. 13.3C).
4. Cover hair with head cover (use beard cover if applicable; see Fig. 13.3D).
5. Put on face mask (see Fig. 13.3E).
6. Cover shoes with protective shoe covers (see Fig. 13.3F).
7. Put on gown with opening in the back (see Fig. 13.3G).
8. Put on sterile gloves (see Fig. 13.3H).

A gowned and gloved technician is shown in Figure 13.3I.

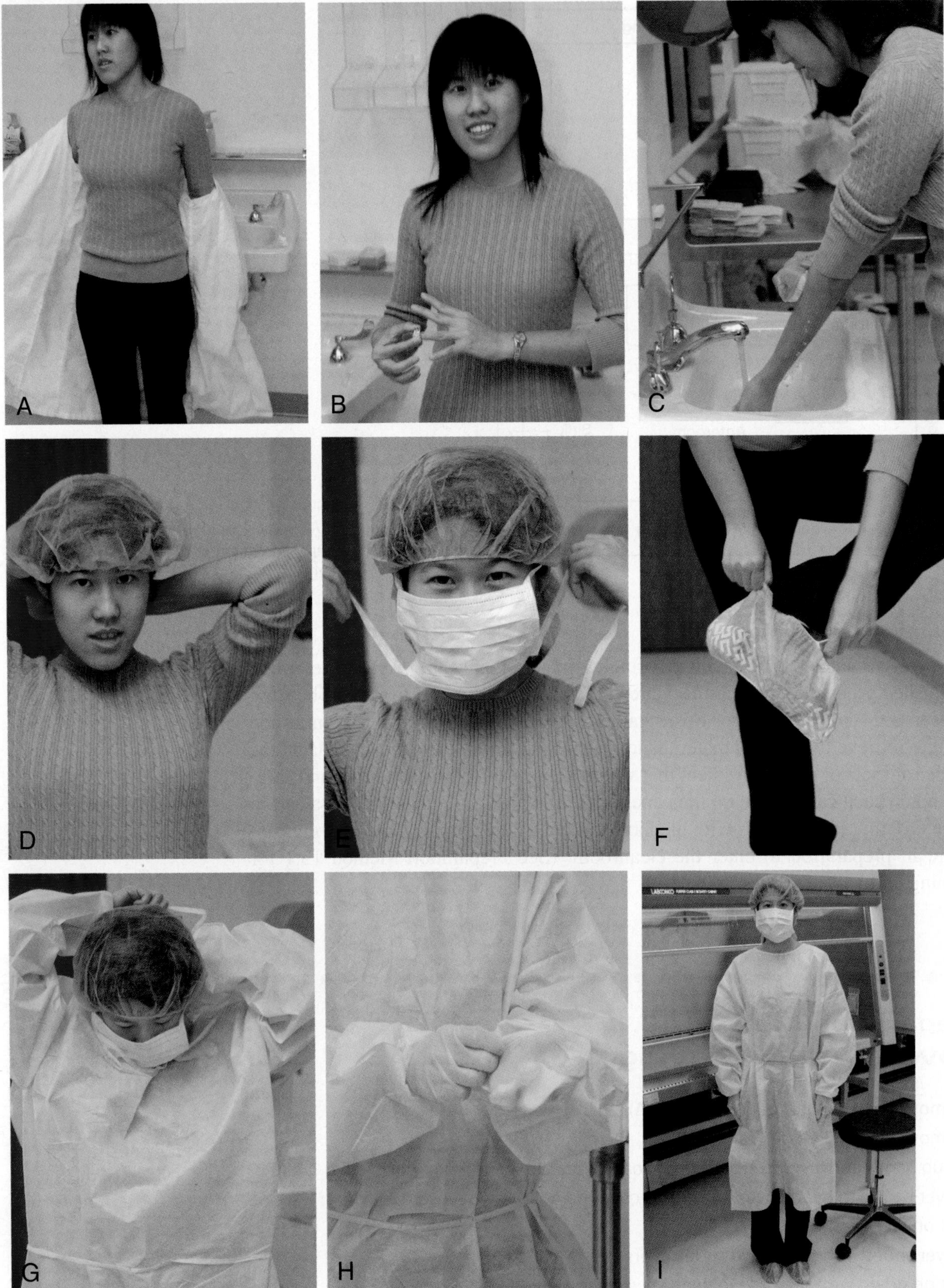

Figure 13.3 The steps for gowning and gloving.

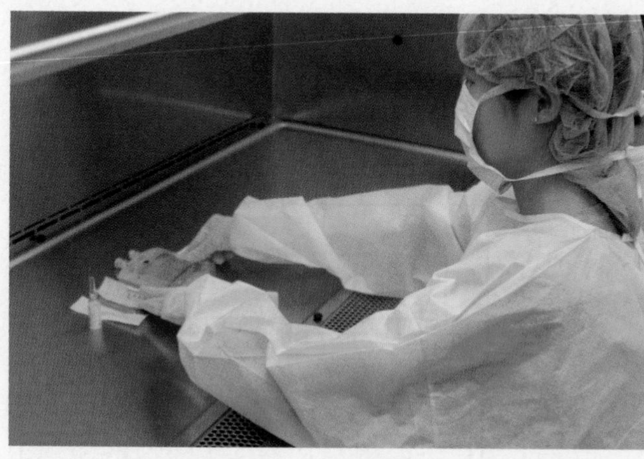

Figure 13.4 Laminar flow hood with setups.

After entering the cleanroom, Susie placed the IV bags, additives, and fluids for reconstitution in the laminar flow hoods in an orderly fashion, keeping each order separate from the others and being cognizant of the airflow in the hood and proper admixture techniques. She asked the experienced technician to check her setups before she began to mix. See Figure 13.4 for an example of a laminar flow hood with the IV setups ready for admixture. After the IVs were prepared, Susie removed them from the hood, applied the appropriate labels, and left them in the checking area with the paperwork, the vials used, and the syringes with the plunger pulled back to the correct mark to indicate the amount of fluid used. See Figure 13.5 for an example of completed IV orders placed in the checking area. After the orders in the cleanroom were completed, the pharmacist would perform the final check and place the finished product in the double-sided cabinet to be delivered to the floors.

laminar flow hood Workbench that provides an environment of air filtered through a high-efficiency particulate air (HEPA) filter to facilitate aseptic work conditions.

total parenteral nutrition (TPN) Intravenous therapy designed to provide nutrition for patients who cannot or will not take in adequate nourishment by mouth.

TPN compounder A compounder that can be programmed to simultaneously pump the four basic ingredients of a TPN and dispense the correct amounts of additives into a TPN bag.

When Susie went to lunch she placed her gown, gloves, and mask in the appropriate container. On returning to the pharmacy, she removed the new orders from the printer and retrieved the materials needed to perform the admixture after calculating the number of vials needed for each order. She placed the materials on the cart, cleaned them with alcohol, and began the hand washing, gowning, and gloving procedure. As Susie re-entered the cleanroom, she reminded herself of the importance of her task and her responsibility to triple-check her work. She knew the significance of aseptic technique and took great pride in her ability to perform this important task.

During her week in the IV room Susie also learned to prepare total parenteral nutrition (TPN). She had observed others programming the TPN compounder

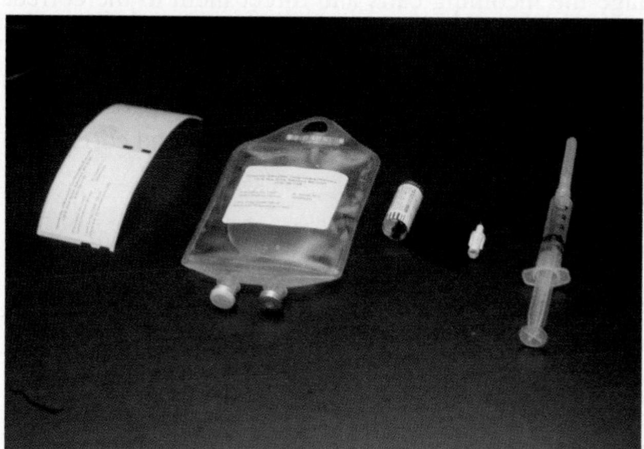

Figure 13.5 IV bags ready for RPh check.

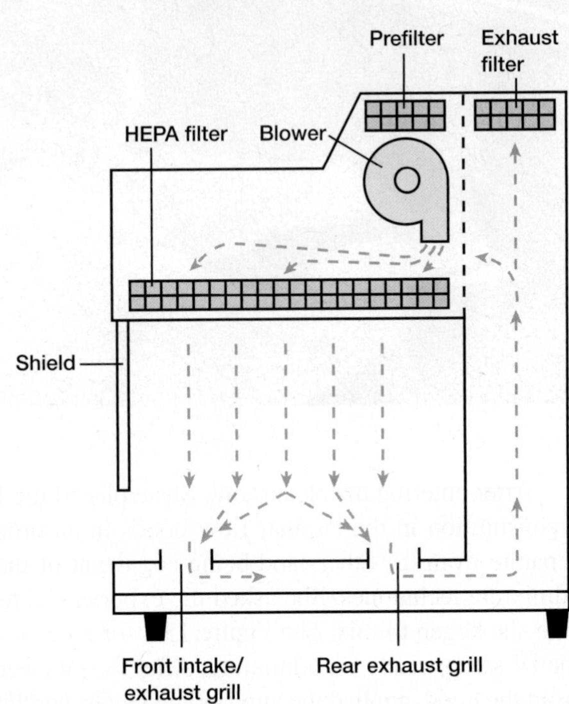

Figure 13.6 Biological safety cabinet. (Reprinted with permission from Thompson JE. A Practical Guide to Contemporary Pharmacy Practice, 2nd ed. Baltimore, MD: Lippincott, Williams & Wilkins, 2004.)

during her experiential time as a student and was now able to perform this task under the supervision of an experienced technician. Refer back to Figure 2.8 for a picture of a TPN compounder. Preparing chemotherapeutic admixtures was reserved for more experienced technicians, but Susie was able to observe the procedure, as well as the procedure for cleaning a hazardous spill. Chemo drugs were prepared in a biological safety cabinet with a vertical airflow, which required a different mixing technique to maintain sterility. See Figure 13.6 for a picture of a biological safety cabinet. Some hospital systems invest in a barrier isolator to eliminate the need to construct a separate cleanroom for USP 797 compliance. See Figure 13.7 for a picture of a barrier isolator.

biological safety cabinet A ventilated cabinet designed to protect the worker, the product, and the environment with a downward HEPA-filtered airflow and a HEPA-filtered exhaust; a vertical flow laminar flow hood used to compound chemotherapeutic agents.

barrier isolator A sealed laminar flow hood that is supplied with air through a HEPA filter, maintaining a Class 5 ISO environment. It allows the compounder to access the work area through glove openings and maintain sterility without the need for a cleanroom or gowning.

Phone Triage

During the following week, Susie worked with the technician assigned to answer the phone and learned to triage the incoming calls and direct them to the correct area. She realized how important her communication skills would be now that she was speaking with healthcare professionals at many different levels. Often the calls were from a nurse concerning a medication that had not arrived on the floor when expected. Susie learned various ways to track the medication order and correct the problem.

Pharmacy Warehouse and Control Room

Susie also had an opportunity to spend time in the pharmacy warehouse. She learned the proper procedure for checking in a pharmacy order and stocking the items on the correct shelf. She was careful to rotate the stock and also learned the procedure for checking items out of the warehouse to fill medication orders. She was trained in the controlled-drug room of the warehouse, where various

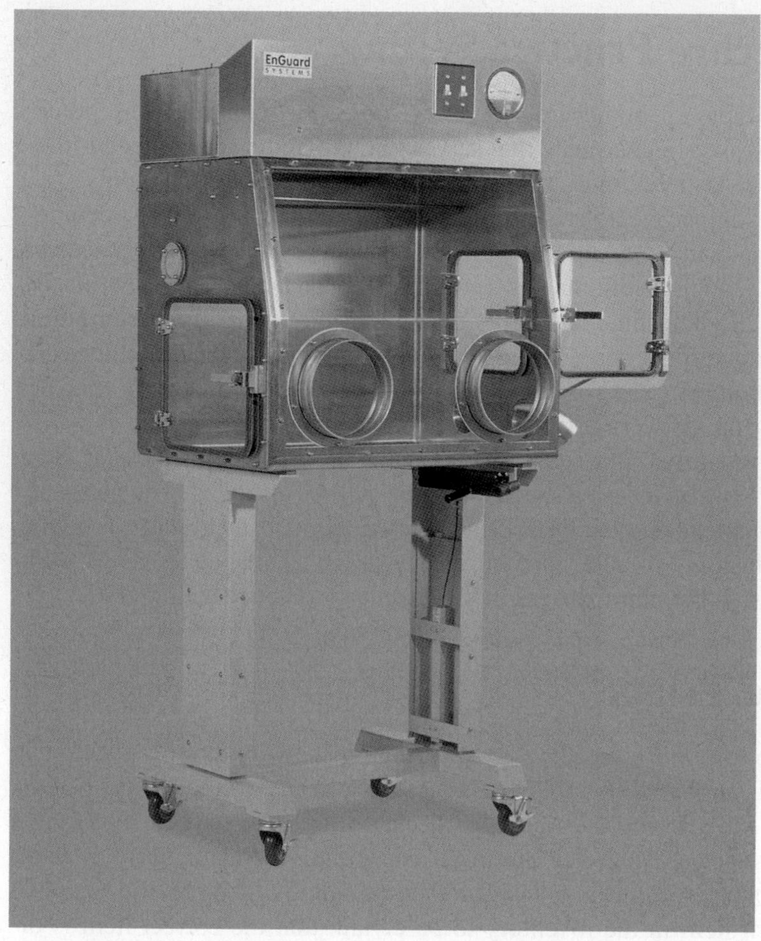

Figure 13.7 Barrier isolator. (Courtesy of Containment Technologies Group, Inc.)

automated dispensing devices were kept in a securely locked room and access was available to one trusted technician each day.

Robot Room

Finally, she spent several days in the robot room. Susie had learned in her classes that there were many types of automated dispensing machines, each with different capabilities, so she was anxious to learn the procedures for operating the robot in her practice setting. Refer back to Figure 2.3 for a picture of an automated robotic dispensing machine.

robot room A room housing a large automated dispensing system capable of dispensing medications using bar-code technology.

TIP

The technician should be familiar with the use and maintenance of all automated dispensing machines used by the practice setting.

After her 2 weeks of orientation, Susie was pleased to see her name on the schedule for the next week. She had developed a preliminary understanding of the workflow process in each area of her practice setting and could take her place as a qualified technician. Rotating through the different work areas would keep the work interesting. Susie also knew that there were opportunities for advancement in other areas of the pharmacy as she continued to grow in knowledge and skill. She would one day be eligible to work in a satellite pharmacy or mix chemotherapeutic drugs. She could advance to a technician educator position or be a technician supervisor.

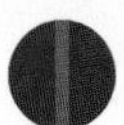

Homecare Practice Setting

There are many types of homecare practice settings, but the workflow process described here involves a pharmacy that serves nursing homes and assisted-living facilities, as well as patient homes that are located within a 100-mile radius of the pharmacy. The pharmacy employs six pharmacists and is a 24-hour operation. There are 16 technicians in addition to a technician supervisor who is responsible for hiring, training, and scheduling, and serves as a liaison between the pharmacists and management. Eight technicians work the day shift, four work the evening shift, and two work the overnight shift. This discussion will focus on the day shift workflow process. All orders called or faxed in to the pharmacy by 5:00 p.m. each day must be ready for the delivery drivers by 7:00 p.m.

Orders received after 5:00 p.m. will be sent the next day unless it is an emergency order, in which case a special delivery will be arranged. The pharmacy also carries a complete line of durable medical equipment, including IV tubing, catheters, and colostomy supplies. It is important for the technician to have a working knowledge of all the items carried in the pharmacy practice setting.

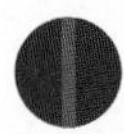

Phone Triage

The phone triage technician has the very important responsibility of ensuring that each phone call is answered in a timely manner and directed to the correct person. Communication skills are vitally important because the caller may be a patient, a physician, a nurse, or a caregiver. Questions concerning the availability of products require the phone technician to have an understanding of the specific sizes and variations of each item in the inventory to be certain that the correct item is ordered. Questions about drugs or drug interactions, or about the suitability of medical equipment for a given patient should be directed to a pharmacist. A nurse or a physician calling in a medication order for a patient should be immediately directed to a pharmacist. The phone technician is the ambassador for the pharmacy and should be adept at handling complaints or courteously directing them to the correct person.

Data Entry Technicians

Many orders for the daily pharmacy delivery will be faxed in to the pharmacy during the evening and early morning hours. The data entry technicians will remove the faxed orders from the fax machine and begin entering the information into the pharmacy software system. Orders called in to the pharmacy during the day are also entered into the pharmacy software. When the labels are printed, they will be checked against the written orders by the pharmacists and distributed to the filling technicians. It is important for the data entry technicians to be knowledgeable about the type of facility ordering the medication because this will determine the amount of medication sent and the correct packaging. Some facilities use medication carts that are exchanged each week so each patient will receive a 7-day supply of medication packaged in unit dose form to fit in the patient drawers. These med carts are filled by the night shift technicians. Others may prefer the 30-day bingo card packaging, and assisted-living facilities may prefer the medication dispensed in prescription vials.

bingo card A heat-sealed card with rows of blister packs designed to hold a 30-day supply of medication.

Order-Filling Technicians

After the labels have been checked against the order sheets by the pharmacists, they are disbursed to the filling technicians. The technicians separate the orders that require extemporaneous compounding and those that are IV admixtures, and place them in the appropriate areas. They complete the medication orders, being careful to package them in the correct manner for the facility receiving them. The completed orders, along with the paperwork, are placed in the checking area for the final check by the pharmacist. After the medication orders are checked, they are placed in the totes assigned to the facility to which they will be delivered and the order summary for that facility is checked to ensure that every order has been completed and placed in the tote.

Exchange Technician

The exchange technician is responsible for delivering medication carts to homes using a 7-day medication cart system for distributing medications to patients. The technician removes the empty cart from the home and exchanges it for a cart that has been filled at the pharmacy. This technician may be responsible for verifying amounts of drugs left in the removed carts and may assist in the billing process. The empty carts are returned to the pharmacy with the medication records and are refilled by the night-shift technicians.

Extemporaneous Compounding Technician

Orders for medications to be compounded are placed in the compounding area and prepared by the extemporaneous compounding technician. The technician will refer to the master formula sheet if the compound is one that has been prepared before. This will give the exact quantities and ingredients in addition to notes about the actual procedure for compounding. If the compound is one that has not been previously prepared in the pharmacy, the technician will calculate the amount of each ingredient needed, gather the correct ingredients, list the steps for compounding the preparation, and have the setup checked by a pharmacist (or another technician, if tech-check-tech is permitted). The compounding technician will then prepare the medication, package it in an appropriate container, apply the prescription label and the necessary auxiliary labels, and leave the paperwork and ingredients for the final check by the pharmacist. The compounding area and equipment should be thoroughly cleaned before another preparation is started. See Figure 13.8 for a picture of a compounding area.

IV Admixture Technician

The IV technician will begin the day by cleaning the laminar flow hood and restocking the supplies needed for the day, being careful to adhere to the provisions of USP 797. When the day's IV orders are received, the technician will gather the needed medications and transfer them to a cart in the anteroom. After the hand washing, gowning, and gloving procedure is completed, the IV tech will transfer the medications into the cleanroom and begin the setups in the hood. Using excellent aseptic technique, the technician prepares each admixture while double-checking each medication and all calculations. The mixtures are then placed on the checking table with the correct labels and auxiliary labels applied and the accompanying paper-

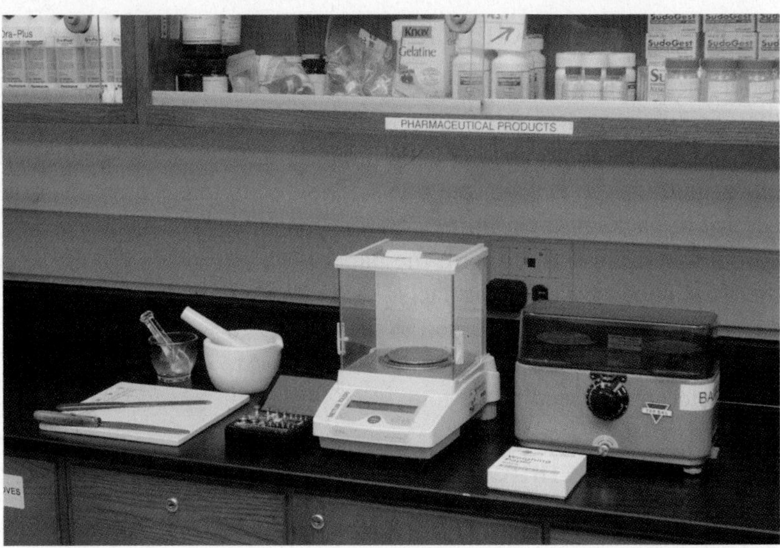

Figure 13.8 Extemporaneous compounding area.

work for the final check by the pharmacist. They are then packed in proper containers for delivery. At the end of the day, the IV technician cleans the laminar flow hood and leaves the cleanroom in proper order.

Each pharmacist and technician in the pharmacy understands the scope and standards of their practice in the homecare setting. They use their knowledge and skills as competent team members to form an efficient workflow process and provide excellent pharmaceutical care for all the patients served by the practice setting. Many, if not all, technicians are cross-trained to assist in providing seamless service during employee sick time and vacations.

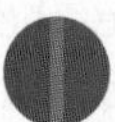

Chapter Summary

- Technician responsibilities at the front window area of an inpatient pharmacy may include processing EDKs, sending drug orders to the floors through a pneumatic tube system, and answering questions from healthcare professionals or directing them to the proper person.
- The technician delivering medications to the floors must be familiar with the layout of the hospital, understand the protocol for delivery and storage of medications, and be familiar with the automated dispensing units used by the hospital.
- A technician working in the IV area of an inpatient or a homecare pharmacy must be trained in USP 797 regulations for aseptic technique, understand the hospital protocols for IV admixture, and establish an efficient workflow process.
- To prepare TPNs, the technician must be proficient at calibrating the automated TPN compounder.
- Chemotherapeutic IV admixture requires a biological safety cabinet with a vertical airflow or a barrier isolator to provide aseptic conditions and protect the technician.
- The technician must be familiar with the procedures for cleaning a hazardous spill when mixing chemotherapeutic drugs.

- It is important for technicians to learn basic compounding skills and the required documentation for formulas and compounding techniques in inpatient and homecare practice settings.
- Technicians must be knowledgeable about all aspects of their practice setting and be able to communicate effectively with healthcare professionals.
- Each facility must devise an efficient workflow process to serve the needs of its patients.

Review Questions

Multiple Choice

Choose the best answer for the following statements.

1. The front window area of an inpatient pharmacy may involve the following technician tasks:
   a. IV admixture
   b. checking emergency drug boxes
   c. answering questions for healthcare professionals
   d. b and c
2. Items that should not be placed in a pneumatic tube system include all of the following except:
   a. unit dose antibiotic tablets
   b. unit dose narcotic tablets
   c. heparin ampules
   d. none of the above
3. IV admixture may be performed in:
   a. a cleanroom
   b. a laminar flow hood
   c. a biological safety cabinet
   d. a barrier isolator
   e. all of the above
4. Medication delivery systems include all of the following except:
   a. a barrier isolator
   b. a Pyxis automated dispensing machine
   c. a medication cart exchange
   d. a pneumatic tube system
5. Unit dose packaging may be accomplished by:
   a. filling and labeling single dose oral syringes in the pharmacy
   b. sending a 16-ounce bottle of liquid to the floor for the nurse to administer each dose
   c. using a packaging machine to package and label tablets in individual doses.
   d. a and c

Fill in the Blank

Fill in the blank(s) with the most correct word(s) to complete the statement.

6. Patients who are unable to take adequate food orally may need a daily IV containing ____________ ____________ ____________.

7. A self-contained glovebox that allows closed-system transfers of wastes and sharps with a built-in system of HEPA filtration for IV admixture is called a ____________ ____________.

8. A schedule outlining responsibilities for the technicians in the workplace is called a ____________ process.

9. ____________ ensures that each technician will be able to perform all of the responsibilities in a practice setting.

10. The ____________ technician delivers filled medication carts to nursing homes and returns the empty carts to the pharmacy.

True/False

Mark the following statements True or False.

11. ________ Although the workflow process differs between an inpatient hospital pharmacy and a homecare pharmacy, many of the basic skills are the same.

12. ________ When mixing IVs in a barrier isolator, the technician must be gowned and gloved.

13. ________ An IV chemotherapeutic admixture can be sent to the oncology unit through the pneumatic tube system.

14. ________ Like the homecare practice setting, the inpatient pharmacy delivers medications to the floor units once a day.

15. ________ Communication skills are important in the homecare setting but not in the inpatient pharmacy setting.

Matching

Match the following terms with the descriptions:

16. _____ biological safety cabinet
17. _____ unit dose machine
18. _____ phone triage
19. _____ cleanroom
20. _____ extemporaneous compounding

A. A method of packaging medications for administration to the patient.
B. A room designed to prevent contamination of sterile products while they are being prepared.
C. Laminar flow hoods with a vertical airflow used for working with hazardous substances.
D. Preparing a medication order in which two or more ingredients are mixed.
E. Answering calls and directing them to the correct person in a timely manner.

LEARNING ACTIVITY

Devise a floor plan for a homecare pharmacy setting. Include placement of the data entry computers, unit dose filling area, compounding area, IV room, and other necessary areas. Plan a workflow process to facilitate delivery of medications to patients in nursing homes and assisted-living facilities. Include the number of technicians needed and the area each will cover. Discuss the results with the class.

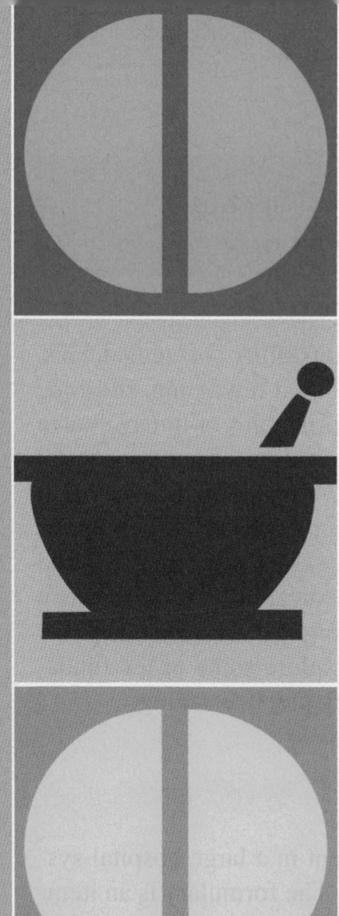

Chapter **14**

Inventory Control

OBJECTIVES

After completing this chapter, the student will be able to:

- Discuss the development and use of a formulary system.
- Outline the responsibilities of a P&T committee.
- Demonstrate knowledge of various ordering systems.
- Outline steps in the receiving process.
- Describe an invoice and order check-in process.
- Detail a process for handling and storage of items.
- Establish an inventory management system.

KEY TERMS

- ACE inhibitors
- average inventory
- computerized inventory management
- double-blind study
- expiration date
- formulary system
- inventory
- inventory budget
- inventory management
- invoice
- min/max system
- Pharmacy and Therapeutics (P&T) committee
- purchase order
- shipper's manifest

- recall
- stock rotation
- therapeutic substitution
- turnover rate
- want book

inventory All of the items a pharmacy has available for sale.

recall Notice that a product must be removed from the shelves due to various problems with the product.

turnover rate The number of times a given item is dispensed in a given time period.

Inventory control is increasingly becoming a responsibility of technicians. Managing the inventory in a large hospital system may be a rewarding, full-time position for a technician who is well versed in business principles or it may evolve as a result of on-the-job training. In a smaller retail organization, inventory control may be just a part of a technician's total responsibilities. Regardless of whether it is a full-time position or a small part of your day as a technician, the principles of inventory control are vitally important for medication safety (checking expired drugs and drug recalls), customer service (having medications in stock when needed by the patient), and the profitability of the organization (keeping the turnover rate at a reasonable level). This chapter will explore some of the fundamentals of inventory control as they apply to a pharmacy practice setting.

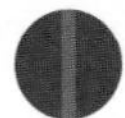

The Formulary System

formulary system A system in which a committee establishes a list of drugs approved for use by an institution.

pharmacy and therapeutics (P&T) committee A group of health professionals who are chosen to research drugs and make decisions about which drugs to include in the formulary of an institution.

A major factor in inventory control and cost management in a large hospital system is the establishment of a hospital formulary system. The formulary is an itemized list of medications that have been approved by the pharmacy and therapeutics (P&T) committee to provide the most cost-effective and efficacious medications for the patients in the system. The P&T committee consists of physicians, pharmacists, nurses, and possibly other health professionals who have been appointed to determine which drugs should be included in the formulary. Following are a number of factors to be considered when reviewing a drug for inclusion in the formulary:

- Effectiveness: Has the drug information literature been reviewed to determine whether the drug is as effective or more effective than other entities already on the formulary?
- Safety: Has there been adequate research in large groups of people to determine an accurate side-effect profile? How serious are the adverse effects?
- Abuse potential: Will the drug create a risk for abuse in the institution?
- Drug interactions: Will there be drug interactions with many of the commonly used formulary drugs?
- Therapeutic duplication: Does it offer any advantages over current formulary drugs in the same therapeutic category?
- Abuse potential: Is this a drug that will present storage concerns because of a risk for abuse?
- Medication errors: Does the drug look or sound like any other drug in the formulary, increasing the risk of medication errors?
- Cost: Does the drug offer a cost advantage over current formulary drugs for the same indication?

Often different members of the P&T committee will be responsible for researching these various factors and reporting to the committee. The committee will then vote to include the drug or exclude it from the formulary. In a large institution the P&T committee may decide to use therapeutic substitution as a way to reduce inventory costs. The committee researches all the drugs in a given class, such as the ACE inhibitors. The committee then chooses one drug from that category that is cost-effective and can be readily substituted for other drugs in the category, such as enalapril. A grid is established to define comparable doses of other ACE inhibitors so that when an order is written for another ACE inhibitor, a comparable strength of enalapril will be substituted. Formulary changes are then announced to healthcare professionals in an information bulletin sent out following a meeting of the committee. Therapeutic substitution is allowable only within the institution where physicians have been informed of the policy and agreed to it. Often there is a disclaimer on the medication order form stating that orders filled in the institution will adhere to formulary guidelines. Generally, there will be a mechanism for ordering a nonformulary drug for a particular patient. A technician involved in inventory control could be an asset to a P&T committee by addressing drug costs and usage and the likelihood of a drug contributing to medication errors.

therapeutic substitution Choosing one drug from a given drug class to be dispensed when any drug in that class is prescribed.

ACE inhibitors Class of antihypertensive drugs that may be chosen for therapeutic substitution.

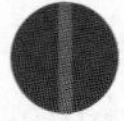

Product Buying Sources

Direct from the Manufacturer

Some manufacturers will sell directly to retail establishments, but the minimum dollar amount of an order may be prohibitive for a small business. In some cases, several pharmacies may join together to form a buying group so they can meet the manufacturer minimums. This can require a great deal of effort to coordinate the ordering date, distribute the order to each pharmacy when it arrives, and calculate payment for each participant in the group. In some instances, the cost savings may be worth the effort. However, because many manufacturers will not sell directly to retailers, a wholesaler would still be required.

Wholesale Buying

As with other businesses, most of the small drug wholesale houses have either ceased to do business or have been bought by the larger companies. Some of the large chain pharmacies have their own warehouses and most, if not all, items are ordered on a regular basis from the company warehouse. The chain may choose a preferred wholesaler to provide items that are not available from the warehouse or are needed at times other than the regular company ordering days.

Hospital systems and small retail pharmacies generally choose a wholesaler and enter into a prime vendor agreement. This involves a contract stating that the pharmacy will purchase a certain percentage of its products from the prime wholesale house in return for pre-established discounts and services to be provided by the vendor. Orders from a prime vendor are generally received the day after they are ordered. Large wholesalers may have an online Web page listing all items available and the number of each item in stock so a pharmacy can determine if it will receive an item in the next day's order. The prime vendor will have a generous return policy for items that have been misordered, are near the expiration date, or are overstocked. The returns may be processed by a representative from the wholesale house, an employee of the pharmacy, or a company that processes returned goods for a fee.

expiration date Date established by the manufacturer of a drug after which the potency of the drug is no longer guaranteed.

Ordering Processes

want book A book kept in some pharmacies to jot down items that need to be ordered.

min/max system An ordering system based on establishing the minimum and maximum levels for each item carried.

purchase order Document originated by an institution listing the items ordered.

The simplest ordering system involves writing items in a want book or tossing empty bottles in a box until the end of the day and then sending an order by phone, fax, or computer modem. Another method, called the min/max system, involves bar-coding the shelves and calculating the minimum and maximum amounts for each drug. The technician then uses a hand-held computerized machine to scan the bar codes of items that need to be ordered. The hand-held device can then be connected to a phone line or a computer modem to transmit the order. Some large wholesale companies may have an online Web page connected to pharmacies by a modem that allows online ordering. In a fully computerized system, each dispensing transaction is automatically subtracted from a perpetual inventory log. All products received are added to the log. When the quantity reaches a predetermined par level, a purchase order is generated. Automated dispensing machines, such as the Pyxis machines placed in decentralized locations in nursing units, are connected to a mainframe computer in the pharmacy that prints a list of medications that need to be restocked.

Schedule II drugs must be ordered using a DEA form 222 filled out in triplicate and hand delivered to the driver, who takes it to the wholesaler. The signature on the DEA form must be the signature of the person authorized to order schedule II drugs for that facility. The form must be filled out completely and accurately with no erasures or words crossed out. The exact drug, strength, dosage form, package size, and quantity of the drug should be listed along with the NDC number.

Receiving Process

shipper's manifest Document presented by the person delivering an order describing the number of boxes included in the order.

The receiving process begins when the order arrives at the pharmacy. The receiving technician should verify each box received from the shipper or delivery person. The delivery person will have a shipper's manifest indicating the number of boxes being delivered. The technician should verify that the correct number of boxes is being delivered. The boxes should be examined for apparent damage. Any damage should be noted on the manifest or the box refused. Products that require special storage, such as refrigeration or freezing, should be noted so they can be processed promptly. Boxes or packages containing controlled drugs may require a pharmacist's signature on the manifest. When the order has been verified, the driver's manifest should be signed without delay so the driver can continue on his or her delivery route.

Checking the Order

invoice Document that accompanies each order and lists the items sent, the quantity, the cost of each item, the total invoice cost, and the terms of payment.

There are two documents that should be consulted when checking in an order. The purchase order and want book or computerized printout of the items actually ordered should be consulted to ascertain that no items were sent in error and that no ordered item is missing. An invoice will accompany the order listing the name, brand, dosage form, package size, strength, and quantity of each item sent. The cost of the item, any discounts, and the terms of payment will also be listed. Each item received should be carefully checked against the invoice for all the above factors and the expiration date should also be checked. Any ordered item that was not received should be reordered for the next day. If the item was needed for an order to be picked up that day, the patient may have to be called or the technician may need to find the item at another pharmacy to assist the patient. Generally, a newly ordered item should have at least 6 months left before the expiration date. On a busy day, items may be needed to fill prescriptions before the order is checked. When an item is removed before being properly checked, the person removing the item should create a written record of the item removed and the initials of the person removing it to prevent discrepancies later. When the order has been completely checked, the invoice should be dated and initialed. It should then be promptly sent on to the accounts payable department or the person responsible for payment so that no available discounts will be lost due to late payments.

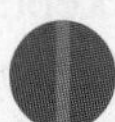

Product Storage and Handling

The checked order can now be placed in stock. The inventory technician may want to check the box for any prescriptions on hold from the previous day awaiting an item in the order. These items can now be placed on the counter with the order for processing. As the order items are placed on the appropriate shelf, it is important for the technician to check the label three times to be certain that it is being placed in the proper spot. Stock rotation will ensure that older products are used before the new items.

Stock rotation Placing items that expire first in front of those with later expiration dates.

CAUTION

Look-alike products that are placed in the wrong place will increase the risk of medication errors.

The manufacturer's packaging often emphasizes the company logo rather than the drug name and strength. Products similar in appearance should be stored separately or in a manner that will enable them to be distinguished from each other. As liquids and injectables are placed in the proper storage area, the technician should note whether they require refrigeration or freezing, and/or protection from light. A quick examination of the color and clarity of the product should be performed.

Expiration Dating

The inventory should be checked regularly (at least monthly) for expired medications. In a large institution the inventory technician should set up a schedule for this task to be performed and documented. Often, each technician will be assigned a certain section of the pharmacy to inspect for expired medications and a pharmacist will document the inspection. There will be a policy concerning when a drug should be removed from the shelf (usually 6–8 weeks before the expiration date). All satellite pharmacy areas and all floor stock must be included in the inspections. Opened liquids and injectables are required to be marked with the date the product was opened. Any floor stock items in bottles that are not properly labeled and dated should be discarded during the inspection. Hospital staff may need to be reminded of storage rules for floor stock medications. Expired medications must be disposed of properly. Unopened bottles may sometimes be returned for credit, which requires the proper forms to be filled out. Most institutions and large chain pharmacies contract with a returned-goods company that will process all their expired products for a fee. The disposal process for controlled drugs is more complicated and can vary from state to state. Be sure to learn the regulations for your state.

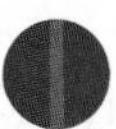 Investigational Drugs

Research for most drugs is conducted in conjunction with hospital pharmacies. Each study will have very specific protocols for the selection of study participants and strict guidelines for the dispensing and return of unused drugs. Investigational drugs may be dispensed through the regular hospital pharmacy system or there may be an investigational drug pharmacy satellite with pharmacists and technicians specially trained to follow the strict protocols established for the drugs during the research study. Inventory management of study drugs is critical because the drugs can be obtained only from the manufacturer and dispensed only to persons enrolled in the study. Any unused drug must be returned and strict records must be kept. Details about the drugs, study protocols, and patients involved are confidential. In a double-blind study, the pharmacy personnel are the only ones who know which participants are taking the study drug and which are taking a placebo.

inventory management An organized method of controlling inventory to optimize profitability while serving the needs of patients.

double-blind study An investigational drug study in which neither the patient nor the physician knows whether the patient is receiving the study drug or a placebo. Only the pharmacy knows.

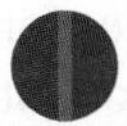 Controlled Drugs

There are special inventory and storage requirements for controlled drugs, and some of these may vary from state to state. Each institution will have established storage policies. In a large institution, controlled drugs are often kept in a locked room with access restricted to certain personnel. There are automated dispensing machines specifically designed to provide extra security for controlled drugs or any drug that may be an item of abuse. In a retail pharmacy, controlled drugs may be distributed alphabetically on the open shelves of the pharmacy. They should not be stored together in a controlled-drug section unless it is inside a safe or locked area. A biennial inventory of all controlled drugs is required, but many facilities keep a daily record of all class II transactions. Schedule II records must be kept separately from other records, and schedules III, IV, and V records must be kept in an area where they can be easily produced on request. State board inspectors often check controlled-drug invoices against daily dispensing records to look for any buying discrepancies. Keeping such records can be a very time-intensive procedure, and a technician can be a vital link in the process.

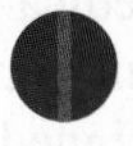 Inventory Management

An effective inventory management process is vital to maintain the profitability of a pharmacy department. The inventory is all of the items a pharmacy has in stock for sale or dispensing to customers or patients. Most pharmacies have an inventory budget established by the institution or the pharmacy owners. This may be between $100,000 and $800,000 depending on the type of pharmacy. A retail pharmacy with daily ordering capability and a high turnover rate would be able to manage with a lower inventory amount, and therefore fewer dollars would be tied up in inventory costs. The turnover rate is the number of times each item in the stock is dispensed and reordered in a year's time. It can be calculated by taking the total cost of goods for the year and dividing it by the average inventory. The average inventory is calculated by taking the beginning inventory in a given time period, adding it to the ending inventory, and then dividing this number by two. Calculating the average inventory and turnover rates can provide a quick snapshot of how well the inventory is being managed. Removing expired drugs from the

inventory budget The amount of money allocated to the pharmacy for the purchase of supplies.

average inventory A figure calculated by adding a beginning inventory and an ending inventory for the desired period of time, and dividing that sum by two.

shelf, promptly sending back recalled drugs, and lowering the amounts on hand for infrequently used drugs are all methods for keeping inventory levels in line. Even with computerized inventory management, the minimum and maximum amounts to have on hand must be adjusted periodically to keep inventory levels well managed. Inventory control requires a great amount of time and effort, but a poorly managed inventory can destroy the profitability of a pharmacy.

computerized inventory management A system that records all purchases and dispensing of items, and produces a purchase order when items reach a certain minimum level.

Chapter Summary

- Inventory management plays an important role in medication safety, customer service, and the profitability of a pharmacy.
- Establishing a formulary system will assist with inventory control and cost management in an institution.
- The P&T committee makes decisions about formulary products for an institution.
- Buying directly from manufacturers can save costs, but it may require a large minimum order.
- Most pharmacies enter into a prime vendor agreement with a wholesaler, which provides generous discounts and return policies in return for an agreement to purchase a large percentage of items from the prime vendor.
- Ordering processes can vary from a simple want-book system to a very advanced computerized inventory management system.
- The receiving process involves checking the shipper's manifest to verify that the correct numbers of boxes are delivered and the boxes are not visibly damaged. Then the shipper's manifest is signed.
- The order must be checked against the invoice and the purchase order to ensure that the items were shipped as ordered.
- The items in the checked order should be placed in the proper storage area to prevent medication errors.
- There are special inventory requirements for controlled drugs and investigational drugs.
- An inventory management process is vital to maintain the profitability of a pharmacy.

Review Questions

Multiple Choice

Choose the best answer for the questions below.

1. Factors considered by the P&T committee in choosing formulary drugs are:
   a. cost
   b. effectiveness
   c. abuse potential
   d. all of the above

2. A prime vendor agreement is made between:
   a. several retail pharmacies
   b. pharmacies and manufacturers
   c. a pharmacy and a wholesaler
   d. none of the above

3. All of the following are associated with the ordering process except:
   a. a want book
   b. rotation of stock
   c. min/max inventory levels
   d. a hand-held bar code scanner

4. Checking in a pharmacy order requires:
   a. consulting the purchase order
   b. checking the name, strength, package size, and quantity of each item sent
   c. calculating the turnover of each item
   d. a and b

5. When an item is needed for a prescription before the order has been checked in:
   a. the customer should be told to return later after the order has been checked.
   b. The item can be removed from the order and a note can be placed in the order describing the item that has been removed.
   c. Items can be removed as needed and the checker will assume the items have all been sent.
   d. None of the above.

Fill in the Blank

Fill in the blanks with the correct term.

6. The group of professionals who make decisions about the drugs included in a hospital formulary is called the ______________________________.

7. The number of times an item is dispensed in a given time period is called the ______________________________.

8. Placing the items with the earliest expiration dates at the front of the shelf is an example of ______________________________.

9. The form required to order schedule II drugs is called ______________.

10. The form listing the items being delivered by the wholesaler is called the ______________________________.

True/False

Mark the following statements True or False. If the statement is False, change it to make it true.

11. __________ The shipper's manifest lists each item included in the order.

12. ________ Products should be removed from the shelf when the expiration date is reached.

13. ________ A prime vendor agreement requires a pharmacy to purchase most of its items from a certain wholesaler.

14. ________ Inventory can be managed by pharmacy technicians.

15. ________ Automated dispensing machines can help with inventory management.

Matching

Match the following terms with the descriptions:

16. _____ Document that lists each item included in the order.

17. _____ Choosing one drug in a class of drugs to be dispensed when any drug in that class is prescribed.

18. _____ A figure derived by dividing the sum of the beginning inventory and the ending inventory by two

19. _____ A system in which certain drugs are chosen to be included in the pharmacy stock by a group of professionals.

20. _____ A document that lists the number of boxes being delivered.

A. Average inventory
B. Formulary system
C. Therapeutic substitution
D. Shipper's manifest
E. Invoice

UNIT V

Extemporaneous Compounding

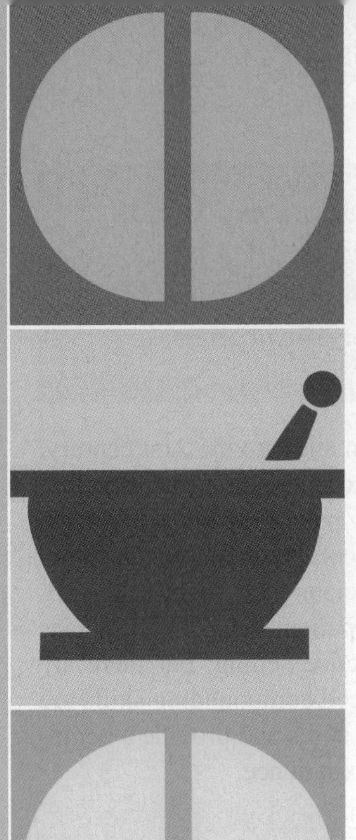

Chapter 15

Compounding Equipment and Use

OBJECTIVES

After completing this chapter, the student will be able to:

- Discuss the rationale and guidelines for extemporaneous compounding.
- Identify compounding equipment used to measure volume.
- Choose the proper volumetric measuring device for a given task.
- Level a prescription torsion balance and demonstrate weighing procedures.
- Tare an electronic prescription balance and demonstrate weighing procedures.
- Identify types of mortars and pestles and discuss the rationale for their use.
- Demonstrate different mixing techniques and equipment.
- Identify patients who would benefit from extemporaneous compounding.
- List dosage forms and routes of administration for compounded products.
- Differentiate between manufacturing and compounding with reference to legal guidelines.

KEY TERMS

- aliquot
- beakers
- calibrate
- capsule filling machine
- conical graduates
- cylindrical graduates
- electronic balance
- filter paper
- levigate
- lozenge mold
- meniscus
- mortars
- ointment mill
- ointment pad
- oral syringe
- ovals
- pestles

- pipettes
- prescription torsion balance
- prescription quality weights
- prescription weights
- spatulas
- spatulate
- stirring rods
- suppository molds
- tare
- weighing boat
- weighing paper

From the early development of the pharmacy profession and into the 21st century, pharmacy professionals considered extemporaneous compounding an important part of the art of pharmacy. With the introduction of patent medicines and the growth of the manufacturing industry, pharmaceutical compounding began to decline. In recent years, however, pharmacists and physicians have realized the advantages of individualizing products to meet specific patient needs. Technicians should possess basic compounding skills for any practice setting, but there are many specialty compounding pharmacies where advanced compounding skills are needed. The following chapters will introduce the basic skills and provide a beginning for technicians who desire further compounding experience.

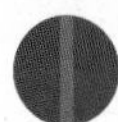

Definition of Compounding

The National Association of Boards of Pharmacy (NABP) defines compounding as "the preparation, mixing, assembling, packaging, or labeling of a drug or device as a result of a practitioner's prescription drug order based on the patient/pharmacist/practitioner relationship in a professional practice." This triangular relationship is vital for determining the legality of extemporaneous compounding that does not require strict regulation by manufacturing standards. Most state pharmacy practice acts have guidelines for compounding in pharmacies. It is important to follow these guidelines, just as it is important to be knowledgeable and careful during the process of calculating amounts of ingredients, weighing, measuring, and compounding procedures.

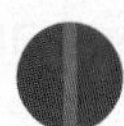

Basic Compounding Procedures

Preparation Method 15.1
Preparing a Compounded Product

1. Examine the prescription or medication order for clarity of ingredients and amounts. Discuss any concerns with a pharmacist.
2. Perform any needed calculations. Have them checked by a pharmacist or another technician.
3. Determine the compounding procedure and gather the ingredients and necessary equipment.
4. Weigh and/or measure each ingredient.
5. If possible, have the setup checked by a pharmacist or another technician.
6. Using correct technique, prepare the product.

7. Choose an appropriate container and package the compound.
8. Apply a label containing pertinent information and the expiration date. Include any necessary auxiliary labels.
9. Document the compounding procedure and ingredients on a master formula sheet.
10. Leave the product with the formula sheet and medication order in the assigned area for a final check by the pharmacist.

Legislation Concerning Compounding

The Food Drug Modernization Act of 1997 addressed the issue of extemporaneous compounding by stating that it must take place in a state-licensed pharmacy or be done by a state-licensed physician. Any bulk substances used must comply with USP or NF standards or be approved by the FDA. No ingredients that have been removed from the market due to safety or efficacy concerns can be used, and there can be no copies of commercially available products. Finally, the compound must be for an individual patient on the order of a prescriber. Practices that indicate a pharmacy is involved in manufacturing procedures include the following:

- bulk compounding of a product for nationwide distribution
- advertising compounded products
- selling at wholesale to other companies

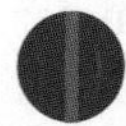

Reasons for Compounding

One of the benefits for the pharmacists and technicians who practice extemporaneous compounding is the professional satisfaction of being able to individualize products to meet specific patient needs. Working with physicians to provide excellent pharmaceutical care for individuals who have not found a commercially available product to meet their needs is very rewarding for the pharmacists and technicians involved. They also have an opportunity to expand their areas of expertise into preparing drugs for research projects or radiopharmaceuticals for special procedures.

Some patient populations that can be well served by pharmacy professionals who are willing to compound special formulations are children and the elderly, who may have difficulty swallowing conventional medications or have special dosing requirements. Patients with difficult dermatologic problems can benefit from the pharmacist and physician working together to formulate a product that will provide relief. An important field of compounding, since the controversy about hormone replacement therapy in menopausal patients has arisen, is the compounding of bioidentical hormones. Hospice patients may have special medication needs as they try to find comfort in the final days of a terminal disease. Also, veterinary medicine has expanded, as science has provided us with the knowledge and technology to provide better care for animals. The need for pharmacists and technicians who are experienced in compounding is again growing and the opportunities for professional development are great. Table 15.1 lists some of the dosage forms that can be formulated to assist patients in finding a product that has been individualized to meet their special needs.

Table 15.1 Compounded Dosage Forms

Suspensions	Freeze pops	Lollipops
Lozenges	Gummy gels	Capsules
Tablets	Tablet triturates	SR capsules
Ointments	Creams	Gels
Lip balms	Topical application sticks	Bioidentical hormones

Compounding Facilities

The pharmacy should have a separate area away from the data entry and dispensing area set aside for compounding. It should be well lighted and ventilated, with adequate shelf space to accommodate the compounding chemicals and equipment. There should also be adequate counter space to perform the compounding procedures. In close proximity to the compounding area should be a sink with hot and cold running water for hand washing and cleaning the compounding area. Trash containers should be nearby and must be maintained on a regular basis.

cylindrical graduates Graduates that have volumetric markings and parallel sides from top to bottom.

conical graduates Graduates with volumetric markings for measuring liquids. The sides of the graduate flare out from the bottom to the top.

meniscus The curved margin formed at the top of a liquid being measured in a graduate. The measurement should be taken at the bottom of the curve.

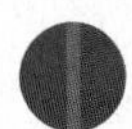

Compounding Equipment

Volumetric Measuring Equipment

Liquids are measured in a pharmacy setting using graduates of various shapes and sizes. Cylindrical graduates have sides that are parallel and are the same diameter from top to bottom. They may be made of either plastic or glass and are considered more accurate than conical graduates. Conical graduates have sides that flare out at the top. A pharmacy should have several sizes and types of graduates to accommodate the measuring needs. The smallest graduate that can measure the amount of liquid needed should be used because this improves accuracy. A 100-mL graduate should not be chosen to measure 20 mL or less.

TIP **When measuring liquids in a graduate, the technician should use the bottom of the** meniscus **as the measuring point, as shown in Figure 15.1.**

oral syringe A syringe intended to administer oral liquids; also used as a measuring device in compounding.

pipettes Thin hollow tubes used for volumetric measuring; they may be either single-volume or calibrated to measure more than one amount.

beakers Glass receptacles that are suitable for mixing liquid preparations but not for accurately measuring volume.

ovals Another name for amber prescription bottles with volumetric markings.

Smaller amounts of liquids can be measured using an oral syringe, which can range in volume from 1 mL to 10 mL. These syringes have markings on the barrel to facilitate measuring and are disposable. To measure small amounts of liquids, there are also pipettes, which are thin glass tubes that can be either calibrated pipettes or single-volume pipettes. See Figures 15.1 and 15.2 for pictures of volumetric measuring devices. Glass beakers are important for mixing liquids and can be used for hot water baths when needed, but they do not have exact graduated markings and are not suitable for volumetric measuring. See Figure 15.3 for a picture of glass beakers.

Graduated prescription bottles, called ovals, are adequate for measuring amounts of manufactured products for dispensing purposes, but should not be used to measure liquids in a compounded prescription.

Weighing Solid Materials

To accurately weigh solid dosage forms or powdered chemicals, a prescription balance is needed. There are two basic types of prescription balances commonly found in pharmacy practice settings. Many state practice acts list the Class A

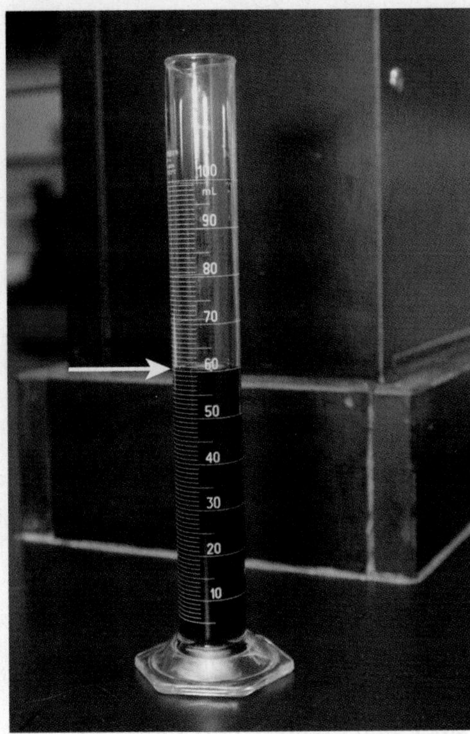

Figure 15.1 Volume is measured at the bottom of the meniscus. This is a cylindrical graduate, which has sides that are parallel. Cylindrical graduates come in various sizes.

prescription torsion balance, which is now called a Class III by the National Institute for Standards and Technology, as the required balance. This balance has a sensitivity requirement of 6 mg and a usual capacity of 15.5 g. Some Class III balances may have greater capacities of up to 60 or 120 g. If this is the case, it will be noted on the balance. See Figure 15.4 for a Class III double pan prescription torsion balance, with the various parts indicated. Only prescription quality weights are to be used to weigh substances for compounded prescriptions. Weights must be stored in a rigid compartmentalized box and should be handled only with forceps to prevent contamination by oils on the hands of the technician. Most prescription weights contain both metric and apothecary weights, but generally only metric weights are used. See Figure 15.5 for a prescription weight set.

prescription torsion balance Class A or class III double pan torsion balance calibrated to specific standards acceptable for prescription compounding.

prescription quality weights Prescription weights that have been checked for accuracy by the Department of Weights and Measures.

prescription weights A set of finely calibrated metric and apothecary weights approved for use in prescription compounding.

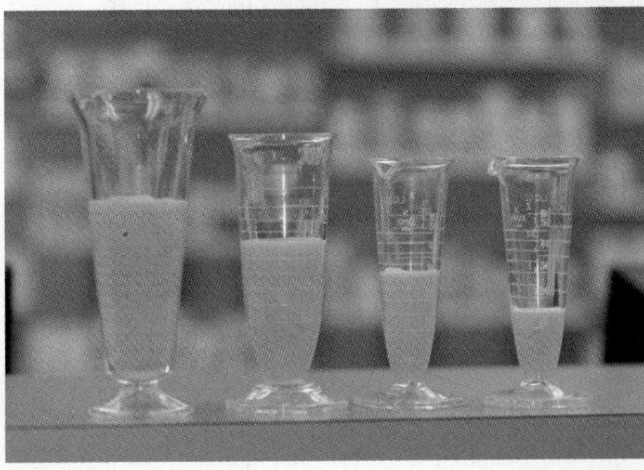

Figure 15.2 Conical graduates, which come in various sizes, have sides that angle outward and increase in circumference at the top.

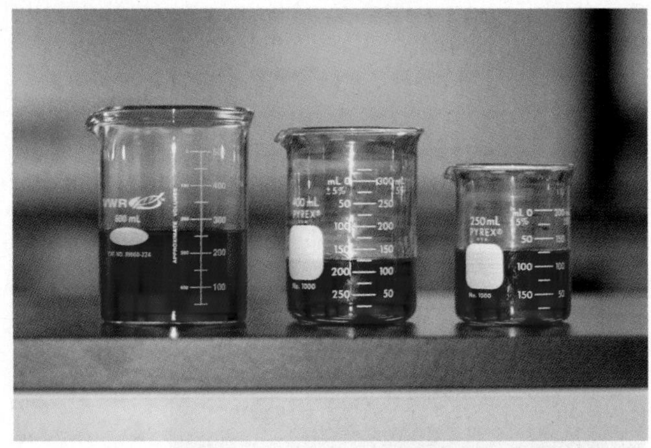

Figure 15.3 Glass beakers may have graduated markings but are not considered accurate for measuring volume.

CAUTION **When both apothecary and metric weights are present, the technician must be extremely careful to select the weight from the correct system.**

weighing paper Coated paper that comes in various sizes and can be creased to form a pocket to hold the substance being weighed.

Substances to be weighed may be placed on a glassine weighing paper that has been folded to form an indentation that will assist in keeping the substance on the paper. For larger amounts of chemicals or thick liquids, a weighing boat is used. Figure 15.6A shows a weighing paper, and Figure 15.6B shows a weighing boat.

CAUTION **Never place the substance to be weighed directly on the balance pan, to prevent corrosive chemicals from damaging the pan and to prevent cross-contamination of drugs as they are being weighed.**

weighing boat Small plastic receptacle used to hold a substance to be weighed.

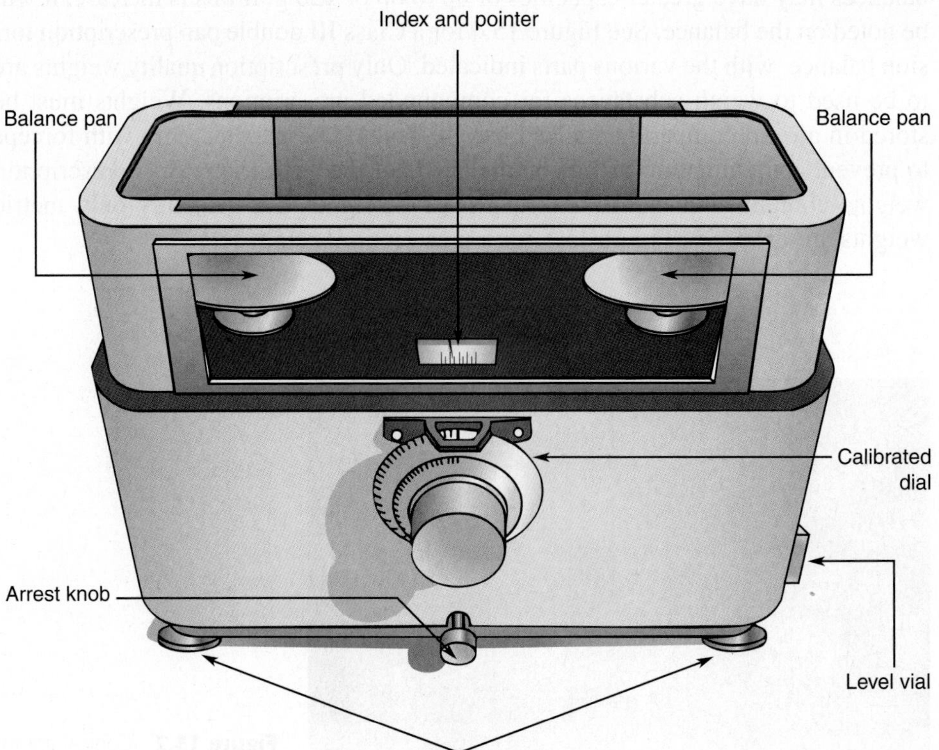

Figure 15.4 The parts of the Class III prescription balance can be adjusted for accuracy. (Reprinted with permission from Mohr ME. Lab Experiences for the Pharmacy Technician. Baltimore, MD: Lippincott, Williams & Wilkins, 2006.)

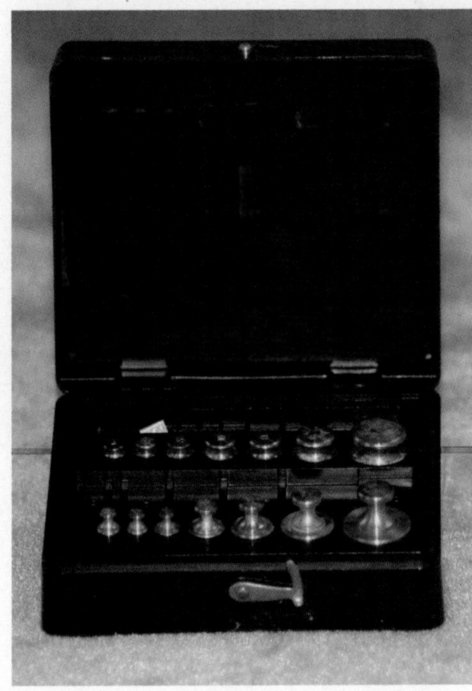

Figure 15.5 Metric prescription weights for use on a prescription balance. (Reprinted with permission from Lacher BE. Pharmaceutical Calculations for the Pharmacy Technician. Baltimore, MD: Lippincott, Williams & Wilkins, 2008.)

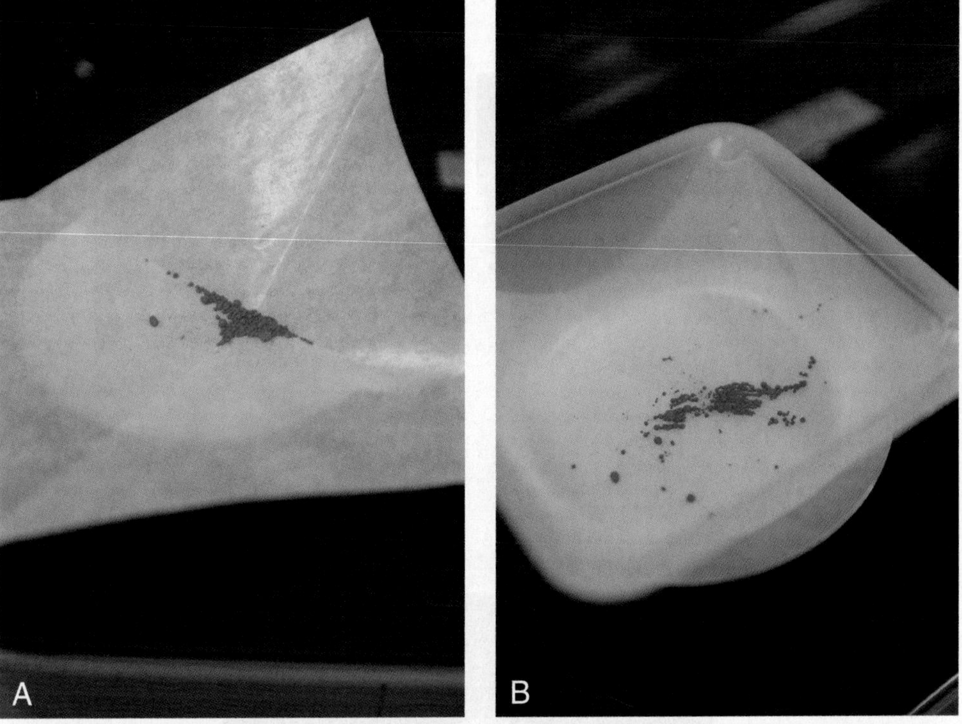

Figure 15.6 Weighing papers and boats are used to protect the surface of the balance from chemical erosion.

See the student CD and website for a video of this procedure.

Preparation Method 15.2
Weighing a Powder on a Prescription Torsion Balance

1. Place the balance on a clean flat surface away from air vents and open windows. Check the balance pans for any residue. Set the calibration dial to zero. (See Fig. 15.7A.)
2. Open the arrest knob and check the index pointer to see if the balance is leveled. (See Fig. 15.7B.)
3. If the pointer is not in the center of the index, carefully rotate the leveling screws in the correct direction to bring the pointer to a level position. Lock the arrest knob. (See Fig. 15.7C.)

TIP **To level the balance, turn the leveling screw on the side of the balance pan that needs to be lowered in a counter-clockwise direction.**

4. Add the correct weight to the pan on the right side of the balance. You may use the calibration dial for amounts less than 1 gram. Turning the calibration dial will add weight to the right side pan of the balance. (See Fig. 15.7D.)

TIP **Be sure to account for the weight of the weighing paper or boat by placing one on each side of the balance before leveling it.**

5. With the arrest knob still locked, add a small amount of the substance to the left pan of the balance. (See Fig. 15.7E.)

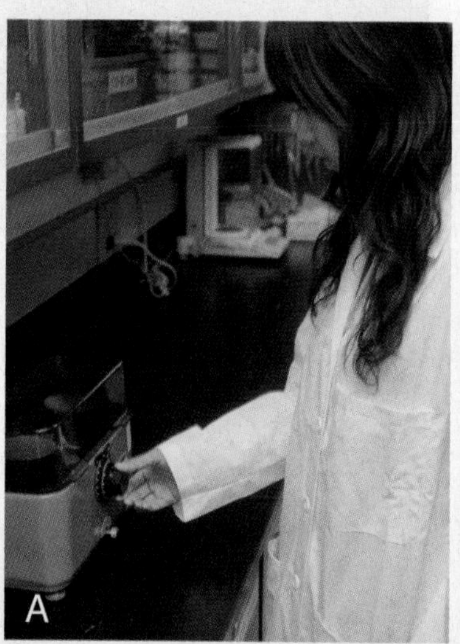
A

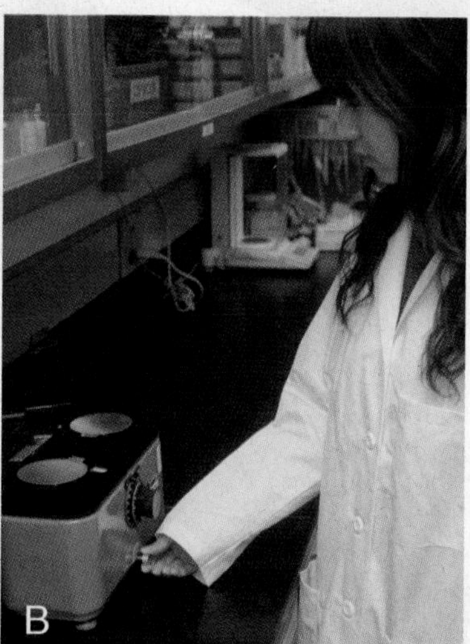
B

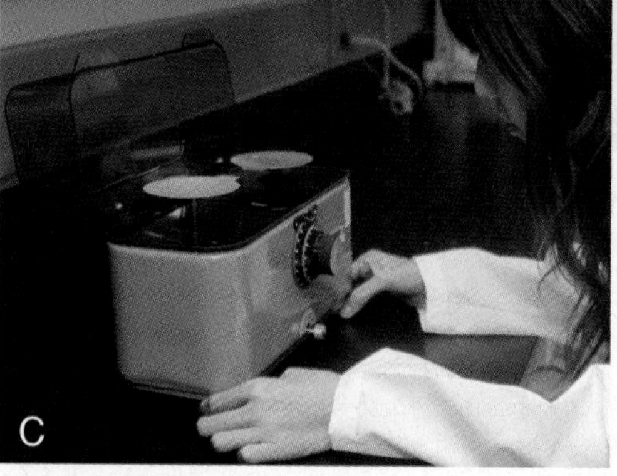
C

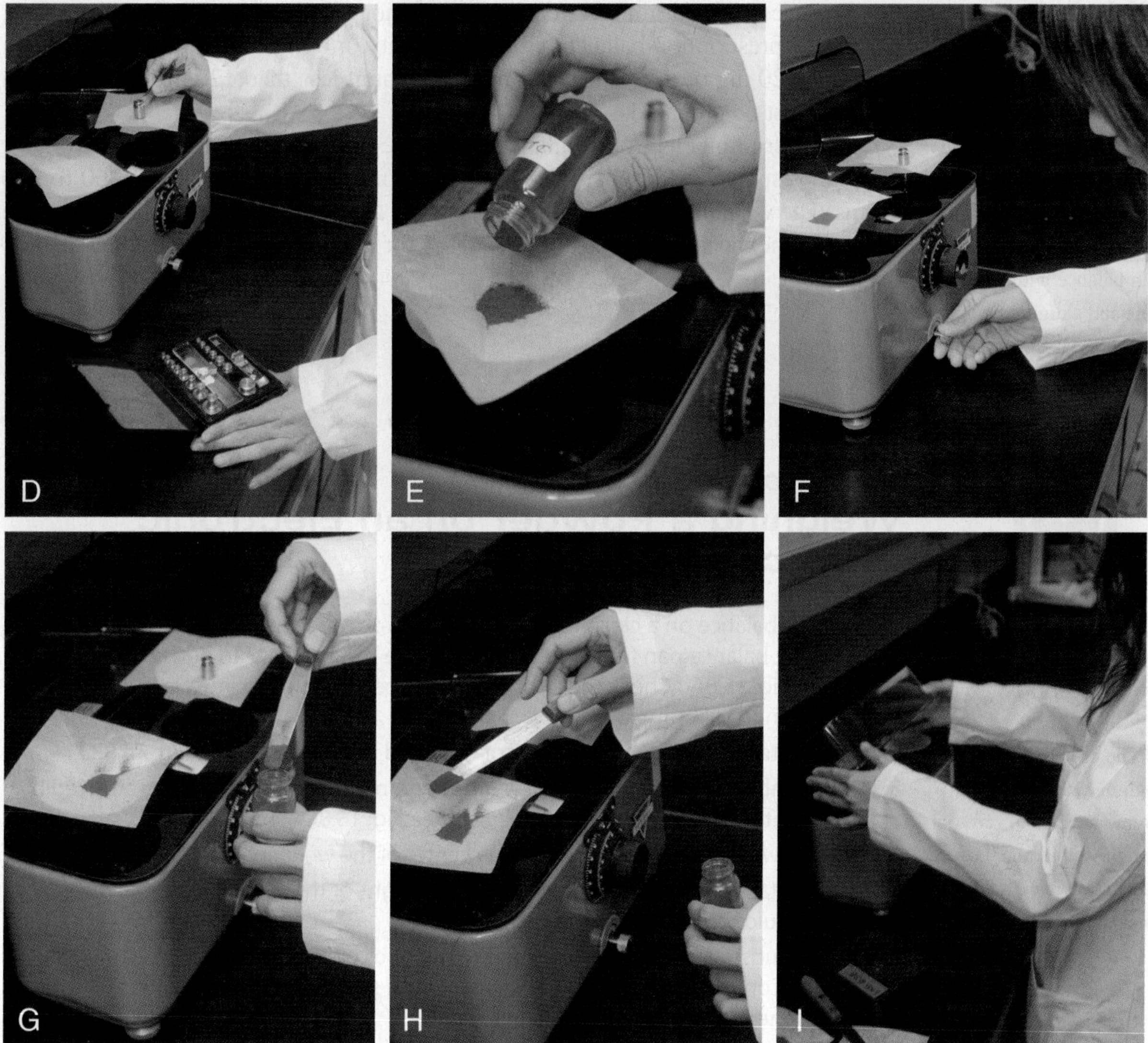

Figure 15.7 Steps for weighing a powder on a prescription torsion balance.

6. Unlock the arrest knob and observe the balance pointer to determine whether the powder added was too little or too much. If the pointer rests to the left of the index center, too much substance has been added. If the pointer is to the right of the center, too little substance has been added. (See Fig. 15.7F.)
7. Lock the arrest knob and add or remove the substance being weighed, opening and closing the arrest knob with each addition or deletion to check the balance. (See Fig. 15.7G.)
8. When the pointer is near equilibrium, it will move back and forth within the index when the arrest knob is released. At this point, you may leave the knob unlocked and add minute amounts of substance by placing a small amount on the spatula and gently tapping the spatula until the balance reaches equilibrium, as indicated by the pointer resting in the center of the index. Lock the arrest knob and remove the weighing paper or boat with the weighed substance. (See Fig. 15.7H.)
9. After completing the weighing process, replace the weights and tweezers in the weight box and close the lid. Clean the balance and pans of any residue and close the balance lid. Clean residue from the spatula and the counters, and return each item to its proper place. (See Fig. 15.7I.)

aliquot An aliquot is produced by adding a diluent to a weighable amount of the drug and weighing the part of the mixture that contains the correct amount of the desired drug.

electronic balance A single pan balance with internal weights and a digital readout display.

The accepted margin of error for prescription compounding is 5%. Therefore, a Class III prescription balance with a sensitivity of 6 mg cannot accurately weigh less than 120 mg of a substance. When an amount less than 120 mg is needed, an aliquot must be prepared.

A prescription electronic balance is a single pan balance with internal weights, a digital display, and a sensitivity of 1 mg. It may have a capacity of 100 to 210 grams. The weighing procedure is simpler with an electronic balance, and some are relatively inexpensive. Refer to Figure 15.8 for a picture of an electronic balance.

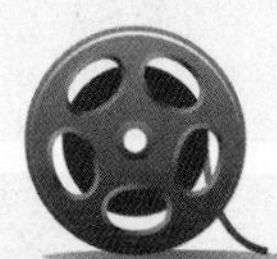

See the student CD and website for a video of this procedure.

Preparation Method 15.3
Weighing a Powder on an Electronic Balance

tare The process of adding a weighing receptacle to an electronic balance to zero out the weight so that the balance will accurately weigh the chemical.

1. Place the balance on a clean flat surface away from air vents or open windows. Check the balance pan for any residue. Plug the balance into an outlet and turn it on. (See Fig. 15.8A.) Check the accuracy of the balance by placing a known weight on the pan to calibrate it.
2. Press the tare button. The digital display should read 0.000 g. (See Fig. 15.8B.)
3. If the numbers on the digital display are changing, the balance is being affected by movements or air currents. Close the lid. (See Fig. 15.8C.)
4. Place the weighing paper or boat in the center of the weighing pan. (See Fig. 15.8D.)
5. Press the tare button again to zero out the weight of the boat. The digital display again should read 0.000 g. (See Fig. 15.8E.)
6. Add the substance to be weighed to the paper or boat on the balance pan of the balance. Continue adding small amounts of the substance until the digital readout reaches the amount needed. (See Fig. 15.8F.)
7. Remove the substance and clean the balance pan. Turn the balance off when weighing is completed. (See Fig. 15.8G.)

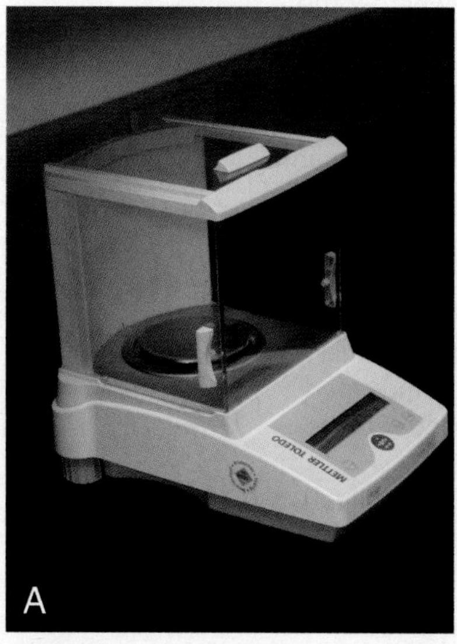

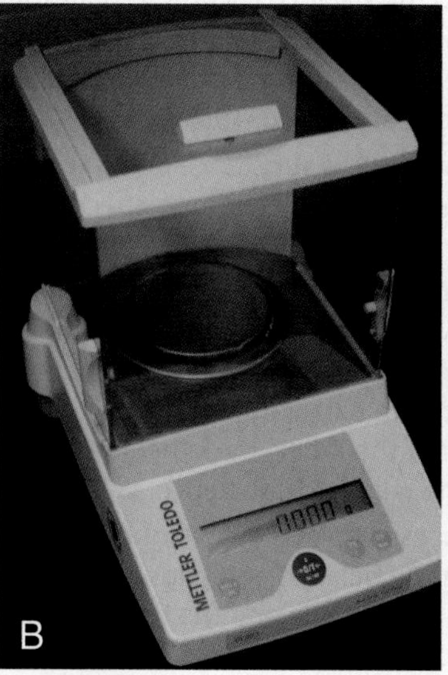

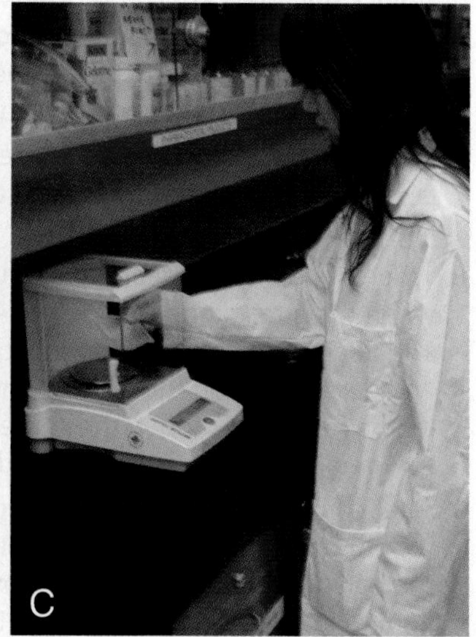

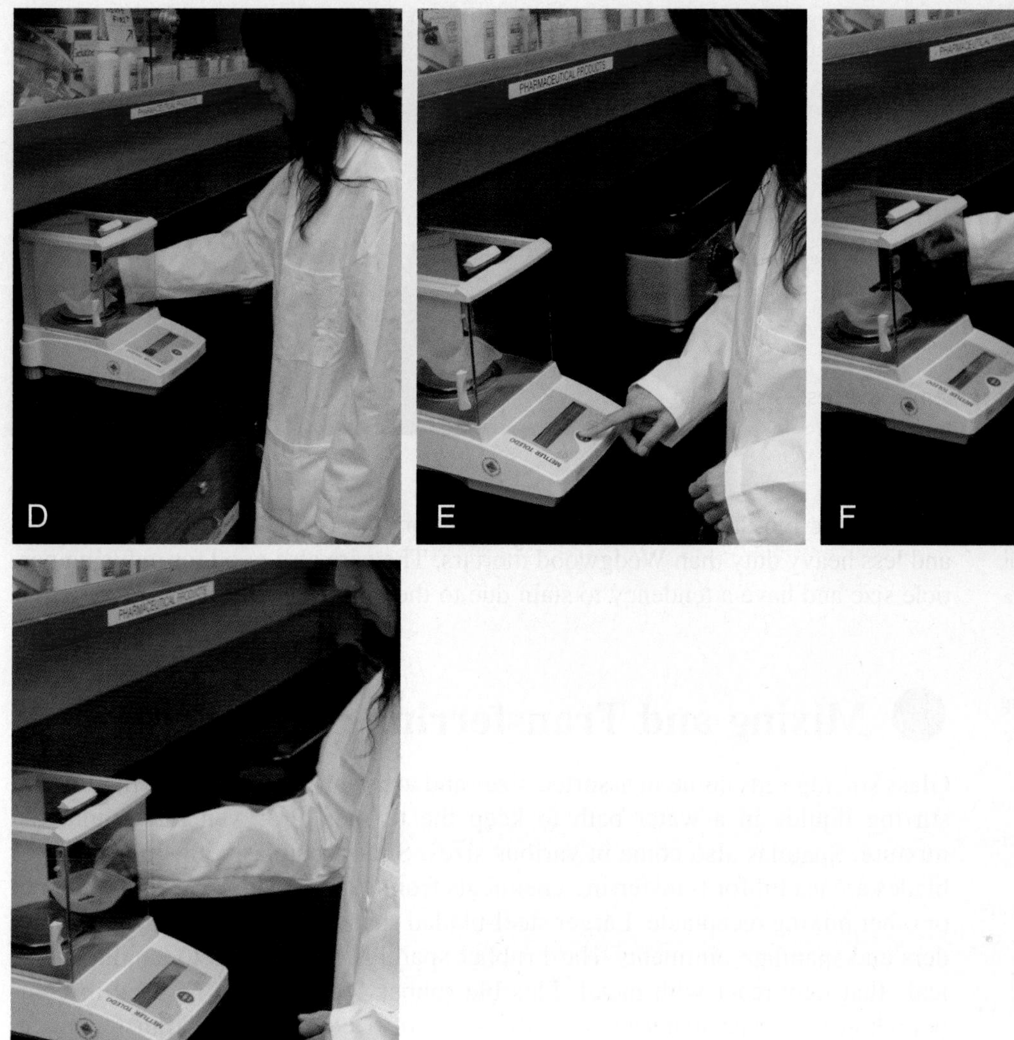

Figure 15.8 Steps for weighing a powder on an electronic balance.

Mortars and Pestles

There are three types of mortars and pestles used in pharmacy compounding. See Figure 15.9 for a picture of mortars and pestles. Clear glass mortars have a smooth, nonporous interior surface. They are available in various sizes and are useful for triturating drugs that might stain a more porous surface, and for very potent drugs. Because of their smooth surface, they are not effective for reducing the particle size of powders.

mortars Pharmacy receptacles used for mixing, triturating, or pulverizing substances.

pestles Devices used with mortars to mix, triturate, or pulverize substances being compounded.

Wedgwood mortars have a rough interior surface that is excellent for reducing the particle size of powders, but they may stain if used for drugs that have a tendency to stain, and the porous surface may retain some of the drug, so they are not suitable for very potent drugs or those used in very small quantities.

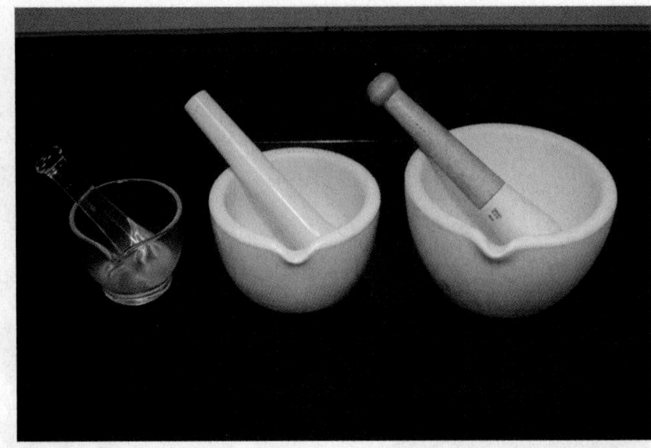

Figure 15.9 Three types of mortars and pestles: porcelain, glass, and Wedgwood.

Ceramic mortars also have a rough interior surface but are somewhat lighter and less heavy duty than Wedgwood mortars. They are also good for reducing particle size and have a tendency to stain due to the porous surface.

stirring rods Thin glass rods of various lengths that are used to mix liquids in a beaker to form a homogenous mixture.

spatulas Tools consisting of a wood or plastic handle and stainless steel or plastic blades of various sizes; used for several functions associated with compounding.

levigate To reduce the particle size of a chemical by triturating or spatulating it with a small amount of liquid in which it is not soluble.

spatulate The process of using a spatula to evenly mix an ointment and eliminate graininess in the final product.

filter paper Porous paper intended to be placed in a funnel to remove unwanted substances from a liquid preparation.

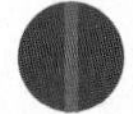

Mixing and Transferring Equipment

Glass stirring rods come in assorted sizes and are valuable for mixing liquids and stirring liquids in a water bath to keep the temperature even throughout the mixture. Spatulas also come in various sizes. Small spatulas with stainless-steel blades are useful for transferring chemicals from a container to a weighing paper or other mixing receptacle. Larger steel-bladed spatulas are used to levigate powders and spatulate ointments. Hard rubber spatulas can be used to handle chemicals that may react with metal. Flexible rubber spatulas may be used in compounding to scrape material from the sides of a container and transferring it. Figure 15.10 shows the various types of spatulas.

Glass or plastic funnels are available in various sizes and can be used to transfer a liquid from one container to another, or they can be fitted with appropriately sized filter paper to filter unwanted chemicals from a liquid. Because the opening in the stem of the funnel is fairly small, funnels are not useful for transferring thick liquids.

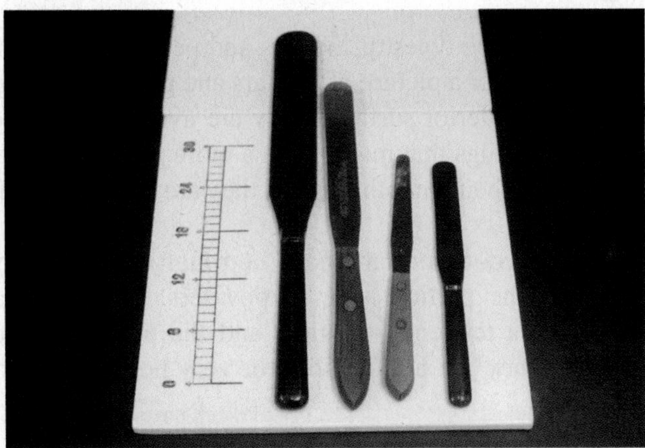

Figure 15.10 Spatulas come in various sizes and may be metal, plastic, or rubber.

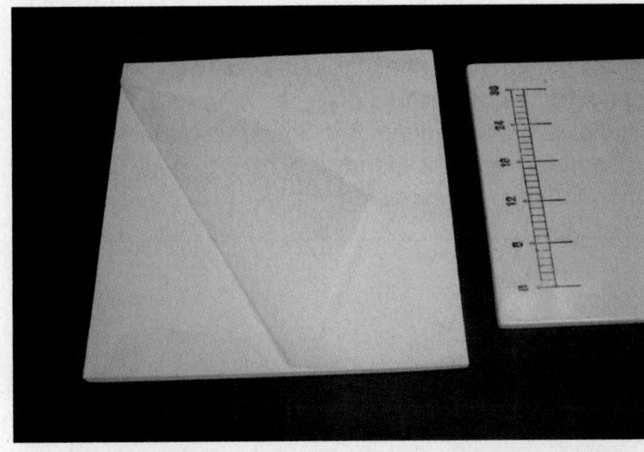

Figure 15.11 An ointment pad of parchment paper may be used instead of an ointment slab.

Ointments are spatulated on either a glass ointment slab or a paper ointment pad. The glass slab is ideal because it is totally nonabsorbent and provides a stable solid platform for mixing. The advantage of the ointment papers is that no cleanup is required, which can save a great deal of time if there is frequent compounding of ointments. The disadvantage is that they can soak up liquids that are being incorporated into ointment bases. Figure 15.11 shows the ointment slab and ointment pad.

Other accessories for a compounding lab will depend on the amounts and types of compounds anticipated. A capsule filling machine is an important device for a pharmacy that frequently compounds capsules. These machines are available in various sizes and feature varying degrees of technology. Lozenge molds and suppository molds are also helpful for compounding these products. More-advanced compounding pharmacies may use homogenizers or blenders to facilitate mixing of larger quantities, and an ointment mill to improve the texture of compounded ointments.

It is important for the technician to learn the correct terms for basic compounding equipment and the rationale for the correct use of each item. Equipment must be thoroughly cleaned and dried after each use and stored correctly to prevent damage to finely calibrated items. Developing competency in basic compounding skills will increase the career opportunities and professional knowledge of a technician.

ointment pad A pad of papers used to spatulate ointments in lieu of a glass ointment slab.

capsule filling machine A device that holds the capsule body while it is being filled with powdered ingredients before it is capped.

lozenge molds Manufactured devices for measuring and dispensing lozenge formulations.

suppository molds Aluminum molds of 1- or 2-mL capacity designed to shape a suppository formulation as it cools and hardens. There are also many types of disposable molds for suppositories.

ointment mill A device used to process ointments to ensure their smooth consistency.

Case Study 15.1

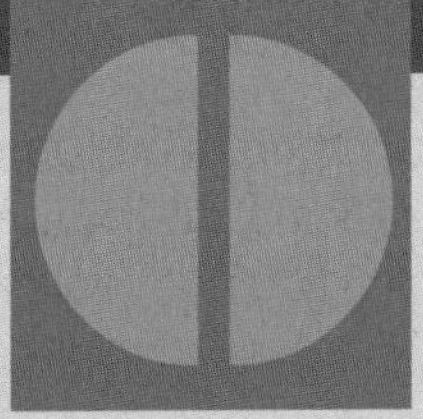

Mandy works in a compounding pharmacy where the pharmacist has formulated an ointment that has been used very successfully to treat various kinds of skin rashes. The pharmacist often suggests the formulation to physicians when they consult with her about a particular patient with a dermatologic problem. Mandy loves her position as a compounding technician and is proud of the pharmacist for developing this very successful ointment. The patients for whom the compound is prescribed often express their appreciation to Mandy for the relief they experience when using the ointment. Mandy is so enthusiastic about the product that she wants to make more people aware of it. The next time Mandy has an appointment with her physician, she takes a copy of the formula for the ointment to let the physician know they have had great results with it. She tells the doctor that they could make the product in bulk and send some to the office as samples for the patients. The doctor seems interested and says he will speak with the pharmacist about it. Mandy is excited to think that she has helped increase the compounding business of the pharmacy.

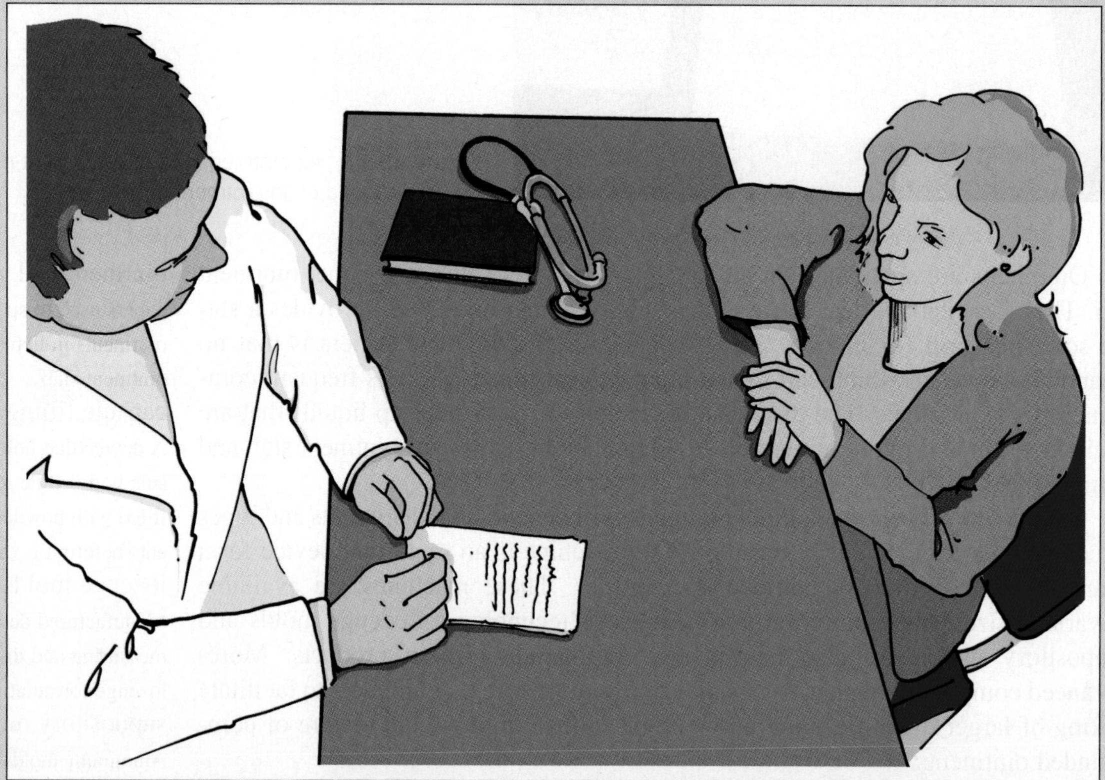

Discuss Mandy's behavior in the above situation. Did she violate any ethical standards? Did she step over the line between compounding and manufacturing? How might the pharmacist deal with this situation?

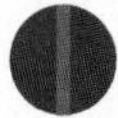

Chapter Summary

- Extemporaneous compounding requires a triangular relationship involving the physician, the pharmacist, and the patient.
- Basic compounding procedures should be followed when preparing a compounded product.
- The Food Drug Modernization Act of 1997 states that extemporaneous compounding must take place in a state-licensed pharmacy or by a state-licensed physician.
- Children, the elderly, and patients with difficult-to-treat dermatologic problems are some of the populations that will benefit from products compounded to meet their specific needs.
- The compounding area of a pharmacy should be a well lighted and ventilated area of adequate size with a sink and disposal facilities located away from the regular dispensing area.

- Pipettes, syringes, and graduates of appropriate sizes should be used to measure liquids for compounding.
- Solid chemicals should be carefully weighed on an electronic prescription balance or a Class III two pan torsion prescription balance using prescription quality weights.
- Mortars and pestles are used to mix and triturate solid materials to attain an evenly dispersed mixture with an appropriate particle size.
- Spatulas may be used in transferring powders from one container to another or to spatulate ointments on an ointment slab.

Review Questions

Multiple Choice

Choose the correct answer to the following statements.

1. Acceptable practices for a compounding pharmacy include:
   a. consulting with physicians to formulate a product to meet a specific patient need
   b. advertising compounded products
   c. bulk compounding for nationwide distribution
   d. selling compounded products at wholesale to other pharmacies

2. Compounded products may include:
   a. bulk substances approved by the FDA
   b. chemicals that comply with USP standards
   c. products removed from the market for efficacy concerns
   d. a and b

3. Compounding equipment used to measure exact amount of liquids include:
   a. conical graduates
   b. mortars
   c. glass beakers
   d. graduated prescription bottles

4. The sensitivity requirement of a Class III torsion prescription balance is:
   a. 120 mg
   b. 60 mg
   c. 6 mg
   d. 15.5 g

5. To level a prescription torsion balance, turn the leveling screw on the side of the balance pan that needs to be lowered
   a. clockwise
   b. counter-clockwise
   c. back and forth
   d. none of the above

Fill in the Blank

Fill in the blanks in the following statements with the correct word or words.

6. When weighing a substance on a prescription torsion balance, the arrest knob should be ___________ when the chemical is being added to the weighing boat.

7. When using an electronic balance, the weight of the weighing boat is accounted for by placing the empty boat and pressing the ________________ button.

8. The best type of mortar and pestle for reducing the particle size of a chemical would be a ___________________________.

9. When mixing very potent drugs or those that may stain, the best mortar to use would be a _________________________.

10. When mixing chemicals that may react with metal, use a __________ spatula.

True/False

Mark the following statements True or False.

11. _________ A paper ointment pad is totally nonabsorbent and good for mixing liquids into ointment bases.

12. _________ Prescription weights must be stored in a compartmentalized box and handled only with tweezers.

13. _________ When measuring liquids in a graduate, the measurement should be taken at the top of the meniscus curve.

14. _________ When pouring a manufactured liquid into a prescription bottle for dispensing, the graduated markings on the bottle can be used for measuring.

15. _________ The calibration dial on a prescription torsion balance can be used to measure quantities up to 5 grams.

Matching

Match the term in column A with the definition in column B.

Column A	Column B
16. _____ pipette	A. A single pan balance with internal weights and a digital readout display.
17. _____ pestle	B. Porous paper used to remove unwanted substances from a liquid.
18. _____ ovals	C. A thin hollow tube used for volumetric measuring of small amounts.
19. _____ electronic	D. Amber prescription bottles with graduated markings.
20. _____ filter paper	E. A device used with a mortar to mix, triturate, or pulverize powders.

LEARNING ACTIVITY

Have the instructor place numbers on the compounding equipment in the pharmacy technician lab. Using the following list, locate each item and indicate the number that corresponds to the item. Learn the correct terminology for the lab equipment and describe the use of each item.

a. ______ beaker

b. ______ conical graduate

c. ______ cylindrical graduate

d. ______ glass stirring rod

e. ______ spatula

f. ______ glass ointment slab

g. ______ funnel

h. ______ weighing boat

i. ______ glassine papers

j. ______ filter paper

k. ______ mortars

l. ______ pestle

m. ______ oral syringe

n. ______ prescription oval

o. ______ prescription vial

Suggested Readings

Allen LV, Popovich NG, Ansel HC. Ansel's Pharmaceutical Dosage Forms and Drug Delivery Systems. Philadelphia: Lippincott, Williams & Wilkins, 2004.

Shrewsbury R. Applied Pharmaceutics in Contemporary Compounding. Englewood, CO: Morton Publishing, 2001.

Thompson J, Davidow L. A Practical Guide to Contemporary Pharmacy Practice, 3rd ed. Philadelphia: Lippincott, Williams & Wilkins, 2004.

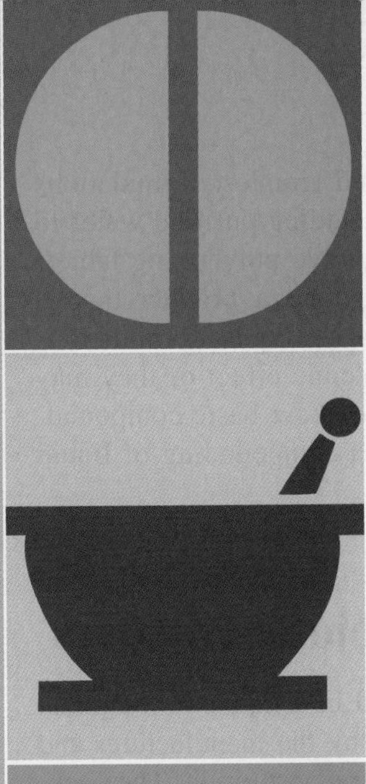

Chapter 16

Solutions, Syrups, and Suspensions

OBJECTIVES

After completing this chapter, the student will be able to:

- List characteristics of solutions, syrups, and suspensions.
- Differentiate between the three types of liquids.
- Provide examples of each of the three types of liquids.
- Describe compounding procedures for each liquid preparation.
- Calculate expiration dates and storage requirements for compounded liquids.

KEY TERMS

- elixirs
- flocculated suspending agent
- isotonic
- miscible
- pharmaceutical elegance
- powder displacement
- reconstitution
- saturated solution
- solubility
- solute
- solvent
- spirits
- suspension
- syrup
- tincture
- vehicle
- viscosity
- wetting agent

Liquid formulations are among the most common and simplest formulations to be compounded. The process may be as simple as adding purified water to an antibiotic powder for reconstitution. Or it may involve pulverizing tablets and adding a suspending agent and flavor to compound a product that is therapeutically effective and pharmaceutically elegant. Liquid formulations may be used for oral administration to produce a systemic effect or they may be topical to provide a local effect. This chapter will explore basic compounding and dispensing considerations for extemporaneous compounding of liquid formulations.

reconstitution Purified water or an appropriate liquid is added to a powder to produce a solution or suspension for oral administration.

pharmaceutical elegance A term used to describe a compounded formulation that is expertly made and packaged to present a pleasing appearance.

suspension A liquid in which particles are not dissolved but are dispersed when shaken.

powder displacement The amount of liquid that is displaced by the powder in a powder for reconstitution.

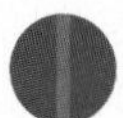

Reconstitution of Oral Antibiotic Powders

Many antibiotics have a limited shelf life when placed in a liquid formulation. These antibiotics are packaged in a unit-of-use bottle by the manufacturer and contain the prescribed amount of antibiotic powder for reconstitution. The package contains instructions for the amount of purified water to be added to attain the concentration listed on the package. The amount of water to be added is always less than the final total volume of the solution or suspension due to the powder displacement of the antibiotic powder in the bottle. Adding a different amount of water (or diluent) to the antibiotic powder will result in a final concentration that differs from that stated on the bottle, and an incorrect dose administered to the patient. See Figure 16.1 for an example of reconstituting a bottle of cephalexin powder for oral suspension.

Preparation Method 16.1
Reconstitution of an Antibiotic Powder

1. Check the label on the bottle for the correct amount of purified water to add.
2. Check the strength listed on the prescription to see that it coincides with the final concentration listed on the bottle.
3. If the final strength listed on the bottle differs from the strength prescribed, perform calculations to determine the amount of purified water to add.
4. Using a cylindrical graduate, measure the total amount of purified water needed to attain the correct concentration.
5. With the lid still intact on the bottle, turn the bottle upside down and tap it on the counter to loosen any powder that may be packed in the bottom of the bottle.
6. Return the bottle to the upright position and let it sit for a minute to allow the powder to settle.
7. Open the bottle and carefully pour half the total amount of the premeasured purified water into the bottle.
8. Replace the lid and shake thoroughly, turning the bottle upside down to ensure that no powder pockets remain on the bottom of the bottle.
9. Remove the lid and add the remaining purified water to the bottle.
10. Replace the lid and shake again. Check to see that all powder particles are evenly distributed.

11. Apply the prescription label and any necessary auxiliary labels indicating the storage requirements, expiration date, and whether it needs to be taken with or without food.
12. Leave the bottle along with the paperwork and any calculations in the checking area for the final check by the pharmacist.

Solutions

A solution is a liquid formulation in which one or more solutes is completely dissolved in a solvent. When compounding a liquid formulation, it is important to know the solubility of any solutes being added to determine whether the formulation will be a solution or whether a suspending agent needs to be added. A solution should be clear with no particles visible in the final product. Solutions may be categorized according to the type of solvent used in the formulation. An elixir is a hydroalcoholic solution in which one or more solutes have been dissolved. (An example of an elixir is Nyquil.) A syrup is a solution in which sugar has been added to form a sweetened solution. A compounding pharmacy will often use simple syrup, which is a saturated solution of sugar in water, or a commercial product, such as Ora-Sweet, that has sugar and flavoring added to make the solution

solute A chemical that is to be dissolved in a liquid.

solvent A liquid that is used to dissolve a solute.

solubility A figure that describes the amount of a solute that will dissolve in a given amount of solvent at a given temperature.

elixir A hydroalcoholic solution that contains one or more dissolved drugs and is sweetened and flavored for oral use.

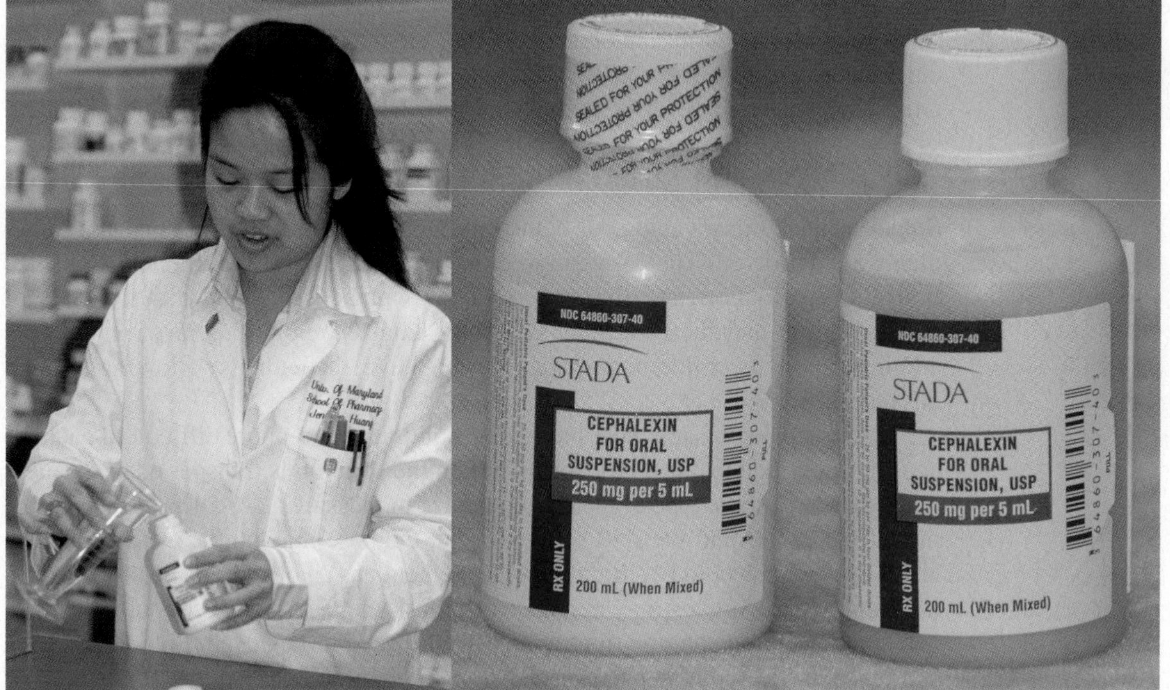

Figure 16.1 **(A)** A pharmacy technician reconstituting an oral powder for suspension. **(B)** On the left is a bottle of cephalexin powder for oral suspension; on the right is a reconstituted bottle of cephalexin ready to be dispensed. (Reprinted with permission from Lacher BE. Pharmaceutical Calculations for the Pharmacy Technician. Baltimore, MD: Lippincott, Williams & Wilkins, 2008.)

syrup An oral solution containing a high concentration of sugar.

saturated solution A solution that has the maximum amount of solute that will dissolve in that amount of solvent at room temperature.

spirits Alcoholic or hydroalcoholic solutions of volatile substances, often used for flavoring.

tincture An alcoholic solution of a drug that is much more potent than a fluid extract (do not substitute one for the other); an alcoholic or hydroalcoholic solution containing vegetable materials or chemicals made by a percolation or maceration process.

isotonic A solution that has equal electrolytes and buffers with the area where it is being used.

more palatable. (An example of a commercial syrup is Robitussin cough syrup.) Spirits are alcoholic or hydroalcoholic solutions of a volatile substance and are often used as flavoring agents (e.g., peppermint spirits). Because of their high alcohol content, these solutions must be stored in tight, light-resistant containers to prevent evaporation of the alcohol and an increase in the potency of the active ingredient. A tincture is an alcoholic or hydroalcoholic solution with chemicals, such as iodine tincture, or vegetable materials.

Solutions may also be categorized according to the route of administration, and the intended route of administration will determine various compounding issues and storing and packaging issues. Oral solutions are liquid preparations that contain one or more therapeutically active ingredients dissolved in a liquid. They often contain flavors, colors, and preservatives. Oral solutions are intended for oral administration to produce a systemic therapeutic effect. Nasal solutions are intended to be sprayed or instilled into the nose, generally for a local action in the nasal passage, although some new medications are administered through the nose for a systemic effect. It is important to ensure that nasal solutions are isotonic in nature to avoid irritating the nasal passages.

Nasal solutions should also be sterile when dispensed. Ophthalmic solutions must be isotonic solutions that are sterile and particle-free. They contain active ingredients that have been dissolved in water with the addition of preservatives, buffers, and other ingredients to adjust tonicity. Compounding ophthalmic solutions requires excellent compounding skills and proper compounding equipment to prevent irritation or infection of the eye. Topical solutions are intended to be applied to the skin or mucous membranes to treat a local condition. Topical solutions can be dispensed in various types of applicator bottles, spray bottles, or flip-top squeeze bottles to aid in administration to the local site. Otic solutions may contain one or more active ingredients dissolved in water, glycerin, and/or alcohol. They are intended for administration into the outer ear. They may also contain other additives, such as buffers and preservatives. Otic solutions should be dispensed in a dropper bottle to facilitate administration.

Advantages and Disadvantages of Solutions

Solutions have the advantage of being completely homogenous because the ingredients are dissolved. The active ingredients are immediately available for absorption and distribution into the system. They can be used by various modes of administration and the dose may be easily adjusted. Solutions provide for easy administration to children or patients who have difficulty swallowing a solid dosage form.

Because solutions are more bulky than solids, they are more difficult to package and transport than solid dosage forms. When the solution is transported, the patient must also carry some type of measuring device to measure a dose. Depending on the measuring device and the skill of the patient, the dose may not be as accurate as a tablet or capsule would be. If the active ingredient has an objectionable taste, flavorings and other additives may be needed to mask the taste. Because most drugs are less stable when in solution, preservatives may need to be added. Solutions have a shorter shelf life and may have special storage requirements.

Compounding Considerations for Solutions

A prime consideration when compounding a solution is the solubility of the active ingredient(s). Reference books are available that list the solubility of various chemicals in various solvents (for example, see *Remington: The Science and Practice of Pharmacy*). The solvent used must be appropriate for the intended purpose of the solution. It is important to note when using solubility tables that solubilities are given in grams of solute per milliliters of solvent and not per milliliter of the final solution. Be cautious when dissolving a chemical in boiling water because you may create a supersaturated solution and the chemical may precipitate out when the solution is cooled to room temperature. Water is the most common solvent, and glycerin and alcohol are also commonly used. Other factors to consider when compounding a solution are how long the drug will be stable in solution, how long it will take to dissolve the drug, and whether preservatives need to be added to prevent bacterial contamination. Stability is also affected by packaging and storage, so most compounds are packaged in tight, light-resistant containers; some may be stored at room temperature, whereas others may need refrigeration. A beyond-use date should be calculated for each compound. Storage and beyond-use dates must be indicated on the label.

Preparation Method 16.2
Compounding a Solution

1. Carefully read the prescription to determine the correct formula for the solution. Perform any necessary calculations and have them checked by a pharmacist or another technician.
2. Check the solubility of any solids in the prescribed solvent.
3. Gather the materials and equipment needed, and place them in the work area.
4. Weigh the solute and put it in a mortar.
5. Triturate the solute to a fine powder to facilitate dissolution.
6. Measure the correct amount of solvent, paying close attention to the meniscus.
7. Pour the solvent into an appropriately sized beaker for mixing.
8. Gradually add the solute while stirring with a glass stirring rod. To hasten solution, the beaker may be placed in a water bath. Continue stirring until all of the solute has been dissolved and the solution is clear.
9. If the solution was heated in a water bath, allow it to cool to room temperature and again check to see that no particles have come out of the solution.
10. Pour into an appropriate container and label with the prescription label and any necessary auxiliary labels, including the storage requirements and expiration date.
11. Place in the checking area for the final check by the pharmacist.

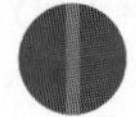

Suspensions

When a liquid formulation is needed for a drug that is not commercially available as a liquid and is not soluble in any solvents that are appropriate for oral administration, a suspension can be formulated in the pharmacy to meet the patient's needs. Topical suspensions often require compounding when physicians formulate special products for a specific patient need. A physician attempting to treat a particular skin condition will often require a dermatologic formulation. The solid ingredients in the suspension should be reduced to finely divided particles of a uniform size to form a smooth, well-dispersed suspension.

Compounding Concerns for Suspensions

Regardless of whether tablets, capsule contents, or powdered chemicals are used for the suspension, the particle size of the drug should be reduced with a mortar and pestle until a fine, even mixture is attained. It may be helpful to pass the ingredients through a mesh sieve to achieve uniformity. If the liquid vehicle is not one that will wet the powder particles easily, a wetting agent may be needed. The triturated powder may be mixed with a small amount of water or glycerin to form a thick paste. It is important to ensure that the solid ingredients do not form a hard cake on the bottom of the bottle after the medication is dispensed. A flocculated suspending agent may be added to the formulation to assist in redispersing the particles when the product is shaken. Two commercially available suspending vehicles are Ora-Plus and Suspendol-S. They form weak bonds with the particles when they are at rest and allow the particles to break apart easily when the product is shaken.

vehicle A liquid (e.g., alcohol, mineral oil, or water) used to dissolve a drug for oral or topical administration.

wetting agent Small amount of liquid added to a powder so it will mix evenly in a suspension ointment.

flocculated suspending agent A viscosity-increasing agent that forms a controlled lacework-like structure of particles that cause the suspension to settle slowly at rest but readily disperse the particles when shaken.

miscible Liquids that can be mixed together and will not separate.

When more than one liquid is used as the vehicle for a liquid preparation, it is important to know whether the two liquids are miscible. If the miscibility is not known, consult a reference book such as *Remington: The Science and Practice of Pharmacy* or the *USP DI Volume III.* Immiscible liquids can sometimes be combined by adding an emulsifying agent and making an emulsion.

Types of Vehicles

Care must be taken when choosing a vehicle for a compounded product. The vehicle should be exactly what is ordered on the prescription formula, and no substitutions should be made without consulting with the prescriber. General terms, such as "water," "alcohol," and "oil," must be clarified and be consistent with the use of the product. The water used in compounding dosage forms must conform to the standards of one of the official USP monograms. Purified Water USP must be processed by distillation or some other suitable method. It is a clear, colorless, odorless liquid that contains no additives and meets all USP standards. It is acceptable for use as a solvent or vehicle for dosage forms for internal or external use, but not for parenteral preparations unless it is sterilized first. Sterile Purified Water USP is purified water that has been sterilized. It can be used for internal and external dosage forms, but is not for parenteral administration. Compounded products to be used for inhalation should be made with Sterile Water for Inhalation USP. Products to be used for irrigation fluid must be made with Sterile Water for Irrigation USP. Using the incorrect type of water in a compound can have disastrous results. The technician should be familiar with the various types of water and double-check that he or she is using the correct type before compounding the product.

When alcohol is ordered in a compounding formula, Alcohol USP must be used unless another type of alcohol is specified. Alcohol USP is ethyl alcohol, 95% v/v. It is a clear, colorless, volatile, flammable liquid with a characteristic odor. It may be used in both internal and external dosage forms. If isopropyl alcohol is specified, the compounded product must be for external use only. Isopropyl alcohol is an effective disinfectant and antiseptic, and mixes well with water, alcohol, glycerin, and propylene glycol, but not with fixed oils or mineral oil.

Glycerin USP is a glycol type of solvent that mixes with water, alcohol, and propylene glycol, but not with ether, fixed oils, or mineral oil. It is a clear, colorless, nearly odorless, viscous liquid that may be used for both internal and external preparations. Propylene Glycol USP is similar in appearance and solubility to glycerin and may also be used for both internal and external preparations. Polyethylene

Glycol NF is a polymer of ethylene oxide and is also known as PEG. There are a number of PEG formulations and all are labeled with a number (ranging from 200 to 8000) indicating the average molecular weight. Peg 400 is the most common liquid PEG and is used as a solvent vehicle for both internal and external dosage forms.

There are a number of oils used as solvent vehicles in compounded preparations, with Mineral Oil USP being one of the most common. It is a colorless, odorless, transparent, oily substance. Mineral oil is insoluble in water and alcohol, soluble in volatile oils, and miscible with most fixed oils (but not with castor oil).

Preparation Method 16.3
Compounding a Suspension

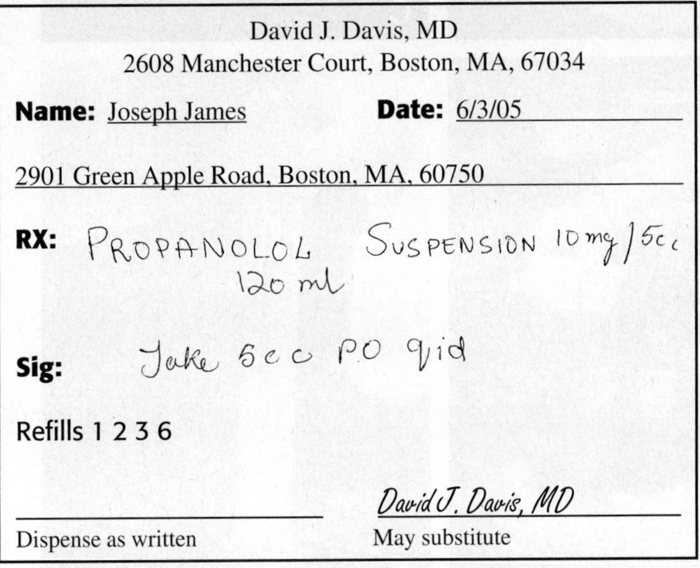

David J. Davis, MD
2608 Manchester Court, Boston, MA, 67034

Name: Joseph James **Date:** 6/3/05

2901 Green Apple Road, Boston, MA, 60750

RX: PROPANOLOL SUSPENSION 10 mg/5cc
120 ml

Sig: Take 5cc PO qid

Refills 1 2 3 6

Dispense as written

David J. Davis, MD
May substitute

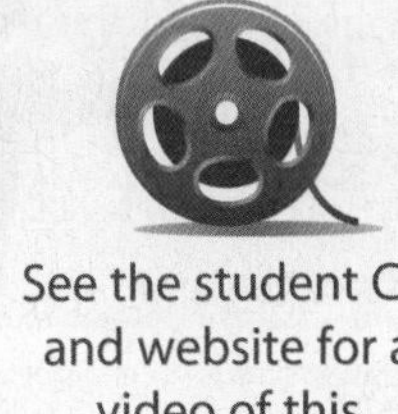

See the student CD and website for a video of this procedure.

(Reprinted with permission from Mohr ME. Lab Experiences for the Pharmacy Technician. Baltimore, MD: Lippincott Williams & Wilkins, 2006.)

1. Technician evaluating the prescription for a compounded suspension. (See Fig. 16.2A.)
2. A compounded prescription using capsule or tablet ingredients or a solid chemical that is not soluble in the liquid vehicle requires that the solid be triturated to fine particles that are relatively even in size. (See Fig. 16.2B.)
3. If the vehicle will not easily wet the powdered ingredients, a wetting agent, such as glycerin, may be used to make the powder into a thick paste. (See Fig. 16.2C.)
4. Add a small amount of a flocculated suspending agent, such as Ora-Plus or Suspendol, and mix well with the powder or paste. (See Fig. 16.2D.)
5. Transfer to a graduate and add a sufficient quantity of the vehicle to reach the required volume. (See Fig. 16.2E.)
6. Stir the product with a glass stirring rod to ensure that the particles are fine enough and will be suspended for a sufficient length of time to administer the correct dose. (See Fig. 16.2F.)
7. Place the suspension in an appropriate container and shake well. Observe the suspension for pharmaceutical elegance. (See Fig. 16.2G.)
8. Apply the prescription label and any auxiliary labels. A suspension must always have a "shake well" label along with any storage requirements and an expiration date. (See Fig. 16.2H.)

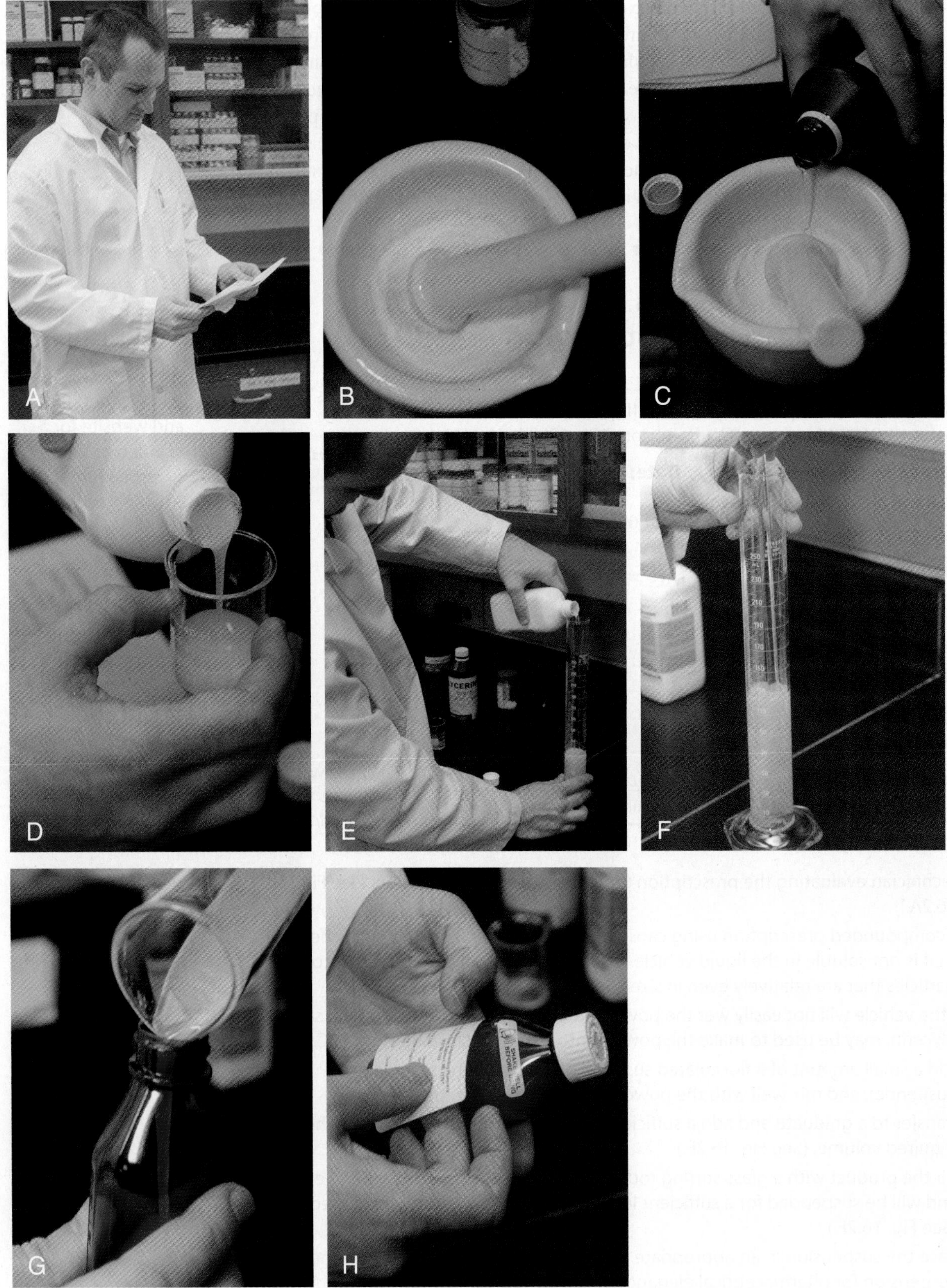

Figure 16.2 Steps for compounding a suspension.

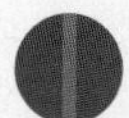

Preservatives

Preservatives are substances that are added to a nonsterile compound to act as an antimicrobial agent and prevent microbial contamination and growth in the product. USP Chapter 1151 states that antimicrobial agents are required for most dosage forms that contain water. Because most microorganisms require water for growth, if no water is present microbial growth is unlikely. Often an antimicrobial, such as alcohol, is already a part of the formula and this negates the need to add another preservative. If the preparation is to be used immediately after preparation and has been compounded with the appropriate technique, a preservative is not required.

Preservatives should not be used in compounded preparations for neonates. CAUTION

The decision about whether to add a preservative, and which preservative to use, require the professional judgment of a pharmacist and should not be made by a technician.

Case Study 16.1

Jill is working as a technician in a retail pharmacy when a customer presents her with a prescription from a local veterinarian. The prescription is for a feline that has been having seizures. It is written for phenytoin chewable tablets 50 mg to give ½ tablet three times a day. The pet owner tells Jill that for some reason, the cat will not take the commercially prepared phenytoin suspension and spits out the tablets even when they are mixed with tuna. The cat is very finicky. Jill consults with Marie, the pharmacist, and together they ask the pet owner if there is a flavor the cat particularly

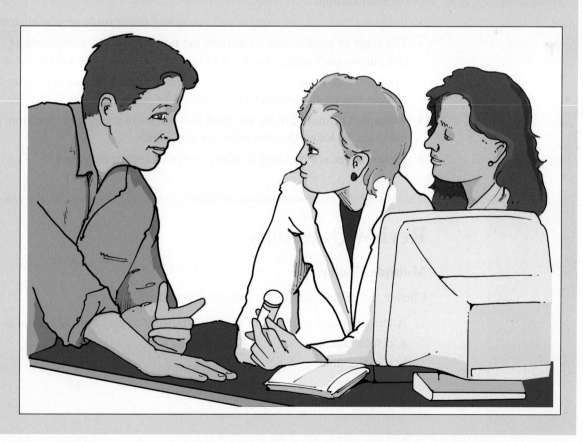

likes. The owner reports that the cat is especially fond of bacon and will run to the kitchen whenever she smells the aroma of bacon being fried. The pharmacy stocks some bacon-flavored concentrate, so Jill and Marie work to devise a compound that can solve this dosage administration problem. When they complete their calculations, they consult with the veterinarian who wrote the prescription.

Using 30 mL of Ora-Plus as a suspending agent and 5 mL of bacon-flavored concentrate, devise a formula for a 30-day supply of phenytoin suspension with a concentration of 25 mg/mL. Use purified water as a diluent.

1. How many phenytoin tablets are needed?
2. Describe the steps and equipment used in the preparation method.
3. What directions, concentration, and expiration date should be on the label?
4. What measuring device would you give the pet owner to administer the dose?

Chapter Summary

- Oral antibiotic powders for reconstitution require the addition of a specified amount of purified water to produce a solution or suspension of the stated strength.
- A solution is a liquid formulation in which one or more solutes have been completely dissolved.
- Solutions may be categorized according to the type of solvent used in the formulation.
- Solutions may also be categorized according to the route of administration.
- The route of administration dictates the type of vehicle, compounding techniques, packaging, storing, and types of additives needed for solutions.
- Compounding products that contain ingredients that are not soluble in the vehicle require the addition of a suspending agent.
- When two or more liquids are used as vehicles in a liquid preparation, it is important to know the miscibility of the liquids.
- Preservatives are required in many compounded preparations.

Review Questions

Multiple Choice

Choose the best answer to the following statements:

1. Adding purified water to an antibiotic powder to make a suspension is called:
   a. displacement
   b. reconstitution
   c. flocculation
   d. suspension

2. The solid ingredients in a compounded solution are called:
   a. solvents
   b. vehicles
   c. solutes
   d. none of the above

3. The following is an example of a solution:
   a. syrup
   b. spirit
   c. elixir
   d. all of the above

4. Advantages of solutions include all of the following except:
   a. completely homogenous
   b. active ingredients are immediately absorbed
   c. difficult to transport and package
   d. easily administered to children

5. Compounding concerns for solutions include:
   a. solubility of the active ingredients
   b. stability of the compound
   c. solvent appropriate for expected use
   d. all of the above

Fill in the Blank

Fill in the blank(s) with the correct word or words.

6. Three common types of vehicles for compounded liquid formulations are ______________, ________________, and ________________.

7. Agents added to a nonsterile compound to act as an antimicrobial are called ________________.

8. A viscosity-increasing agent that causes a suspension to readily disperse the particles when shaken is a ____________________________________.

9. The amount of liquid displaced by the powder in a liquid preparation is the ____.

10. The dose range in which a drug is effective but not toxic is the ____.

True/False

Mark the following statements True or False.

11. ________ To reconstitute an antibiotic powder for suspension with a final volume of 200 mL, the technician should carefully measure 200 mL of purified water and add it to the bottle.

12. ________ A flocculated suspending agent will keep the solid particles in suspension when added to a liquid compound.

13. ________ Oral solutions are liquid preparations intended for oral administration to produce a systemic effect.

14. ________ Nasal solutions must be isotonic to keep from irritating the nasal passages.

15. ________ Preservatives should always be added to a compound intended for use in neonates.

Matching

Match the term in column A with the definition in column B:

Column A	Column B
16. _____ Ora-Plus	A. Liquid in which particles are not dissolved but will disperse when shaken.
17. _____ emollient	B. Oral solutions containing a high concentration of sugar.
18. _____ suspension	C. Flocculated suspending agent.
19. _____ syrup	D. Term indicating the consistency of a substance.
20. _____ viscosity	E. Agent used to soften and lubricate.

Suggested Readings

Allen LV, Popovich NG, Ansel HC. Ansel's Pharmaceutical Dosage Forms and Drug Delivery Systems. Philadelphia: Lippincott, Williams & Wilkins, 2004.

Gennaro, AR, ed. Remington: The Science and Practice of Pharmacy. Baltimore, MD: Lippincott, Williams & Wilkins, 2006.

Lacher BE. Pharmaceutical Calculations for the Pharmacy Technician. Baltimore, MD: Lippincott, Williams & Wilkins, 2008.

Shrewsbury R. Applied Pharmaceutics in Contemporary Compounding. Englewood, CO: Morton Publishing, 2001.

Thompson J, Davidow L. A Practical Guide to Contemporary Pharmacy Practice. 3rd ed. Philadelphia: Lippincott, Williams & Wilkins, 2004.

United States Pharmacopia. 43rd ed. National Formulary. 39th ed. Rockville, MD: United States Pharmacopeial Convention.

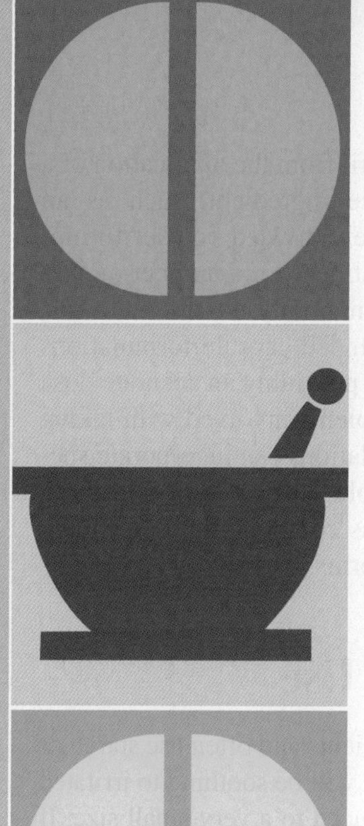

Chapter **17**

Dry Powders, Capsules, and Lozenges

OBJECTIVES

After completing this chapter, the student will be able to:

- Describe the topical effect of chemicals used in dry powder formulations.
- Discuss the reasons for triturating topical dry powders into fine, evenly mixed particles.
- Describe the use of a fine mesh sieve to obtain evenly sized particles.
- List the advantages of using capsules as a compounded dosage form.
- Demonstrate the punch method of making capsules.
- Compare the punch method with the use of a capsule machine.
- Describe three ways to make lozenges as a dosage form.

KEY TERMS

- anesthetic
- antibacterial
- antifungal
- antipruritic
- capsule body
- capsule lid
- comminution
- demulcent
- dispersion
- eutectic mixture
- geometric dilution
- levigating agent
- mesh sieve
- mucilage
- protectant
- spatulation
- trituration
- tumbling

There are many dermatologic conditions that can benefit from the application of a dry powder formulation. The addition of an active ingredient, such as an antifungal, antibacterial, or antipruritic agent, to a finely divided powder formulation can provide a soothing and effective topical treatment for a number of skin conditions. Bulk powders can also be administered internally to dose antacids, bulk laxatives, and antidiarrhea medications. Compounded capsule formulations can facilitate the administration of oral medications by providing an accurate dose of more than one medication and eliminating the problems involved with taking unpalatable medications. Compounded lozenge formulations can incorporate specific medications for a patient and provide a palatable dosage form with both topical and systemic effects. This chapter will discuss compounding issues and preparation methods for these types of solid dosage forms.

antifungal Agent used to treat fungal infections.

antibacterial Agent used to inhibit the growth of bacteria.

antipruritic A drug or chemical that reduces itching.

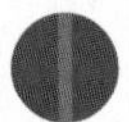

Bulk Powders for External Use

Topical powders may contain one or more active ingredients and often use starch or talc as the diluent to provide a smooth, soft product that will be soothing to irritated skin. The particles in the solid ingredients must be reduced to a very small size. If one or more of the ingredients might form a eutectic mixture, the compounder must either force the mixture to liquefy before adding the remaining dry ingredients or add a protectant, such as starch, to each of the possible eutectic formers to prevent clumping when the mixture is complete.

eutectic mixture Two or more chemicals that change from a solid form to a liquid when mixed together.

protectant An agent, such as starch or talc, that is added to ingredients that may form a eutectic mixture if triturated together (prevents two or more chemicals from reacting when mixed).

Particle Size Reduction

Because most chemicals cannot be purchased in the finely ground form needed for compounding powders, the compounder must use a number of procedures and equipment to reduce the particle size, in a process known as comminution. The most common method is trituration, which involves placing the solid in a mortar and continually grinding the chemical between the mortar and the pestle using a firm, downward pressure. The powder must be frequently scraped from the sides of the mortar to ensure that all particles are evenly reduced and mixed. A levigating agent, such as glycerin, may be added to the solid and processed by either continued trituration or by placing the mixture on an ointment slab and using spatulation to wet the solid and further reduce the particle size. A small mesh sieve can be used to determine the prevalent particle size of a powder after it has been triturated. Standard U.S. sieves are numbered according to the number of openings per linear inch; the larger the mesh number, the smaller the particles that will pass through it. See Figure 17.1 for a picture of a mesh sieve.

comminution The process of reducing particle size.

trituration The process of reducing particle size using a mortar and pestle.

levigating agent A substance added to slightly wet powdered ingredients.

spatulation The process of mixing an ointment on an ointment slab with a spatula to ensure uniformity of particles.

mesh sieve Sieve that has a number of small holes to allow a certan size of powders to pass through.

Preparing a Homogenous Mixture

Some of the same processes used to reduce particle size are also used to mix solid particles into a homogenous mixture. Powders that have been blended with a protectant to prevent the formation of a eutectic mixture must be mixed carefully with little to no pressure. Spatulation, or the mixing of particles with a spatula on an ointment slab, will result in a light, well-mixed powder without interfering with the protectant. Trituration serves the dual purpose of reducing particle size and mixing powders. It is especially effective for mixing small quantities of potent

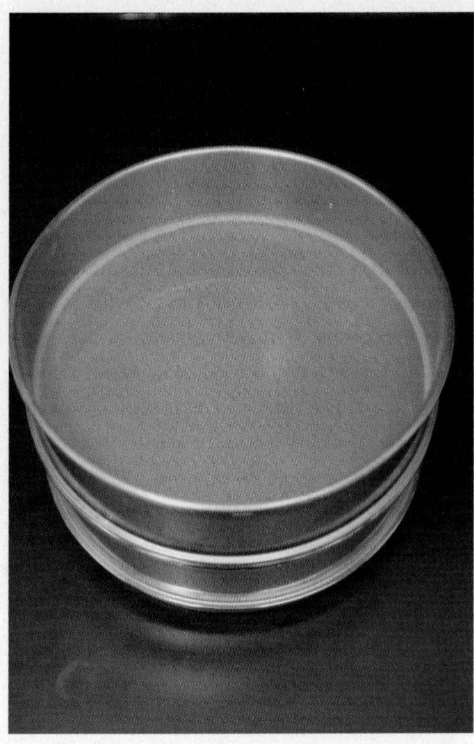

Figure 17.1 Mesh sieve used to determine particle size when compounding dry powders for topical use.

drugs with larger amounts of diluent. Hazardous substances can be effectively mixed by a process called tumbling. The powders are sealed in zipper-sealed bags or clear bottles with a lid and tumbled until they are well mixed. The addition of a coloring agent can assist in determining when the mixture is homogenous. When the powders being combined are unequal in quantity, geometric dilution is the preferred method for mixing them. Begin by placing the powder with the smallest quantity in the mortar and adding an equal amount of each of the other powders. Continue adding each powder in an amount that is equal to the powder in the mortar and triturate well after each addition to form a homogenous mixture. To mix powders of equal volumes, add small, equal amounts of each powder and mix well after each addition. Equal dispersion of each ingredient is important to provide the proper therapeutic effect.

tumbling Mixing powders by placing them in a plastic bag or large jar and rotating it until mixing is completed.

geometric dilution The process of mixing two solid chemicals together by taking equal parts of each in small amounts, mixing them thoroughly, and continuing to add small, equal parts of each until both are thoroughly mixed.

Packaging Dry Powders

Bulk powders for external use (sometimes called dusting powders) are often dispensed in a shaker-top container to facilitate topical application. They may also be dispensed in a wide-mouth jar or a plastic container with a flip-top lid. The jar or plastic container can be closed tightly and provides increased stability and protection from light and moisture, especially for compounds that contain volatile ingredients.

Bulk powders intended for internal use should be dispensed in an amber, wide-mouth powder jar with a tight-fitting lid. They should be accompanied by an appropriately sized dosing spoon or cup and adequate directions for removing and administering a correct dose. Internal bulk powders should be labeled with the concentration of the active ingredient per dose (e.g., potassium chloride 600 mg per tablespoonful).

Divided dry powders are packaged in individual doses and dispensed in either folded papers or plastic bags. If the individual dose of the compound is below the minimum weighable quantity of the prescription balance being used, or is so small in mass that it will be difficult for the patient to handle, a diluent should be added to make the dose more manageable. This can be accomplished by preparing an aliquot to attain the proper concentration. Folded powder papers are very time-consuming and rarely used. Plastic bags that either have a zipper closure or can be heat-sealed are more frequently used to package individual doses of dry powders for internal use. Amber bags are available for products that are light-sensitive, and the filled bags can be dispensed in a light-resistant container. Dry powder dosage forms can be a convenient means of administering a capsule or tablet to a patient who has difficulty swallowing. The capsule contents can be emptied into a small plastic bag or the tablet can be crushed and placed in a small bag.

Preparation Method 17.1
Dry Powders

James Anderson, MD
2901 Church Street, Brooks, IN 47604
Phone: (356) 443-0098 Fax: (356) 444-9800

Name: Sammy Smitz **Date:** 05-03-07

Address: 2603 South Hampshire Road, Brooks, IN 53706

RX: Menthol .1 grams
Salicylic acid .1 grams
Starch qs ad 30 grams
Sig: Apply to callous on bottom of feet daily

Refills 3

Dispense as written

James Anderson, MD
May substitute

(Reprinted with permission from Mohr ME. Lab Experiences for the Pharmacy Technician. Baltimore, MD: Lippincott, Williams & Wilkins, 2006.)

1. Weigh the camphor, salicylic acid, and 29.8 g of starch.
2. Camphor and salicylic acid will form a eutectic mixture, so place them in a glass mortar and triturate them together until they liquefy.
3. Place the starch in a Wedgwood mortar and triturate it by applying downward pressure in a circular motion with the pestle to reduce the particle size. Periodically scrape the powder from the sides of the mortar and continue to triturate until the particles are a fine, even size and any clumps have been removed.
4. Place an amount of starch approximately equal to the amount of liquefied eutectic mixture into the glass mortar and allow the starch to adsorb the liquid.

5. Using geometric dilution, continue adding an amount of starch equal to the amount of mixture in the glass mortar, triturating after each addition, until all the starch has been added and the mixture is blended into a fine homogenous powder.
6. Run the powder through a mesh sieve and triturate again, if necessary, to achieve an appropriate particle size.
7. Place the powder in a shaker-top container and apply the prescription label and any auxiliary labels.
8. Place the ingredients used, the paperwork, the master formula sheet (including any calculations used), and the final labeled product in the checking area for the final check by the pharmacist.

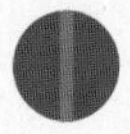

Capsules as an Extemporaneous Compound

A capsule is a solid dosage form in which the active ingredients and diluents are contained in a two-piece hard shell, usually made of gelatin. Gelatin capsules are available in various sizes and colors. See Figure 17.2 for capsule sizes. The double-zero size is the largest size for oral use in humans, although the zero size is more commonly used. The zero-size capsule has a capacity of 0.5 to 0.8 grams of powder depending on the density of the chemical being used. Hard-shell capsules consist of two pieces: the body and the cap (see Fig. 17.3). After the two pieces are separated, the body piece is filled with the dry powder ingredients and the cap is then replaced. The smallest capsule that will hold the ingredients should be chosen for the compound. When several ingredients are being inserted into the capsule, a powder that is near the average weight of all the ingredients should be chosen to determine the capsule size that will best accommodate the ingredients in a slightly packed form. Reference books can be used to find the approximate capsule capacities for some common chemicals. If the amount of drug needed for a single dose is below the minimum weighable quantity, a diluent should be added. If the single dose is too large for a capsule that can reasonably be swallowed by the patient, a diluent should be added and the dose divided into two capsules.

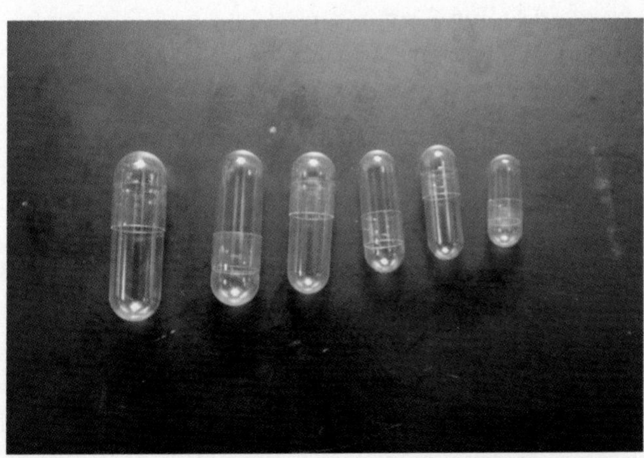

Figure 17.2 Capsule size 00 is the largest capsule used for human oral preparations, and size 5 is the smallest.

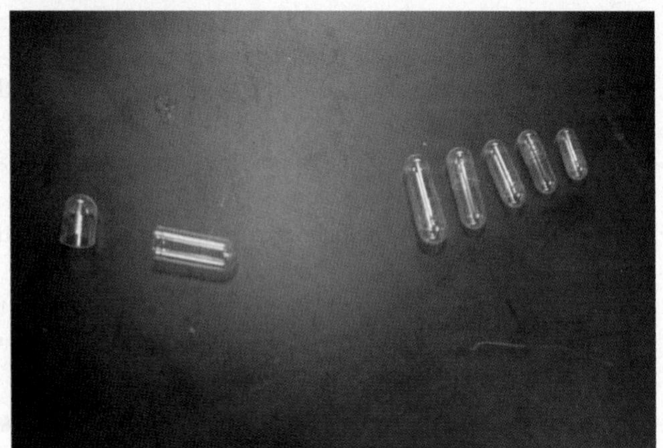

Figure 17.3 The cap of the capsule fits snugly over the body of the capsule after the capsules are filled.

Preparation Method 17.2
Hand-Filling Capsules

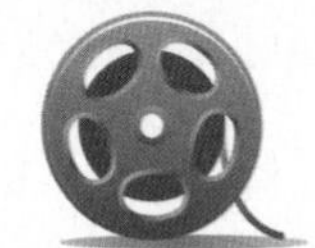

See the student CD and website for a video of this procedure.

Michael Angelo, D.O.
806 Cherry Creek Plaza, Denver, CO 50620
702-317-5030

Name: Sally Sue Sullivan **Date:** 10/19/06

Address: 6072 Denver West Dr., Boulder, CO

RX: Acetominophen 325mg
Ibuprofen 100 mg
mix and prepare 12 capsules

Sig: Give one capsule qid for pain and fever

Dispense as written

Michael Angelo, D.O.
May substitute

(Reprinted with permission from Mohr ME. Lab Experiences for the Pharmacy Technician. Baltimore, MD: Lippincott, Williams & Wilkins, 2006.)

1. Calculate the amount of each powder ingredient needed to compound the total number of capsules to be dispensed. Determine whether the single dose for each capsule will be above or below the minimum weighable quantity, and include a diluent if necessary. (See Fig. 17.4A.)
2. Add enough of each ingredient to make one or two extra capsules to account for any loss that may occur during the compounding process. (See Fig. 17.4B.)
3. Triturate each ingredient to reduce the particle size and add them together using the geometric dilution technique. (See Fig. 17.4C.)

4. When a homogenous mixture has been prepared, place the powder on an ointment slab or pad and form a rectangular block using a spatula. The height of the block should be slightly shorter than the length of the capsule body to facilitate filling the capsule using the punch method. At this point, the compounder should put on disposable gloves. Using bare hands can result in fingerprints on the finished capsule or a slight melting of the gelatin capsule, and is not considered sanitary. (See Fig. 17.4D.)

capsule body The bottom part of the capsule shell that contains the solid ingredients.

5. Prepare the balance by placing a weighing paper on each side of a properly leveled balance and adding an empty capsule and the correct amount of weight to the right-hand pan of the balance. (See Fig. 17.4E.)
6. Remove the cap from one of the capsules to be filled and begin punching the body of the shell repeatedly into the block of powder until the capsule feels full or begins to offer resistance. (See Fig. 17.4F.)
7. Replace the cap on the capsule and place it on the left pan of the balance. Add or remove powder from the capsule according to whether the index pointer is to the left or right of the center. Continue until the pointer moves an equal distance from the left and the right of the center. Repeat this process for each capsule until all are filled. As you progress, you will begin to get a feel for how many times you should punch the capsule and how much resistance should be felt from the powder as the capsule body is filled. The margin of error for each capsule should be no more than ±5%. (See Fig. 17.4G.)
8. If you are using an electronic balance to weigh the capsules, place an empty capsule shell in a weighing boat on the balance pan. Press the tare button to zero the balance with the weight of the capsule and the weighing boat. Remove the empty capsule and place each completed capsule in the weighing boat to determine the weight of the powder in the capsule. (See Fig. 17.4H.)
9. When all capsules are completed and the weights are acceptable, use a soft tissue to remove any particles of powder and place the capsules in a prescription vial for dispensing. Prepare the prescription label and any auxiliary labels, document the compounding procedure and calculations on a master formula sheet, and place the finished product in the checking area for the final check by the pharmacist. (See Fig. 17.4I.)

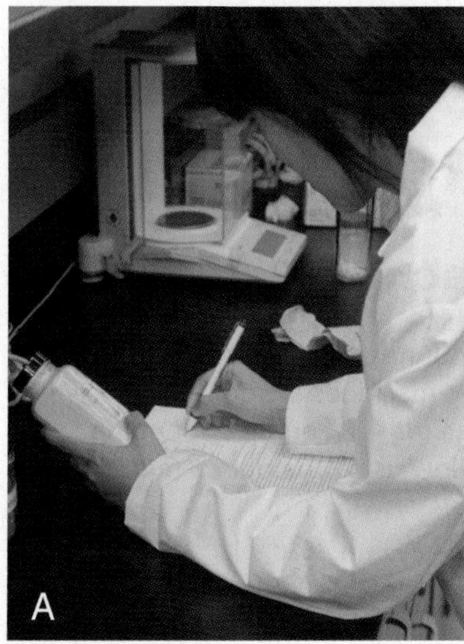
A

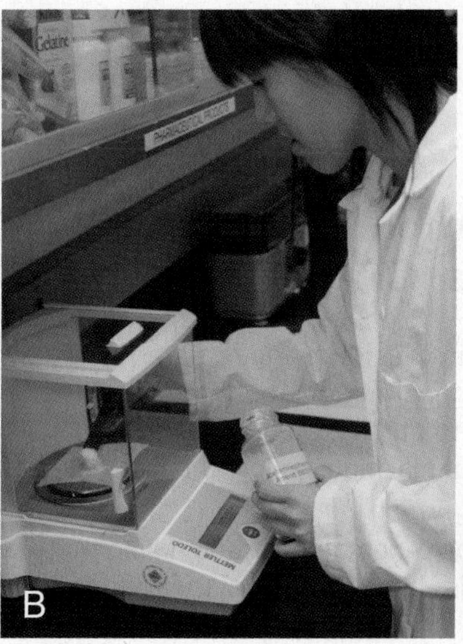

B

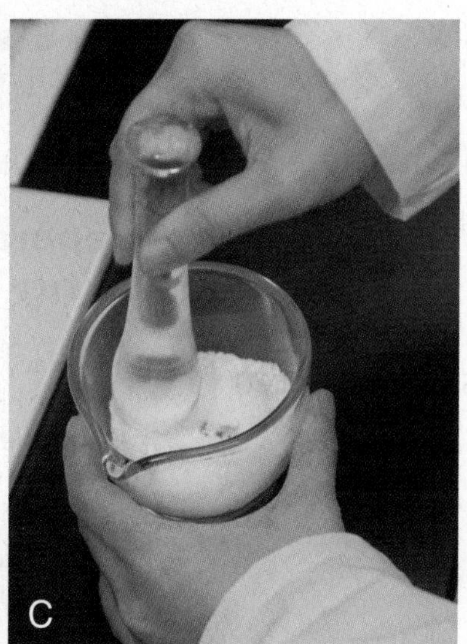
C

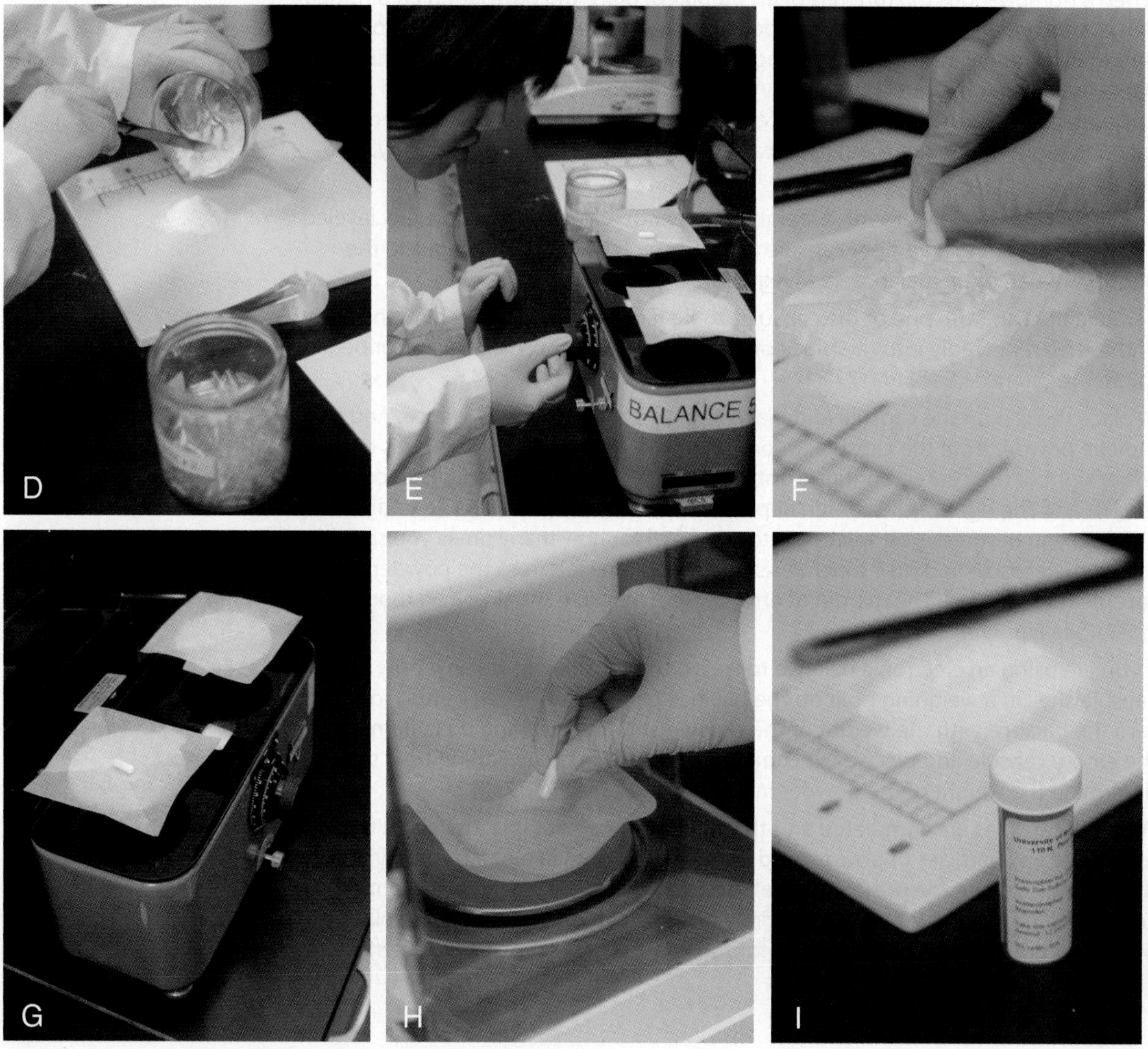

Figure 17.4 Steps for hand-filling capsules.

Preparation Method 17.3
Using a Capsule-Filling Machine

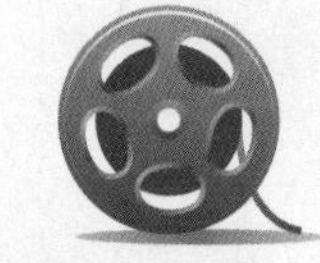

See the student CD and website for a video of this procedure.

A pharmacy in which capsules are frequently compounded may invest in a capsule-filling machine. Although automated capsule-filling machines are quite expensive, it is possible to purchase a non-automated machine for $20 and up depending on the type of machine. Follow the instructions below using the punch method for capsules.

1. Using a non-automated capsule-filling machine (See Fig. 17.5A), place the bodies of the capsules into the holes of the machine (See Fig. 17.5B.)

2. Pour the prepared powder ingredients over the top of the capsules and use a special spatula to direct the powder into the capsules. A tamper is provided with the machine to press the powder into the capsule compactly (See Fig. 17.5C.)
3. When each capsule has been filled, lower the platform of the capsule machine so that the capsule lid can be applied. These machines can usually accommodate 100 capsules at a time and are most efficient when used to compound the full quantity of 100 capsules. (See Fig. 17.5D.)
4. After applying the capsule lids, randomly select 10 completed capsules for weighing and document the weight for quality control. If all 10 capsules are within the range of 85% to 115% of the labeled amount of the drug per capsule, the capsules are considered to be satisfactory. (See Fig. 17.5E.)

capsule lid The top part of a two-piece gelatin capsule that fits over the capsule body.

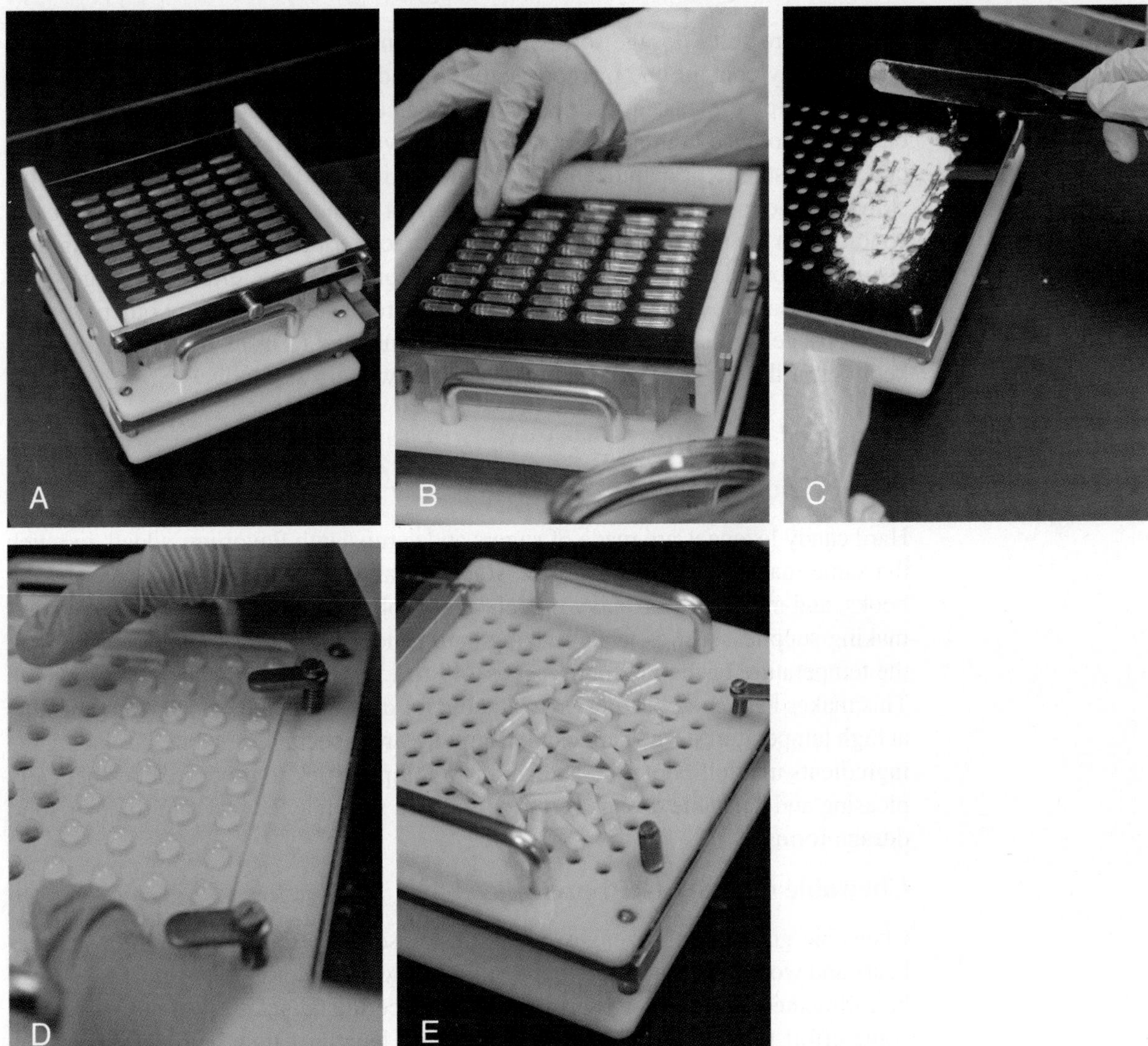

Figure 17.5 Steps for using a capsule-filling machine.

Advantages of Capsule Formulations

Capsules are a convenient dosage form in which an individual dose can be accurately measured. They are easily packaged and transported, and can be easily administered to the patient. Compounded capsules can be filled with a precise dose for a specific patient that may not be available commercially or may be available only in another form. They can contain ingredients that may be unpalatable or toxic to the touch. Two or more active ingredients can be combined into a single capsule dosage form, improving patient compliance. One or more commercially manufactured tablets can be inserted into a capsule with the addition of a diluent, such as lactose, to facilitate dosing. Capsules can be compounded easily in the pharmacy and offer many advantages to patients.

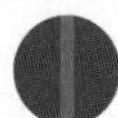

Compounded Lozenges

Lozenges are solid dosage forms that are intended to be dissolved slowly in the mouth. They contain one or more active ingredients and are flavored and sweetened so as to be pleasant tasting. They are generally used for their topical effect, but may also have ingredients that produce a systemic effect. A lozenge may contain an anesthetic, a demulcent, or an antiseptic. The fact that lozenges dissolve slowly in the mouth enhances the topical effect because the medication will be in contact with the mouth and throat tissues for a longer period of time. The drug may also be absorbed in the mouth or swallowed for a systemic effect. Lozenges provide a pleasant dosage form for patients who are unable to swallow other types of solid dosage forms. Because lozenges are formulated to taste good, they must be kept out of the reach of children, who may view them as candy.

Types of Lozenges

Hard Candy Lozenges

Hard candy lozenges are made of sugars and syrups with flavorings added, in much the same manner as candy is made. Recipes can be gathered from candy-making books, and molds, sticks, and wrappers can be obtained from stores that sell candy-making supplies. Just as when making hard candies, it is imperative to ensure that the temperature of the mixture reaches 149 to 154°C (called the hard crack stage). This makes hard candy lozenges unsuitable for drugs or chemicals that are unstable at high temperatures. The hard candy formulas are especially suitable for placing the ingredients in a lollipop mold and adding a lollipop stick to produce an esthetically pleasing and palatable dosage form for children who may be resistant to other solid dosage forms.

Chewable Gummy Gel Lozenges

Chewable gummy gel lozenges began to be used as a dosage form after gummy bears and worms became very popular as a candy for children. The gummy base can be formulated in the lab or pharmacy using glycerin and gelatin, but it does require some effort to heat the mixture for the proper length of time and add the correct amount of flavorings to mask the bitter taste of glycerin. A simpler way to prepare gummy gel lozenges is to use a commercial gummy gel base (available from compounding supply companies) or actual gummy bears, which can be melted in a beaker and a water bath, and add the active ingredients. The liquid can then be placed into molds to solidify because the flavorings and color are already present.

Preparation Method 17.4
Compounding Gummy Gel Lozenges

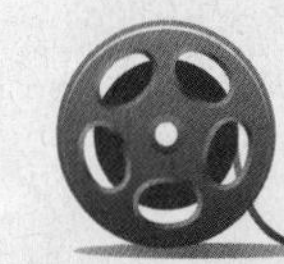

See the student CD and website for a video of this procedure.

Michael Mordo, MD
3798 Golden Rodeo Drive
Palo Alto, CO 80634

Name: Marcia Marathon **Date:** 04-25-06

1223 Dallas Drive, Hoboken, IL 46304

RX: Clotrimazole 100mg
Flavor and color additives as needed
Lozibase qs

Dispense 10 lozenges containing 10mg each of active ingredient

Sig: Dissolve one lozenge in mouth Bid x 5 days

Refill 0 1 2 3

Michael Mordo, MD

Dispense as written May substitute

(Reprinted with permission from Mohr ME. Lab Experiences for the Pharmacy Technician. Baltimore, MD: Lippincott, Williams & Wilkins, 2006.)

1. Place the lozenge mold on the balance pan and tare the balance to zero out the weight of the mold. (See Fig. 17.6A.)
2. Melt the gummy gel base in a beaker placed in a water bath (See Fig. 17.6B).
3. Add enough of the melted gummy base liquid to nearly fill each of the cavities of the mold and place on the balance pan. (See Fig. 17.6C.)

TIP **An oral syringe can be used to fill each of the cavities in the mold without overflowing them.**

4. Record the weight of the base. (See Fig. 17.6D.)
5. Place the base back in the water bath and add the correct weight of solid ingredients for the number of lozenge cavities in the mold. (See Fig. 17.6E.)
6. Place the liquid back in the mold, filling each cavity equally, and reweigh the mold with the liquid to be certain that it contains the correct weight for the base plus the active ingredients. (See Fig. 17.6F.)
7. Allow the liquid to solidify. (See Fig. 17.6G.)
8. Remove the lozenges from the mold and weigh them individually to ensure that they are within the acceptable margin of error. Either return them to the mold or package them appropriately for dispensing. (See Fig. 17.6H.)
9. Apply the prescription label and any necessary auxiliary labels, document the calculations and compounding procedures on the master formula sheet, and leave for the final check by the pharmacist.

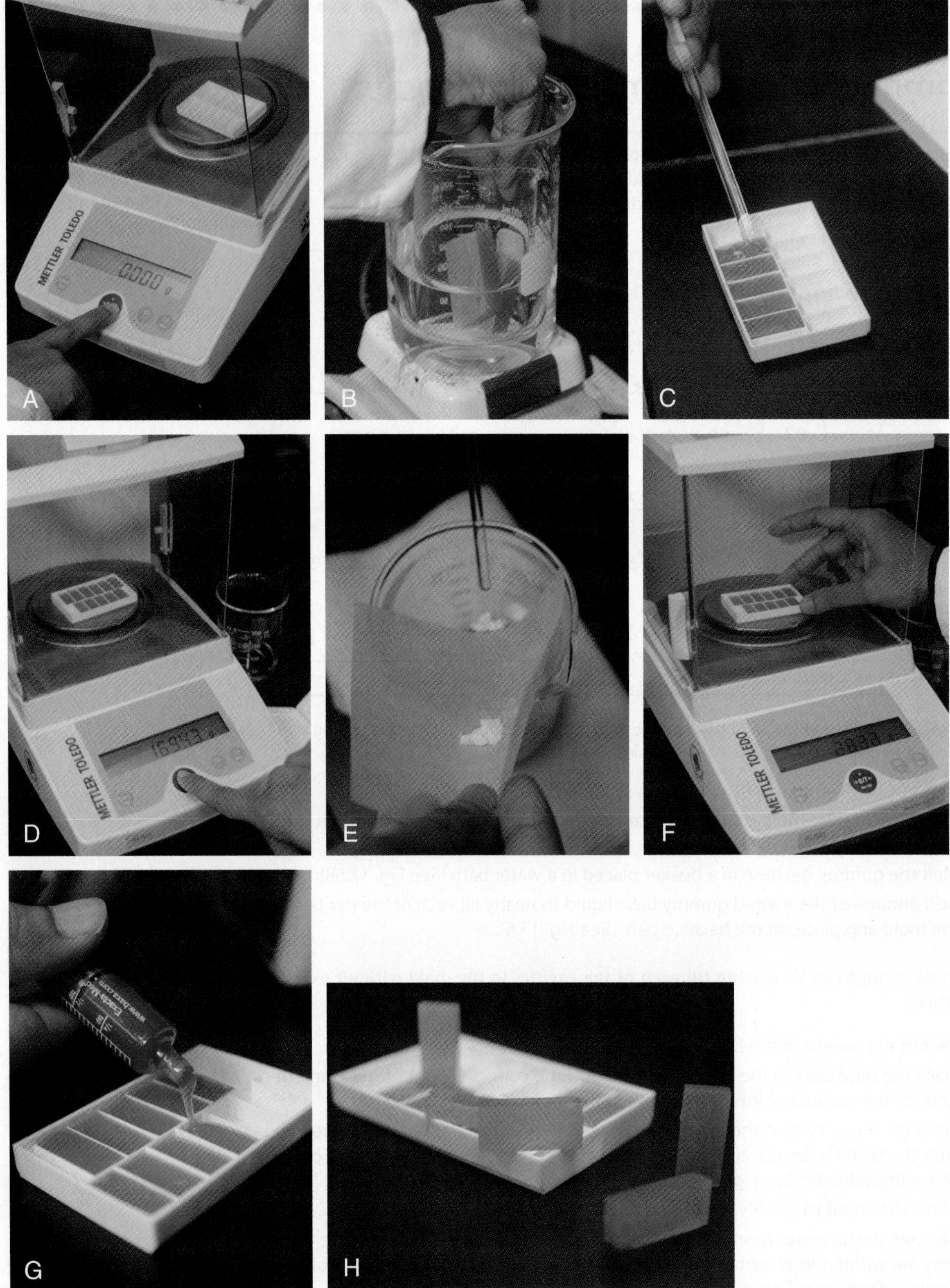

Figure 17.6 Steps for compounding gummy gel lozenges.

Hand-Rolled Lozenges

Hand-rolled lozenges require a few simple ingredients and only basic compounding equipment. However, it does take some experience on the part of the compounder to produce a pharmaceutically elegant lozenge. Even when they are well made by an experienced compounder, hand-rolled lozenges will not have a professional appearance like that of a hard candy or molded lozenge.

Preparation Method 17.5
Compounding Hand-Rolled Lozenges

See the student CD and website for a video of this procedure.

Michael Mordo, M.D.
3798 Golden Rodeo Drive
Palo Alto, CO 80634

Name: Marcia Marathon **Date:** 4-25-06

1223 Dallas Drive, Hoboken, IL 46304

RX: Clotimazol 100mg
Acacia 0.7g
Powdered sugar 10g
Purified water qs
Cherry flavor 5drops
Red food coloring 5 drops
Dispense 10 lozenges containing 10mg each of active ingredient

Sig: Dissolve one lozenge in mouth Bid x 5 days.

Michael Mordo, MD

Dispense as written May substitute

(Reprinted with permission from Mohr ME. Lab Experiences for the Pharmacy Technician. Baltimore, MD: Lippincott, Williams & Wilkins, 2006.)

1. Calculate and weigh of each ingredient needed for the total number of lozenges weighing 2 grams each plus two extras to account for material loss during mixing. (See Fig. 17.7A.)
   10 mg of clotrimazole × 12 lozenges = 120 mg clotrimazole
   22.18 g of powdered sugar
   1.7 g of acacia
   Total weight of ingredients = 24 g/12 lozenges = 2 g/lozenge
2. Place acacia in mortar with 2 ml water, food coloring, and flavor (See Fig. 17.7B)
3. Mix the weighed active ingredient and powdered sugar together using geometric dilution. Sift the mixture before adding it to the mucilage to form a light, homogenous mixture. (See Fig. 17.7C.)

mucilage A mixture used to hold powders together when compounding lozenges.

4. Gradually add the powdered sugar mixture to the acacia mucilage in the mortar and triturate until it is evenly mixed and dough-like. Wearing gloves, use a spatula to help form the dough mass into a cylinder on the ointment pad. (See Fig. 17.7D.)
5. Measure the cylinder with a ruler and divide into 12 even pieces. Each piece should weigh 2 g for an individual lozenge. (See Fig. 17.7E.)
6. Calculate the percent weight variation from the prescribed amount for each lozenge. Use the lozenges closest to the correct amount and discard the two extra lozenges. (See Fig. 17.7F.)
7. Wrap each lozenge in a foil wrapper and place in a vial. Apply the prescription label with the weight of active ingredient in each lozenge and the expiration date on the label. (See Fig. 17.7G.)
8. Apply any auxiliary labels. Document the compounding procedure and calculations on the master formula sheet and leave for the final check by the pharmacist.

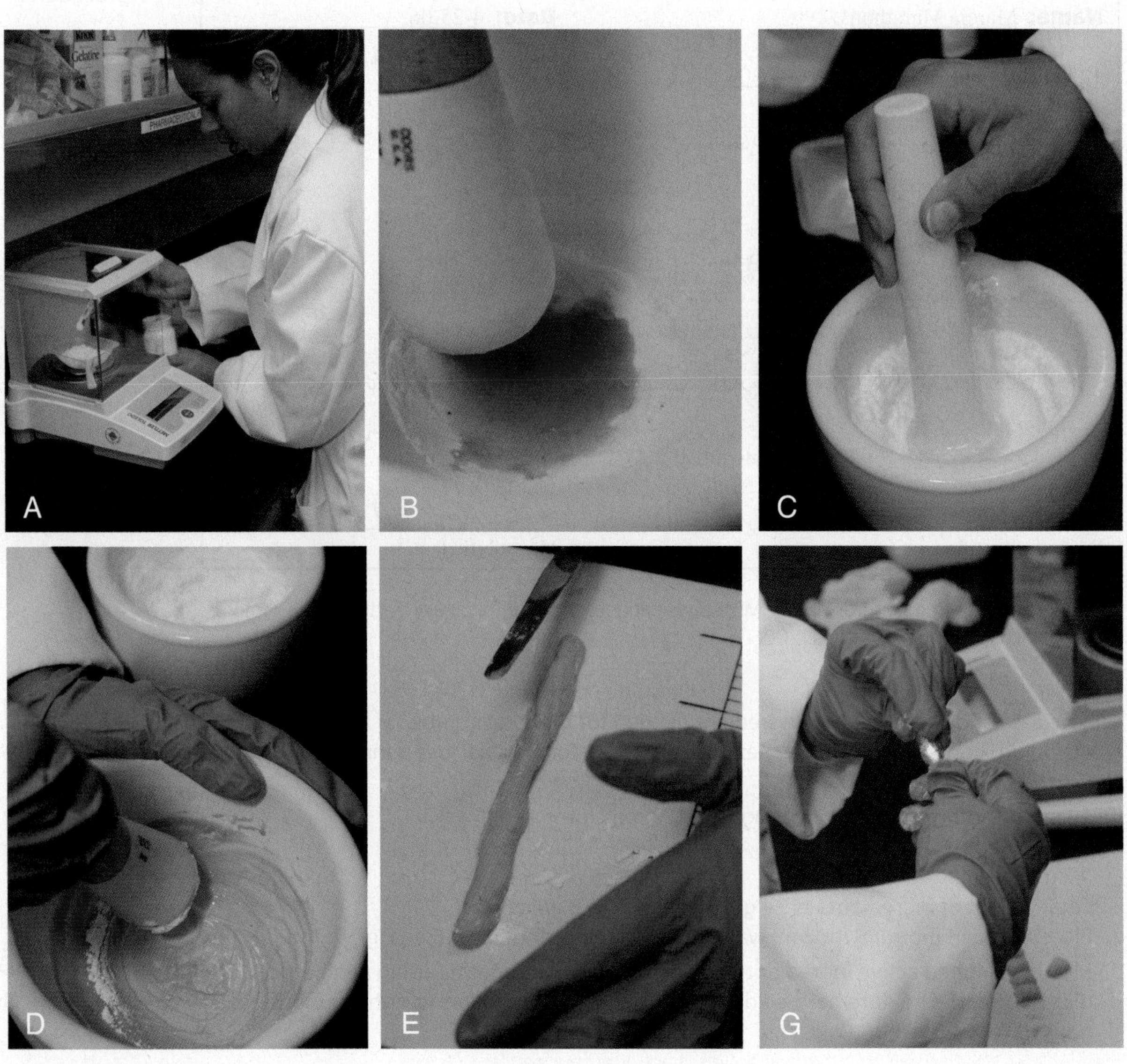

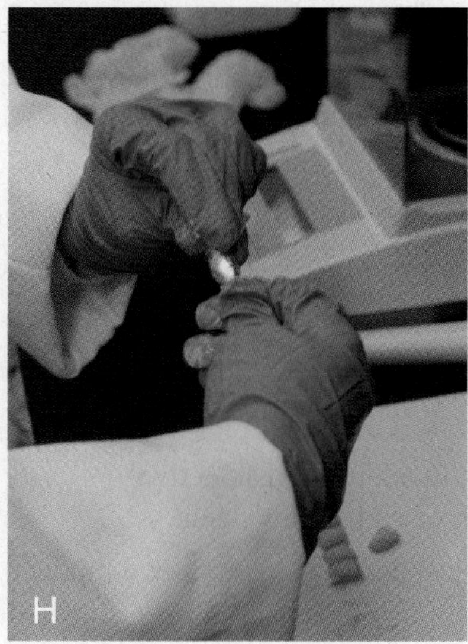

Figure 17.7 Steps for compounding hand-rolled lozenges.

Pharmacies are constantly developing new methods of administering solid dosage forms to serve the needs of individual patients. This chapter has presented some of the basic types of formulations to introduce the fascinating world of extemporaneous compounding. The professional technician should practice basic compounding techniques and become proficient.

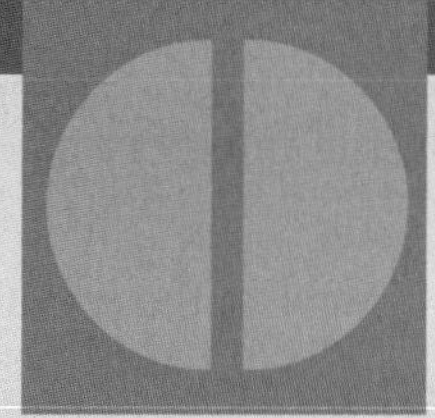

Case Study 17.1

Mr. Joseph arrives at the pharmacy with prescriptions for ketoprofen 25 mg, metformin 500 mg, and glyburide 5 mg. Each medication is to be taken two times a day. Mr. Joseph is an elderly male and states that he has trouble keeping track of three different medicines. He doesn't like having to swallow three tablets and wishes there could be one dosage form for all his medical needs. Jim, the pharmacy technician, conveys Mr. Joseph's concerns to the pharmacist.

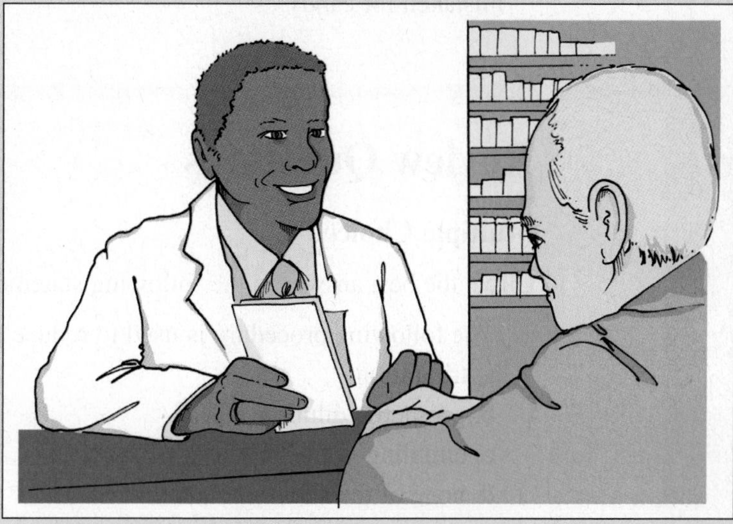

1. What dosage form could they compound to make medication administration more convenient for the patient and possibly improve compliance?
2. Describe a preparation method that would produce a single dosage form for these three medications.

Chapter Summary

- Topical powders usually contain starch or talc in addition to an active ingredient, such as an antifungal, antibacterial, or antipruritic agent.
- It is important to reduce the particle size of topical powders to produce a product that will be soothing to irritated skin.
- Comminution processes include trituration, levigation, and spatulation.
- Mixing powders to form a homogenous mixture can be accomplished by spatulation, tumbling, and geometric dilution.
- Dry powders can be packaged in shaker-top containers, wide-mouth jars, and individually in small plastic bags or folded powder papers.
- Hard-shell gelatin capsules have a body and lid that can be separated to add active ingredients and diluents.
- The punch method for hand-filling capsules involves placing a homogenous mixture of powders in a rectangular block on an ointment slab and punching the body of the capsule until it is filled.
- Each compounded capsule should be weighed for accuracy.
- Capsule-filling machines can facilitate compounding for large numbers of capsules.
- Lozenges are solid dosage forms intended to be dissolved slowly in the mouth.
- Lozenges can be effective for both topical and systemic effects.
- Lozenges must be kept out of the reach of children because they may be mistaken for candy.

Review Questions

Multiple Choice

Circle the best answer to the following statements.

1. The following procedure is used to reduce the particle size of powders:
   a. trituration
   b. geometric dilution
   c. tumbling
   d. none of the above

2. Preparing a homogenous mixture of powders can be accomplished by
   a. spatulation
   b. geometric dilution
   c. tumbling
   d. all of the above

3. Which of the following powders would not be used as a diluent in a topical powder formulation?
   a. starch
   b. salicylic acid
   c. talc
   d. none of the above

4. If the amount of an ingredient needed for a compounded solid dosage form is less than the minimum weighable quantity of the balance, the technician should
   a. call the prescriber and ask to change to a different ingredient
   b. double all the ingredients and save half for the next refill
   c. prepare an aliquot using the required ingredient and a diluent
   d. none of the above

5. Methods for compounding lozenges include all of the following except
   a. hand rolling
   b. the punch method
   c. using a gummy gel base
   d. using a hard candy base

Fill in the Blank

Fill in the blanks with the correct word(s) to complete the sentence.

6. The ________________ ________________ is the largest capsule size used orally in humans.

7. When using the punch method to fill capsules, the rectangular block of powder should be ______________________(higher) or (lower) than the height of the capsule body.

8. The advantages of compounded capsules include the following: _____________, ___________________, and __________________.

9. Lozenges include ________________ and sweeteners to make them more palatable.

10. The weight of an extemporaneously compounded lozenge is usually_______________.

True/False

Mark the following statements True or False.

11. ________ Bulk powders can be administered internally to dose antacids, bulk laxatives, and antidiarrheals.

12. ________ Trituration is one way to achieve comminution of dry powders.

13. ________ With a mesh sieve, the larger the mesh number, the larger the particles that can pass through it.

14. ________ In geometric dilution, the powder with the largest quantity is placed in the mortar and the powders with smaller quantities are added slowly; mixing is repeated after each addition.

15. _____ Bulk powders for internal use are sometimes called dusting powders.

Matching

Match the terms in column A with the definitions in column B.

Column A	Column B
16. _____ levigating agent	A. Particle size reduction.
17. _____ demulcent	B. Agent such as starch or talc added to ingredients that may form a eutectic mixture when mixed together.
18. _____ dispersion	C. Substance such as mineral oil or glycerin added to slightly wet powdered ingredients before mixing.
19. _____ protectant	D. Uniform distribution of each ingredient in a powder mixture.
20. _____ comminution	E. Agent used topically to soothe irritated tissue in the mouth and throat.

Suggested Readings

Allen LV, Popovich NG, Ansel HC. Ansel's Pharmaceutical Dosage Forms and Drug Delivery Systems. Philadelphia: Lippincott, Williams & Wilkins, 2004.

Shrewsbury R. Applied Pharmaceutics in Contemporary Compounding. Englewood, CO: Morton Publishing, 2001.

Thompson J, Davidow L. A Practical Guide to Contemporary Pharmacy Practice, 3rd ed. Philadelphia: Lippincott, Williams & Wilkins, 2004.

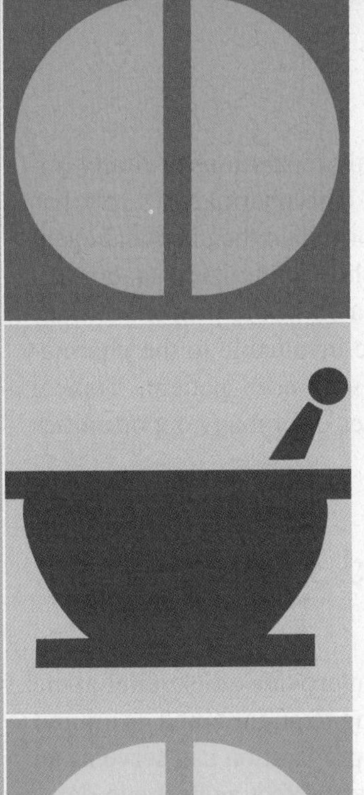

Chapter **18**

Ointments, Creams, Gels, Pastes, and Suppositories

OBJECTIVES

After completing this chapter, the student will be able to:

- Discuss the advantages and disadvantages of topical preparations.
- Differentiate between the available bases according to their physical properties and uses.
- Define compounding techniques used in extemporaneous compounding of ointments, creams, and suppositories.
- Discuss beyond-use dating for topical preparations.
- Demonstrate the ability to evaluate topical formulations for consistency, stability, and pharmaceutical elegance.
- List some factors to consider when preparing a suppository formulation.
- Describe the relationship between the route of administration and the size of the suppository.

KEY TERMS

- absorption bases
- cream
- emollient
- eutectic mixture
- gels
- geometric dilution
- levigation
- lubricant
- O/W emulsion
- occlusive
- ointment
- oleaginous
- paste
- protectant
- spatulation
- systemic
- topical agent
- trituration
- W/O emulsion

Competence in extemporaneous compounding of topical preparations is vitally important in the changing world of pharmaceutical care. The pharmacist's role has become one of consultation with the medical team to formulate the chemical agent that will provide the most effective therapeutic action while minimizing adverse effects. A knowledgeable technician who has been educated in the proper methods and techniques of pharmaceutical compounding will be invaluable to the pharmacist in formulating preparations specific to the needs of each patient. Topical preparations such as ointments, creams, and suppositories offer many opportunities for patient-specific compounding.

ointments Semisolid formulations containing one or more active ingredients intended to be applied to skin or mucous membranes.

creams Semisolid dosage forms containing one or more drug substances dissolved or dispersed in a water-removable base.

emollient A chemical used to soften and lubricate the skin.

lubricant Agent that softens the skin and reduces friction when a suppository is inserted.

protectant An agent, such as starch or talc, that is added to ingredients that may form a eutectic mixture if triturated together (prevents two or more chemicals from reacting when mixed).

systemic A drug intended to be absorbed into the bloodstream and have an action away from the site of administration.

topical agent An agent intended to be applied to the skin or mucous membranes.

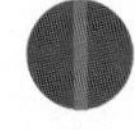

Advantages of Compounded Topical Preparations

Extemporaneously compounded topical preparations can provide quick relief at the site of application. The base can be immediately soothing to an inflamed or injured area before the active ingredient is even absorbed. The preparation can serve as an emollient, a lubricant, or a protectant (e.g., zinc oxide to protect against sun damage). It may have a drying agent to aid in treating rashes with exudates. The active ingredient can target only the affected area with little or no systemic absorption. This allows for a therapeutic action with a low incidence of adverse effects. The type of base used in the product will determine the speed in which the active ingredient can be absorbed. The area covered by the topical agent and the length of time it is in contact with the skin affect the amount of absorption. Because topical preparations provide soothing relief with few side effects, patient compliance is relatively high.

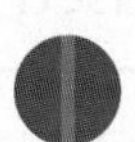

Disadvantages of Compounded Topical Preparations

Topical preparations can be messy to apply and inconvenient to transport. Because they often have a low amount of systemic absorption, they may not solve the underlying problem. This route of administration is also limited in the amount of active ingredient that can be absorbed in a short period of time. This will be a critical factor if systemic absorption is needed to correct the problem.

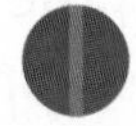

Therapeutic Uses of Compounded Topical Preparations

There are many manufactured dermatologic formulations on the market today, both prescription and over the counter (OTC). However, this field presents a great opportunity for formulating products specific to individual patients to treat skin conditions of known or unknown origin. Keratolytic agents are commonly formulated in concentrations recommended by the prescriber for foot problems such as corns, calluses, and warts. Antifungals are also frequently prescribed alone or in various combinations with corticosteroids, and may include zinc oxide for its protectant effect. These preparations are suitable for athlete's foot, diaper rash, and yeast infections. Antibiotics and antiseptics are often used for minor skin infections or to prevent infection after an injury. Antihistamines will help with allergic skin reactions.

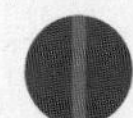

Ointments

Ointment Bases

When choosing an ointment base, it is important to understand the therapeutic use of the ointment and the properties of the various bases, as well as the physical properties of any active ingredients involved. The site of application should also be considered. There are five basic types of ointment bases. Table 18.1 lists the five types, important characteristics of each, and an example of each type.

Compounding Equipment for Ointments, Creams, and Pastes

The following list shows the basic equipment required for routine compounding of ointments, creams, gels, and pastes:

- A Class A prescription balance for weighing ingredients.
- Prescription weights.
- Glassine papers or weighing boats to weigh ingredients.
- A glass ointment slab or parchment ointment pad for mixing. Glass is preferred because it provides a more stable surface. Some ingredients may be absorbed by the parchment, but the pad provides for easier clean up.
- Spatulas of various sizes depending on the amount of ointment being prepared. Metal spatulas are preferred, but plastic may be used if the product will react with metal.
- Mortars and pestles for pulverizing solids.

gels Ointment bases that are semisolid systems of organic or inorganic particles penetrated by a liquid.

paste An ointment base to which a sizeable amount of powder has been added.

Table 18.1 Characteristics of the Five Types of Ointment Bases

Base type	Water affinity	Water-washable	Consistency	Use	Example
oleaginous base	hydrophobic	no	stiff, greasy	lubricate, protect	white petrolatum
absorption base	hydrophilic	no	stiff	lubricate, protect	Aquaphor
water in oil emulsion	hydrophilic	slightly	spreads easily	cleanse, lubricate	Eucerin
oil in water emulsion	hydrophilic	yes	spreads easily	lubricate	Dermabase
water -soluble	hydrophilic	yes	spreads easily, nongreasy	vehicle for active ingredient	polyethylene glycol

Preparation Methods for Ointments, Creams, and Pastes

The following preparation methods deal with ointments, creams, and pastes. Please note the following:

When a liquid is to be added to the ointment base (e.g., see Preparation Method 18.2), care must be taken to ensure that the ointment base will absorb the type and amount of liquid being used. Although only minute amounts of aqueous solutions can be incorporated into an oleaginous base, a considerably larger amount can be added to a hydrophilic base. Alcoholic solutions will readily combine with oleaginous bases. Some thicker liquids may require the addition of a levigating agent before they can be added to the ointment base. Consult the USP and *Remington: The Science and Practice of Pharmacy* for specific guidelines.

oleaginous A base in which the oil is the external phase; usually greasy and non-washable.

Incorporating a solid into an ointment base (e.g., see Preparation Method 18.3) requires proper preparation of the solid particles to ensure an acceptable finished product. If possible, the powdered form of the solid should be used rather than the crystals. If the form is specified by the prescriber, the indicated form should be used unless the prescriber is contacted by the pharmacist to authorize the change. Be sure to document the form and technique used on the master formula sheet so the product can be duplicated in the future.

Solid ingredients can be prepared for incorporation into an ointment base using one or more of the following techniques:

- Trituration: Crystals or powders with coarse particles should be placed in a mortar and triturated with the pestle until the particles are fine and even in size.
- Levigation: To attain a smooth, elegant product, it is often necessary to combine the powdered solid with a levigating agent and triturate until it is no longer grainy. The amount of the levigating agent should be small (a few drops to 1 mL) to avoid changing the concentration and consistency of the final product. If a larger amount is needed, it must be accounted for in the formula.
- Eutectic mixture: Some crystals (e.g., camphor and menthol) will liquefy when they are combined. This facilitates the production of a smooth, non-grainy final product.
- Spatulation: Some solids are available in very fine powders that can be incorporated into a smooth ointment by rubbing small amounts together with small amounts of the ointment base, using a spatula to reduce any graininess.
- Dissolution: Some solids are difficult, if not impossible, to reduce to a fine powder, and even after a considerable amount of time spent on trituration, levigation, and spatulation they will not yield an acceptable topical product. In this case, dissolving the solid in a suitable solvent before combining it with the ointment base may be the best procedure. Reference books such as *Remington: The Science and Practice of Pharmacy* and the USP provide solubility information to aid in the choice of a suitable solvent.

trituration The process of reducing particle size using a mortar and pestle.

levigation The process of reducing the particle size of a chemical by triturating or spatulating it with a small amount of liquid in which it is not soluble.

spatulation The process of mixing an ointment on an ointment slab with a spatula to ensure uniformity of particles.

occlusive Covered in a manner that does not allow penetration by air or moisture.

Creams are sometimes considered to be forms of ointments because they are also semisolid preparations intended for topical application. The main difference between ointments and creams is the base used for compounding. Creams are generally more fluid in consistency and more easily applied. They are not as protective, not occlusive, and are easily water-washable. Because of their ease of application and nongreasy feel, they are more acceptable to patients. The compounding techniques used for ointments apply also to creams.

Pastes are ointment bases that have one or more solid ingredients added in a quantity that will render the final product very thick and stiff. They are somewhat difficult to apply, but once applied are quite protective and occlusive. One example is zinc oxide paste, which is a commonly used product that can protect the diaper area from wetness and rash, and also provide protection from the sun in sensitive areas, such as the nose.

Gels (or jellies) are also grouped in the broad ointment category, but they contain a high amount of water and are easily applied. They are nongreasy, nonocclusive, and easily washed off with water. Gels may be applied topically or inserted into a body cavity, such as the nose or vagina.

Preparation Method 18.1
Mixing Two Ointments, Creams, or Pastes

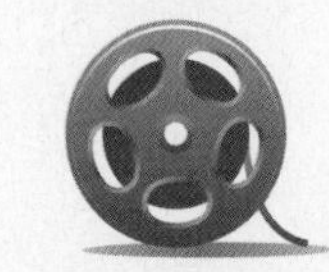

See the student CD and website for a video of this procedure.

1. Weigh each of the ingredients separately and place in separate mounds on the ointment pad or slab to be used for mixing. (See Fig. 18.1A.)
2. With the spatula, divide a small amount of each and mix together by spatulation in the center of the slab until evenly mixed. (See Fig. 18.1B.)
3. Continue adding small, relatively equal portions of each ingredient and spatulate until the entire amount of each ingredient has been combined to produce a final product that is even in color and consistency. (See Fig. 18.1C.)
4. Transfer the compounded ointment to the proper-size ointment jar, fill out the master formula sheet, apply the labels, and leave the completed product along with the paperwork for the final check by the pharmacist. (See Fig. 18.1D.)

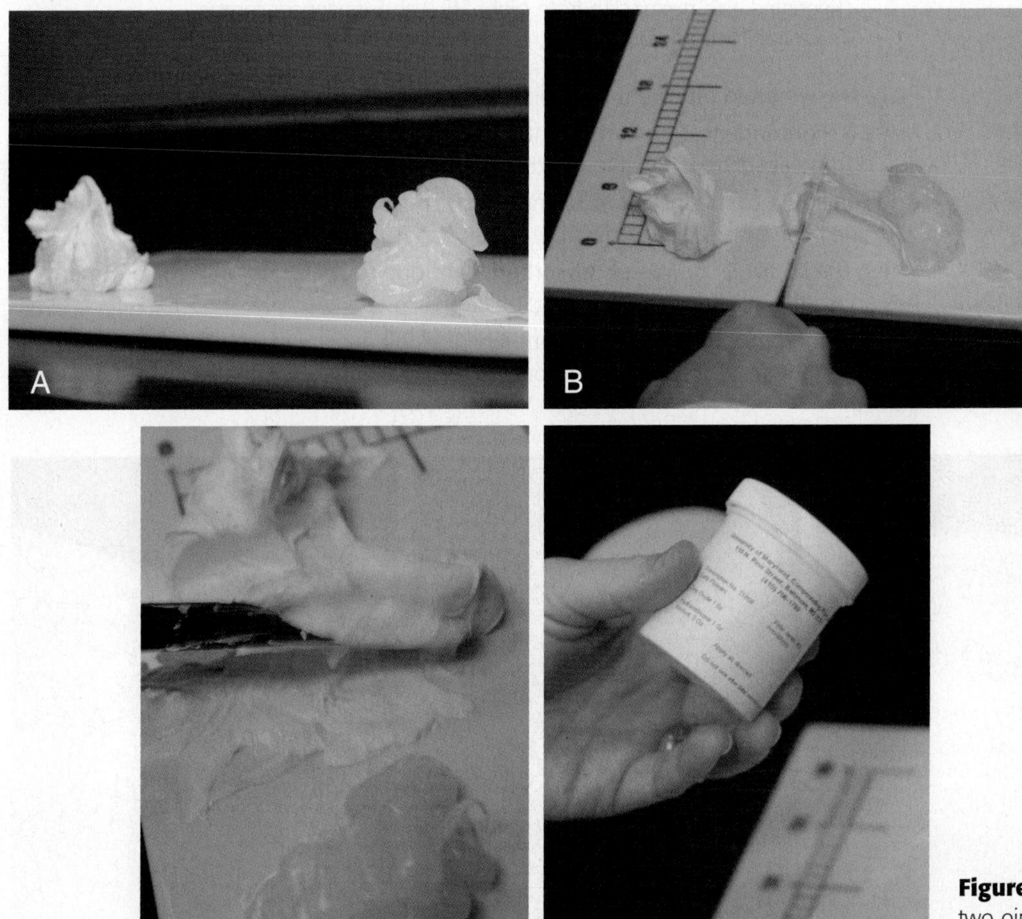

Figure 18.1 Steps for mixing two ointments, creams, or pastes.

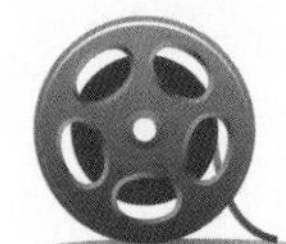

See the student CD and website for a video of this procedure.

Preparation Method 18.2
Mixing an Ointment With a Liquid

Joseph Sorbonne, MD
2802 E. Hardwick
Anycity, Alaska

Marie Shivvers **Date** 10-19-06

806 North 6th Pontoon Lake, Alaska

RX: Povidone-Iodine solution 5ml
White petrolatum 60GM
Mix & Dispense

Sig: Apply to injured area on knee after cleaning with Peroxide bid.

Dispense as written — Joseph Sorbonne, MD — May substitute

(Reprinted with permission from Mohr ME. Lab Experiences for the Pharmacy Technician. Baltimore, MD: Lippincott, Williams & Wilkins, 2006.)

geometric dilution The process of mixing two solid chemicals together by taking equal parts of each in small amounts, mixing them thoroughly, and continuing to add small, equal parts of each until both are thoroughly mixed.

1. Place the weighed ointment base on the ointment slab. (See Fig. 18.2A.)
2. Make a slight indentation in the center of the ointment, adequate to contain the liquid to be absorbed. (See Fig. 18.2B.)
3. Add the liquid to the indentation and begin combining small amounts of the liquid with the base using geometric dilution and spatulation. (See Fig. 18.2C.)
4. When the liquid is completely absorbed, continue to spatulate until the ointment has an even consistency and color. (See Fig. 18.2D.)
5. Place in an appropriate-size ointment jar, label, fill out the master formula sheet, and leave the product and paperwork for the final check by the pharmacist. (See Fig. 18.2E.)

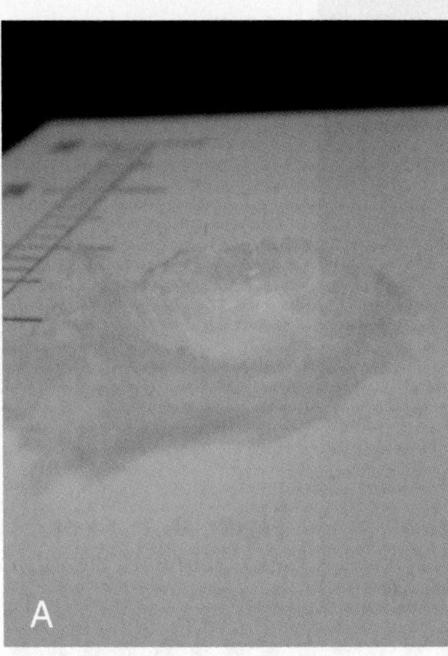
A

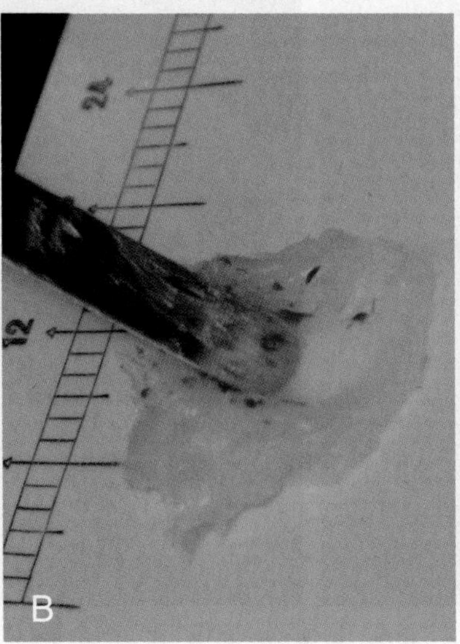
B

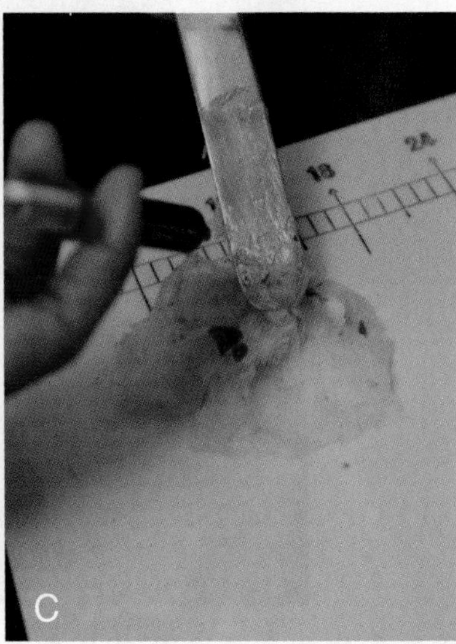
C

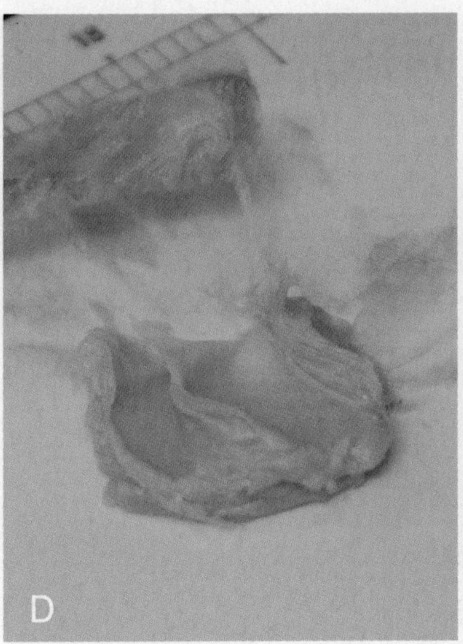

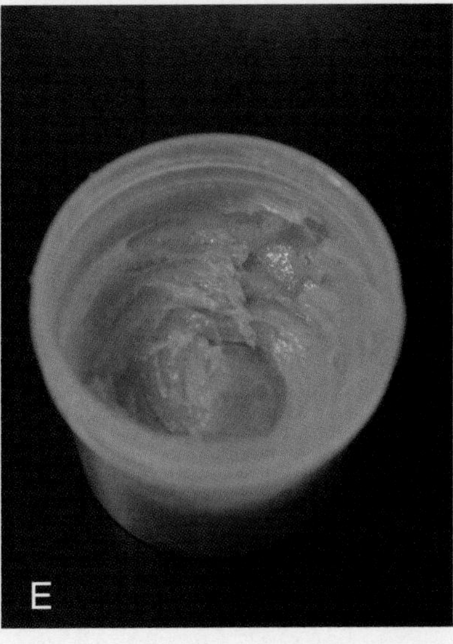

Figure 18.2 Steps for mixing an ointment with a liquid.

Preparation Method 18.3
Mixing a Solid Into an Ointment

See the student CD and website for a video of this procedure.

John Schickel, DO
1801 Lawanna Way
Lansing, MI

Mary Steinhut **Date** 1-15-06

1276 E. Aurelius Road, Masonville, MI

RX: Precipitated Sulfur 300mg
Dermabase 30gm
Apply to affected area bid
John Schickel, DO.

Sig:

Dispense as written — May substitute: *John Schickel, DO*

(Reprinted with permission from Mohr ME. Lab Experiences for the Pharmacy Technician. Baltimore, MD: Lippincott, Williams & Wilkins, 2006.)

1. Triturate the weighed solid into fine particles. (See Fig. 18.3A.)
2. Add a small amount of levigating agent and mix to form a smooth paste. (See Fig. 18.3B.)
3. Spatulate small amounts of the solid mixture into the ointment using geometric dilution. (See Fig. 18.3C.)
4. Continue to spatulate until all ingredients are well mixed. (See Fig. 18.3D.)
5. Place the compound in an appropriate-size ointment jar, label, fill out the master formula sheet, and leave the product along with the paperwork for the final check by the pharmacist. (See Fig. 18.3E.)

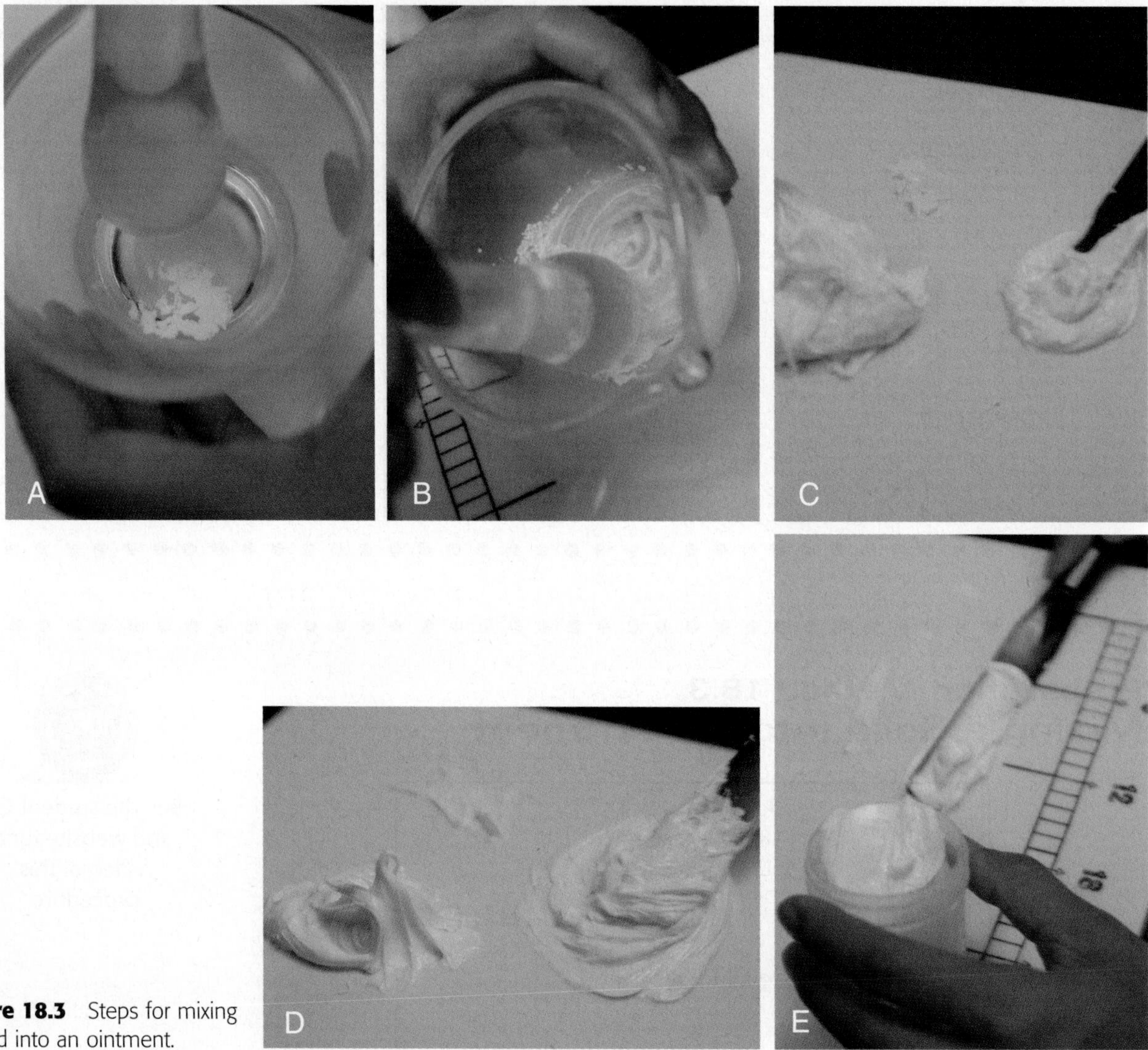

Figure 18.3 Steps for mixing a solid into an ointment.

Packaging and Storage of Compounded Topical Preparations

Extemporaneously compounded ointments, creams, pastes, and gels are packaged in wide-mouth ointment jars with tight-fitting lids or in tubes made of metal or plastic that are crimped at one end and closed at the other end with a tight-fitting lid. It is important to keep them enclosed to prevent contamination, and the container should be light-resistant to ensure protection for any light-sensitive ingredients. Cool temperatures are vital to prevent separation of the ingredients, melting, or other damage from heat.

Labeling and Documentation

A master formula sheet must be completed for each compounded product and kept in a permanent file. See Figure 18.4 for an example of a formula sheet. The manufacturer's expiration date for each ingredient should be noted and an expiration date for the compound should be calculated. There are several methods for

MASTER FORMULA SHEET

Compound ______________________ Quantity __________ Exp Date __________

Student Name __________________ Instructor __________ Date __________

INGREDIENT	NDC #	LOT #	QUANTITY	EXP DATE

Notes:

Figure 18.4 Example of a master formula sheet.

determining an acceptable expiration date. The expiration date is an indication of the length of time that the compounded item may reasonably be expected to remain stable and have the same properties as when it was dispensed. USP Chapter 795 outlines the basic guidelines for establishing beyond-use dating for nonsterile compounds. When a USP or NF substance is the source of one of the ingredients, the expiration date should be no more than 6 months from the date of compounding. When one or more manufactured drug products are used, the expiration date of the final product should be not more than 25% of the time left on the manufacturer's listed expiration date or 6 months, whichever comes first. In some cases, there may be stability problems with the formulation that will dictate a shorter expiration date. Consult appropriate references for this information. The pharmacy should have expiration dating protocols listed in its policy and procedure manual.

The finished compound will require a prescription label listing the ingredients and amounts, the expiration date, and the pertinent information required on all prescription labels. See Figure 18.5 for an example of the prescription label. Any necessary auxiliary labels, such as "For External Use Only" or "Store in a Cool Place," should be applied to the container.

MY Pharmacy
6032 W. Compound Lane
Anycity, Anystate, 60342

RX 1234567 Dr. Killjoy
Marrianna Hope 8/02/07

Apply a thin film to the affected area on leg three times a day until gone
Zinc oxide 2% in White Petrolatum 30 Gm
Expires after 2-20-08

RPh MEM

Figure 18.5 Example of a prescription label.

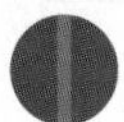

Lip Balms and Topical Application Sticks

Advantages of Lip Balms and Topical Application Sticks

Lip balms and topical application sticks provide a convenient means of applying topical lubricants, protectants, or formulations with various active ingredients. They are very portable and patient acceptance is high. They are often cooling and soothing to the affected area, so there is immediate relief on application.

Disadvantages of Lip Balms and Topical Application Sticks

Lip balms and topical application sticks require storage in a cool place to prevent melting. Because the amount of systemic absorption is minimal, the therapeutic action is primarily topical.

Therapeutic Uses of Compounded Lip Balms and Topical Application Sticks

Compounded lip balms may contain antivirals, camphor, menthol, or thymol to aid in healing cold sores. Adding zinc oxide provides protection from the sun. The emollient base, alone or in combination with other agents, can alleviate chapped lips.

The addition of a hardening agent, such as wax, makes the product suitable for a larger topical application stick. It may contain an anti-inflammatory for arthritis pain, methyl salicylate for a cooling application for muscle pain, or simply cocoa butter to act as a lubricant.

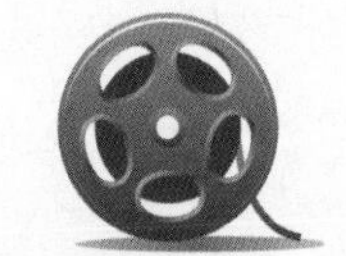

See the student CD and website for a video of this procedure.

Preparation Method 18.4
Compounding Lip Balms and Topical Application Sticks

Peter James, MD
6417 Lily Drive, Fairview, WI 65034
Phone: 642-562-1943

Name: Sally Flowers **Date:** 01-15-06

Address: 7560 West Grant Boulevard, Fairview, WI 65033

RX: Menthol 1%
Thymol 1%
Lip Balm Base qs to make lip balm stick (15gm)

Sig: Apply to sore on lip prn until gone.

Dispense as written

Peter James, MD
May substitute

(Reprinted with permission from Mohr ME. Lab Experiences for the Pharmacy Technician. Baltimore, MD: Lippincott, Williams & Wilkins, 2006.)

1. Prepare the active ingredient(s) by weighing and triturating the menthol and thymol until they liquefy and form a eutectic mixture. (See Fig. 18.6A.)
2. Prepare a water bath by heating water in a large beaker and placing a smaller beaker inside. Be careful to keep the temperature low enough to avoid altering the ingredients. (See Fig. 18.6B.)
3. Weigh 15 g of lip balm base and place it in the smaller beaker. Stir with a glass stirring rod until the base is melted and add the prepared powdered ingredients or liquefied eutectic mixture and mix until clear. (See Fig. 18.6C.)
4. Using an oral syringe, carefully transfer the mixture into a lip balm container. Overfill slightly because the center will recede as it cools. Prop the lip balm tube in an upright position until the balm solidifies. (See Fig. 18.6D.)
5. Clean any excess from the top of the stick and create a pharmaceutically elegant product. Store the finished product in the refrigerator or a cool place. Lip balm can also be poured into a small ointment jar and cooled. (See Fig. 18.6E.)
6. Apply a prescription label including directions for use and storage, and the expiration date. The lip balm tube can either have a flagged label or be placed in a large prescription vial with the complete label and a small label with the prescription number applied to the tube.

eutectic mixture Two or more chemicals that change from a solid form to a liquid when mixed together.

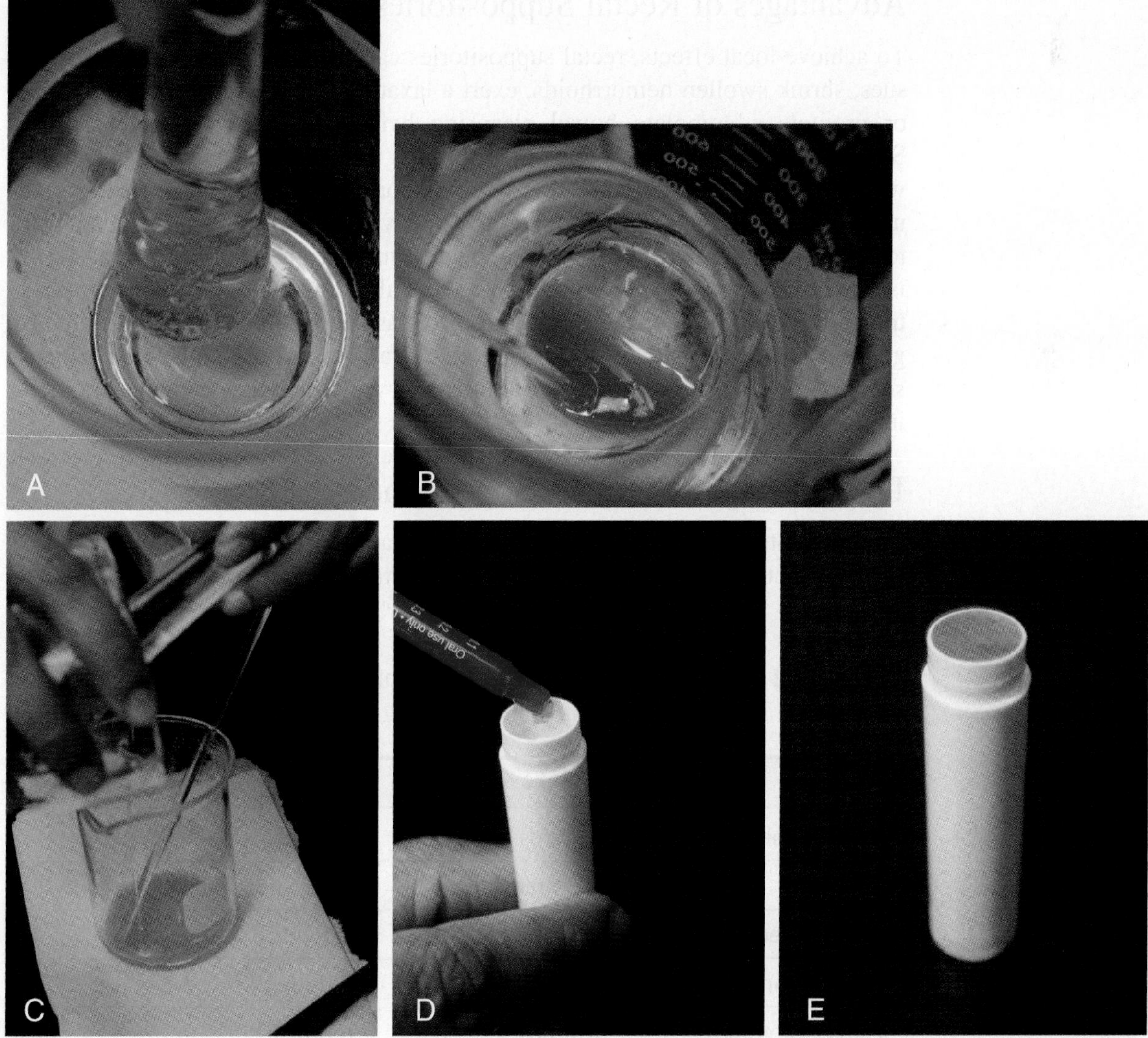

Figure 18.6 Steps for compounding lip balms and topical application sticks.

7. Prepare a master formula sheet and leave the product and paperwork for the final check by the pharmacist.

Larger topical application sticks can be prepared in much the same way using cocoa butter and a small amount of wax to harden the product and facilitate application. Such sticks might contain, for example, acyclovir for application to an area of shingles, or a corticosteroid to apply to an inflamed area. A master formula sheet must be completed for each of these compounded formulations and initialed by the compounding technician and the verifying pharmacist.

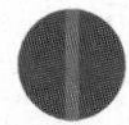

Suppositories

Suppositories are dosage forms that are meant to be inserted into a designated body cavity. The size and shape of the suppository are determined by the administration route and the size of the patient. Table 18.2 gives approximate sizes and uses of some suppository formulations.

Advantages of Rectal Suppositories

To achieve local effects, rectal suppositories can be used to soothe inflamed tissues, shrink swollen hemorrhoids, exert a laxative effect, act as a stool softener, or promote a complete bowel cleansing before diagnostic tests or surgery. Systemic effects can also be attained through the rectal route of administration with suppositories. A patient who is vomiting or unconscious can benefit from the use of a rectal suppository containing an active ingredient. Pain medication for terminal cancer patients is often compounded into a suppository for rectal administration when swallowing becomes too difficult. Drugs that may be destroyed in the gastrointestinal tract or have a high first-pass metabolism in the liver are also good candidates for incorporation into a rectal suppository. Infant or pediatric suppositories may be administered to infants or children who are unable or unwilling to take oral medication.

Disadvantages of Rectal Suppositories

Most patients prefer another route of administration. Rectal suppositories are very inconvenient to use and are not easily transportable for administration away from

Table 18.2 Approximate Sizes and Uses of Some Suppository Formulations

Type	Weight	Use
Adult rectal	2 grams	hemorrhoids
Vaginal	2–5 grams	vaginal yeast infection
Pediatric rectal	1 gram	antipyretic
Male urethral	4 grams	urethritis
Female urethral	2 grams	urethritis

home. The patient is required to lie still for a period of time to prevent expulsion of the suppository, and the suppository may also have a tendency to leak after administration. Although suppositories may contain an active ingredient for systemic absorption, the rate and degree of absorption can be unpredictable.

Administration of Rectal Suppositories

Rectal suppositories are administered as follows:

1. Wash hands and remove the foil wrapping from the suppository.
2. Lubricate the pointed end of the suppository with either K-Y jelly or a small amount of water.
3. Lie on one side with the lower leg straight and the upper leg bent toward the stomach.
4. Lift the upper buttocks and insert the suppository until it passes the rectal sphincter (about 1 inch).
5. Hold the buttocks together and remain lying down for 15 minutes.
6. Wash hands and avoid excessive movement for an hour.

Vaginal Suppositories

Advantages of Vaginal Suppositories

Vaginal suppositories have several advantages as a route of administration. The suppository can be inserted high in the vaginal tract with a vaginal applicator. As the suppository melts, the medication can spread over the vaginal tract. The topical effect of the medication is optimized because it stays in contact with the affected area and can be absorbed through the mucous membrane. The drug also tends to break down more slowly than with the oral route. If the patient has a sensitivity problem with the drug, it can be more easily retrieved.

Disadvantages of Vaginal Suppositories

The vaginal route of administration tends to be inconvenient and messy. Suppositories are usually inserted at bedtime and a sanitary napkin should be worn to absorb any medication leaks. The patient needs to remain somewhat motionless to prevent the suppository from being accidentally expelled. Absorption of an active ingredient is variable because the conditions of the vaginal tract may differ among patients.

Uses of Vaginal Suppositories

Vaginal suppositories are commonly used for treatment of vaginal yeast infections. They are available in 7-day and 3-day dosage forms and have been transferred to OTC status to accommodate patients who have recurring problems with yeast infections and are familiar with the symptoms. Vaginal suppositories can also contain antibiotics for bacterial infections, anti-inflammatory agents, or contraceptives, and be used to adjust the pH of the vaginal mucosa. Different combinations and concentrations of these agents provide many opportunities for extemporaneous compounding.

Administration of Vaginal Suppositories

The steps for administering vaginal suppositories are as follows:

1. Wash hands and unwrap the vaginal suppository.
2. Apply a small amount of K-Y jelly or water.
3. Insert the suppository into the end of the applicator with the plunger extended.
4. Lie on the back and insert the applicator into the vagina.
5. Push the plunger into the vagina as far as it will go and deposit the suppository.
6. Remove the applicator and lie still with legs together as the suppository melts.
7. Wash hands and rinse the applicator.

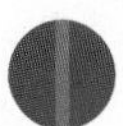

Urethral Suppositories

Urethral suppositories are rather uncommon and rarely encountered. They are usually cylindrical in shape. The size of the suppository depends on the sex of the patient (male suppositories are longer than those used for females).

Factors in Choosing a Suppository Base

The choice of a suppository base is dependent on a number of factors. The first consideration is the route of administration. Fatty-type bases are less irritating to rectal tissue and will be more comfortable for the patient. Polyethylene glycol (PEG) bases are preferred for vaginal and urethral suppositories because they have a lesser tendency to stain clothing when they leak. Fatty bases have fewer compatibility and stability problems when combined with an active ingredient. They are formulated to melt at body temperature and must be stored at controlled room temperature or refrigerated. Systemic absorption of drugs from suppositories is difficult to predict with any base, so the therapeutic effect should be monitored carefully when suppositories are used, and drugs with a narrow therapeutic margin generally should not be used. If a local emollient effect is desired, a fatty base may be the better choice.

Types of Suppository Bases

Cocoa butter is a fatty base that is slightly yellow in color, with a mild cocoa odor and a bland taste. It is insoluble in water and does not absorb significant amounts of water. Some drugs, such as chloral hydrate, phenol, and thymol, will lower the melting point, and wax must be added to maintain the product as a solid. Cocoa butter is an emollient and is non-irritating to sensitive membranes. It is readily available and is easy to pour into suppository molds. Suppositories made from cocoa butter must be stored at controlled room temperature or in the refrigerator to prevent melting. Care must be taken when heating cocoa butter to prevent overheating, which will result in melting at room temperature. The release of drugs from cocoa butter suppositories can be erratic, so it is important to check reference books to determine whether the drug is compatible with cocoa butter.

Other fatty bases include cocoa butter substitutes made from various vegetable oils. Witepsol is a whitish, waxy solid that is odorless and will absorb a small amount of water. There are a number of different grades of this commercial product and pharmacists have reported varying degrees of satisfaction with it. Fattibase is another commercial cocoa butter substitute. This white, waxy, odorless solid offers the advantage of a less-sensitive melting point, but it also has some of the same incompatibilities as cocoa butter.

Glycerinated gelatin bases are similar to gummy gel bases. They are difficult to work with and can only be used for vaginal administration because of their soft rubbery consistency. They need to be stored in a refrigerator.

Nonfatty suppository bases are made with PEG along with surfactants. A commercial PEG base is Polybase. Suppositories made with PEG do not melt at body temperature. They are designed to melt in the body cavity fluids and release the active ingredients. They do not require storage at controlled temperatures, but they tend to be irritating to sensitive body tissues. They have a long list of incompatibilities, including a reaction with polystyrene, so they should not be dispensed in plastic prescription vials unless they are first wrapped with foil. Although suppositories can be a very beneficial dosage form, compounding them requires a certain amount of skill and the release of active ingredients in the body is unpredictable.

Preparation Method 18.5
Preparation Method for Suppositories

1. Calculate the amount of base needed for the prescribed number of suppositories plus two extra to account for loss during compounding.
2. Weigh the active ingredients and triturate them to a fine homogenous powder.
3. Shave the cocoa butter into small pieces and melt it in warm water bath.
4. Dissolve the powder ingredients in melted cocoa butter.
5. Pour the contents into a suppository mold and allow them to cool.

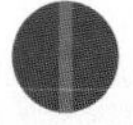

Chapter Summary

- Topical preparations such as ointments, creams, and suppositories provide opportunities for patient-specific compounding by a knowledgeable technician.
- Compounded topical preparations are advantageous because they have an emollient effect, are soothing to inflamed skin, provide protection from the sun or other irritants, target the affected area, have little systemic absorption, cause few side effects, and result in good patient compliance.
- Disadvantages include the facts that they are messy to apply and difficult to transport, and low absorption may result in the underlying problem not being solved.
- Compounded topical formulations can be used as keratolytics, antifungals, antiseptics, emollients, antihistamines, antibiotics, or combinations directed specifically toward the needs of the patient.
- Ointment bases should be chosen according to the properties that would best accomplish the intended use of the final product.
- Creams are forms of ointments made with a base that is more fluid in consistency, easily applied, and water washable.

- Pastes are made by adding large amounts of solid ingredients to make a thick, stiff final product.
- Compounded lip balms and topical application sticks provide a convenient dosage form for application of topical lubricants, protectants, or therapeutic active ingredients to the lips or skin.
- Suppositories can provide local or systemic effects to patients who are unable to take oral medications.

Review Questions

Multiple Choice

Choose the most correct answer to the following statements.

1. Advantages of compounded topical preparations include:
   a. low systemic absorption
   b. immediately soothing to inflamed skin
   c. few side effects
   d. all of the above

2. Disadvantages of compounded topical preparations include all of the following except:
   a. inconvenient to transport
   b. high patient compliance
   c. messy to apply
   d. may not solve the underlying problem

3. Therapeutic uses of compounded topical preparations include:
   a. treatment of fungal infections
   b. antiseptic to minor skin irritation
   c. antibiotic for systemic infection
   d. a and b

4. The following compounding techniques may be used to prepare a compound of a solid chemical in an ointment base:
   a. trituration
   b. levigation
   c. spatulation
   d. all of the above

5. Which of the following characteristics does not describe a cream?
   a. less protective than ointments
   b. water-washable
   c. occlusive
   d. slightly fluid in consistency

Fill in the Blank

Fill in the blanks with the word or words that best complete the statements below.

6. ______________________ have an amount of powder added to an ointment base that makes them stiff in consistency.
7. Two solid ingredients that form a liquid when triturated together are called a ______________________________.
8. ______________________________ contain a high amount of liquid, are nonocclusive, and are easily washed off.
9. The ______________________ is an indication of the length of time a product may be expected to remain stable and retain the same properties as when it was dispensed.
10. Dosage forms that are intended to be inserted into a body cavity for a therapeutic effect are called ______________________.

True/False

Mark the following statements True or False.

11. ________ White petrolatum is an example of an oleaginous ointment base.
12. ________ A person who is vomiting may benefit from a rectal suppository dosage form.
13. ________ Systemic effects cannot be achieved by using a rectal suppository with an active ingredient.
14. ________ Fatty-type suppository bases are less irritating to rectal tissue than PEG bases.
15. ________ Cocoa butter used in compounding suppositories should be melted at a high temperature.

Matching

Match the terms in column A with the definitions in column B.

Column A

16. ______ geometric dilution
17. ______ O/W emulsion
18. ______ cream
19. ______ trituration
20. ______ spatulation

Column B

A. Semisolid dosage form containing one or more drug substances dissolved or dispersed in a water-removable base.
B. The process of reducing particle size using a mortar and pestle.
C. Mixing solid chemicals together by taking equal parts of each in small amounts and mixing thoroughly until all are mixed.
D. Process of mixing an ointment on an ointment slab with a spatula to ensure uniformity of particles.
E. Emulsion in which oil is the internal phase and water is the external phase.

LEARNING ACTIVITY

Using the following prescription for a compounded ointment, describe the preparation and compounding process. Include the following:

- equipment needed
- calculations
- ingredients
- detailed compounding procedure
- documentation
- packaging
- labeling

Joseph James, M.D.
2432 N. Tuxedo Junction
Alexandria, VA 46321

Laverne Wilson 06/07/XX
5672 Larel Lane, Alexandria, Virginia, 46354

RX:

Camphor		3%
Menthol		3%
Hydrocortisone powder		200 mg
White Petrolatum	qs ad 60 g	

Sig: Apply to rash on leg bid

Dispense as written — Joseph James, MD — May substitute

Suggested Readings

Allen LV, Popovich NG, Ansel HC. Ansel's Pharmaceutical Dosage Forms and Drug Delivery Systems. Philadelphia: Lippincott, Williams & Wilkins, 2004.

Gennaro AR, ed. Remington: The Science and Practice of Pharmacy. Baltimore, MD: Lippincott, Williams & Wilkins, 2006.

Shrewsbury R. Applied Pharmaceutics in Contemporary Compounding. Englewood, CO: Morton Publishing, 2001.

Thompson J, Davidow L. A Practical Guide to Contemporary Pharmacy Practice, 3rd ed. Philadelphia: Lippincott, Williams & Wilkins, 2004.

UNIT VI

Compounded Sterile Products

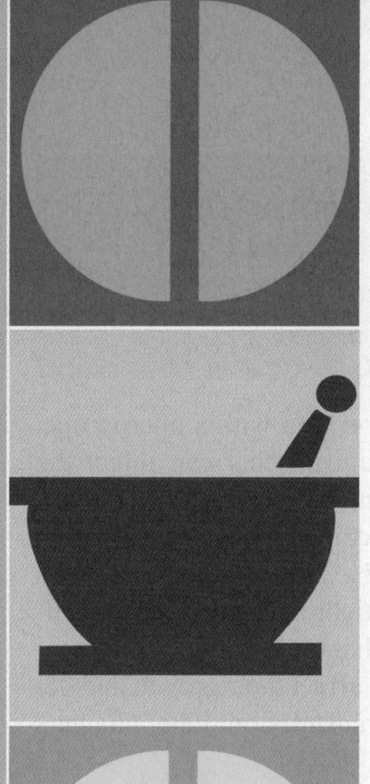

Chapter **19**

Introduction to Microbiology and Aseptic Technique

OBJECTIVES

After completing this chapter, the student will be able to:

- Define microbiology and explain the importance of understanding the relationship of microbial contamination and aseptic technique.
- Differentiate between types of infective agents.
- Describe differences between prokaryotes and eukaryotes.
- Discuss how microbial oxygen use and temperature affect the viability of an organism.
- List portals of entry and transmission methods for microbial contamination.
- Define human microbe relationships.

KEY TERMS

- aerobe
- anaerobe
- antiseptic
- asepsis
- bactericidal
- bacteriostatic
- binary fission
- commensalism
- disinfectant
- endotoxins
- eukaryotes
- exotoxins
- facultative anaerobes
- flagella
- fomites
- fungicide
- Gram staining
- microaerophiles
- microbiology

- microorganisms
- morphology
- mutualism
- normal flora
- nosocomial
- obligate aerobes
- oligate anaerobes
- parasitism
- pathogens
- prokaryotes
- symbiosis
- synergism

microbiology The study of microscopic organisms.

microorganisms Minute living bodies that are visible only with the aid of a microscope.

Microbiology is the study of organisms that can only be seen with a microscope. This includes bacteria, fungi, viruses, and other organisms that can infect the human body. A basic understanding of microbiology and the various forms of microbial contamination that can occur is essential for technicians who are about to begin training in the preparation of parenteral products. The administration of a contaminated parenteral product into the veins of a patient may cause serious illness and may result in the death of the patient. This chapter introduces the common pathogenic microorganisms, discusses factors that affect their growth and development, and describes portals of entry for disease transmission. Later chapters will discuss asepsis in the work environment.

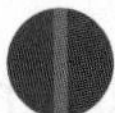

Classifications of Bacteria

morphology The size, shape, and arrangement of bacteria.

flagella Hairlike appendages on bacteria that create movement.

obigate aerobes Organisms that require an atmosphere with oxygen to survive.

microaerophiles Organisms that need only 5% oxygen to survive.

Bacteria are classified in a number of different ways. Morphology pertains to the size, shape, and arrangement of bacteria. Most bacteria range between 0.2 and 10 micrometers in size. Circular-shaped bacteria are called cocci and may occur in pairs of two (diplococci), clusters (staphylocci), or long chains (streptococci). Bacteria that are shaped like a rod are called bacilli and may appear as diplobacilli (a pair of two) or streptobacilli (forming a long chain). Other bacteria may be curved or spiral-shaped and are called spirilla, vibrio, or spirochetes. See Figure 19.1 for pictures of bacteria shapes. Another characteristic of bacteria is their growth rate when cultured on an agar plate in the laboratory. The growth rate of bacteria is determined by the number of organisms present, rather than an increase in the size of the organism. Another identifying characteristic of bacteria is their ability to move, and the method of movement. Bacterial movement is called motility and is accomplished by means of fine hairlike structures called flagella or by axial filaments.

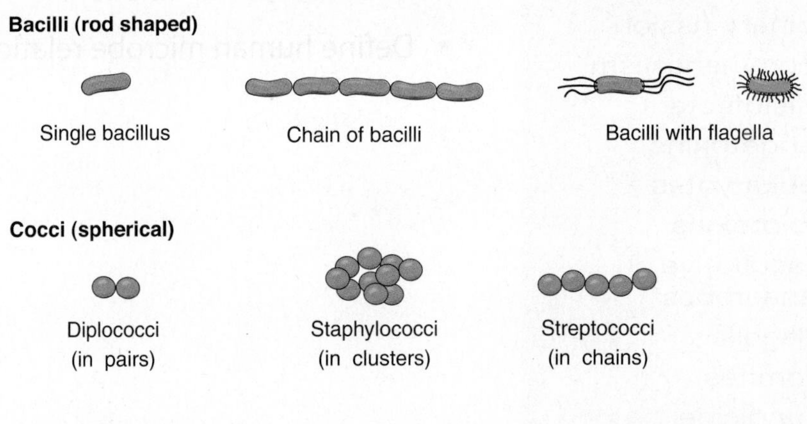

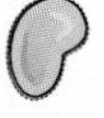

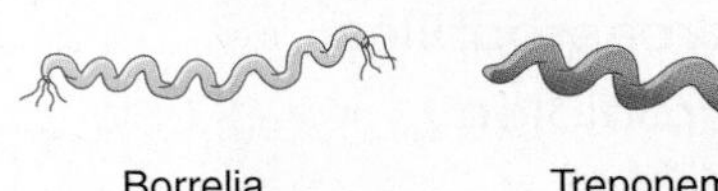

Figure 19.1 Bacteria shapes: cocci, bacilli, spiral. (Reprinted with permission from Sakai J. Practical Pharmacology for the Pharmacy Technician. Baltimore, MD: Lippincott Williams & Wilkins, 2008.)

Bacteria are classified as either aerobes or anaerobes depending on the amount of oxygen needed. Obligate aerobes need a level of oxygen similar to that of room air (usually around 20%), whereas microaerophiles need only about 5% oxygen to survive. Obligate anaerobes require an atmosphere with no oxygen, and facultative anaerobes function with or without the presence of oxygen. Most bacteria grow best in a moderate temperature and a neutral pH, and prefer darkness and moisture. The most important classification of bacteria in a healthcare setting is whether they are pathogenic or nonpathogenic. Pathogenicity can occur by several means. The bacteria may secrete enzymes called exotoxins that can damage the host cell. Some bacteria may cause direct damage to the host cell. When the bacterial cell dies, the cell wall may be lysed and release endotoxins. The degree to which an organism is pathogenic is described as its virulence.

Gram staining is another method of classifying bacteria. It has proved to be very useful for identifying pathogens and determining the specific antibiotic that will provide an effective treatment. The bacteria is first stained with a violet stain and then counterstained with a red stain. Gram-positive bacteria will retain the violet stain. Gram-negative bacteria will assume the red stain.

Bacterial infections are treated with antibiotics. Antibiotics may be bactericidal, meaning they kill the bacteria. They may be bacteriostatic, meaning they inhibit the growth of the bacteria.

oligate anaerobes Organisms that require an atmosphere with no oxygen to survive.

facultative anaerobes Organisms that can function with or without oxygen.

exotoxins Enzymes secreted by bacteria that can damage the host cell.

endotoxins Toxic substances released when a bacterial cell dies and the cell wall is lysed.

Gram staining Laboratory procedure used to identify bacteria.

pathogens Microbes capable of causing disease.

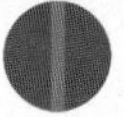

Prokaryotes and Eukaryotes

Bacteria classified as prokaryotes have less-complex cells than eukaryotes. They have a cell wall but no true nucleus, and the cells divide by binary fission. They move by a rotating motion produced by simple flagella. See Figure 19.2 for a drawing of a prokaryotic cell.

Eukaryotes are more complex cells. They include algae, fungi, and all plant, animal, and human cells. They contain a true nucleus and nucleolus, and cell division is accomplished by mitosis. They have a simple cell wall and complex flagella, so they move with a wavelike motion. See Figure 19-3 for a drawing of a typical eukaryote cell.

prokaryotes Less complex cells, including bacteria.

binary fission Manner of cell division of prokaryotes.

eukaryotes Complex cells, including fungi and all plant and animal cells.

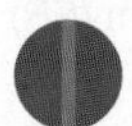

Pathogen Transmission

Pathogens can survive for long periods of time before being transferred to a host. The pools of pathogens are called fomites and they may be living or inanimate objects. Living fomites include animals, insects, and humans. Insects can transmit disease through the bite of an infected insect. Eating infected meat or coming into contact with an animal infected with a transmittable disease can cause disease in humans. Inanimate objects can be reservoirs of pathogens, so it is important to be careful with hospital equipment, linens, and clothing that may be infected with blood or body fluids. Bacteria can be removed from inanimate objects by cleaning with an antiseptic. Disease can be spread by food prepared by a contaminated person or a person infected with hepatitis who does not thoroughly wash his or her hands after using the restroom. Someone who touches an infected person or a contaminated object without either wearing gloves or thoroughly washing his or her hands after exposure can spread disease by direct contact. A person who has come into contact with blood and body fluids (especially if the patient has a cut or open

fomites living or inanimate cells that harbor pathogens

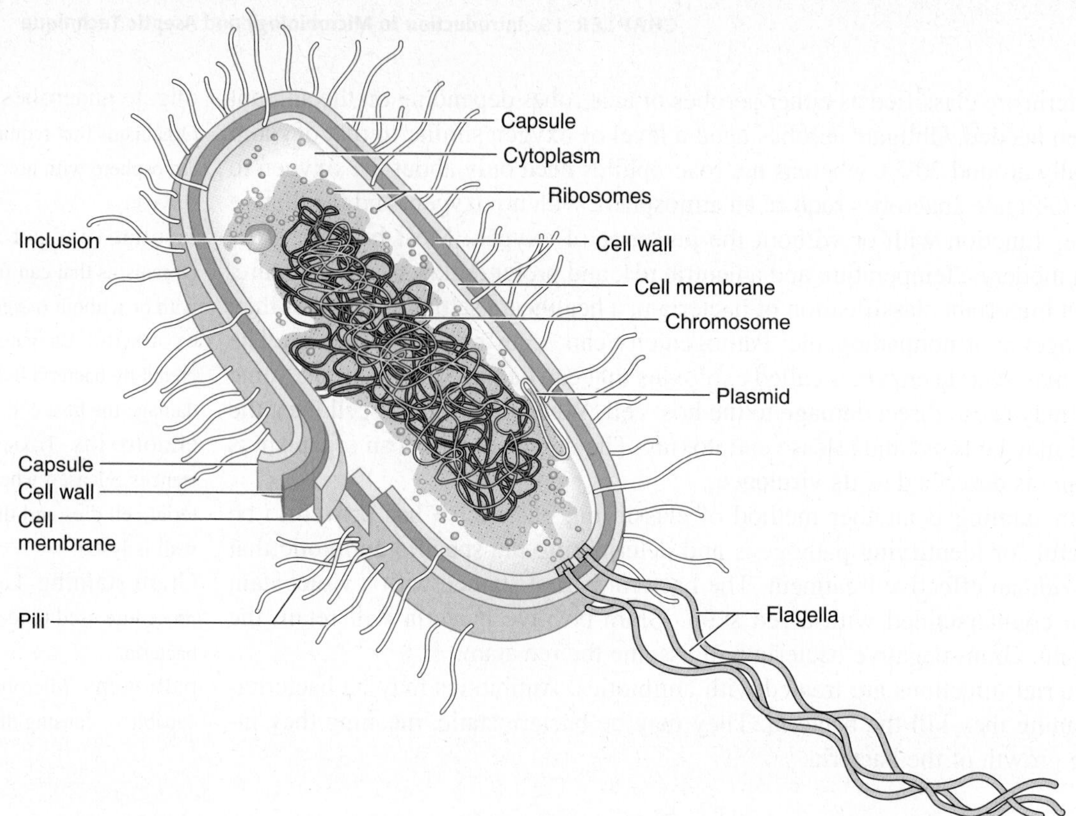

Figure 19.2 Prokaryotic cell. (Reprinted with permission from Engelkirk PG, Burton GRW. Burton's Microbiology for the Health Sciences. 8th ed. Baltimore, MD: Lippincott, Williams & Wilkins, 2006.)

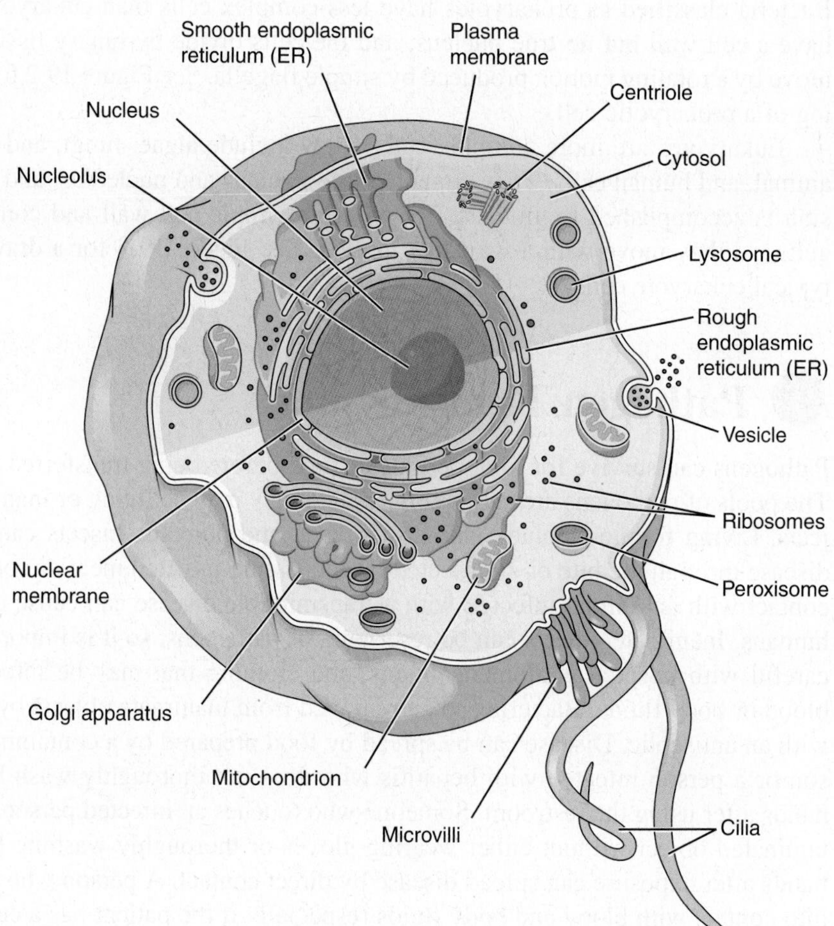

Figure 19.3 Eukaryotic cell. (Reprinted with permission from Cohen BJ. Memmler's The Human Body in Health and Disease. 10th ed. Baltimore, MD: Lippincott, Williams & Wilkins, 2005.)

wound) or with air droplets expelled through sneezing by an infected person can spread disease by direct contact.

 Portals of Entry and Exit

There are various ways in which organisms can gain entrance to the body. The skin is the largest organ in the body, and intact skin is the body's best line of defense against infection by a pathogenic organism. Some organisms can penetrate intact skin, but most need some opportunity for entrance, such as a cut or open wound, an injection, or even an insect bite. In some cases, even the sweat glands and pores of the skin are enough to provide a portal of entry for a pathogen. Mucous membranes line the respiratory tract, gastrointestinal tract, genitourinary tract, and even the eye. These membranes are much easier to penetrate than intact skin and are often the preferred site of entry for pathogenic organisms. Some organisms secrete enzymes that help them gain entry to the skin. Some form a capsule around the cell wall to increase their virulence by making them less susceptible to the body's defenses. Once an organism gains access to the body tissues, it can begin its pathogenic processes.

Just as there are portals of entry into the body, there are also portals of exit through which the organisms leave the host and become available to contaminate another host. Portals of exit include blood and body fluids, fecal matter, saliva, and respiratory secretions. Proper handling of these contaminants is essential to avoid introducing the pathogens into another host. This is particularly true in a hospital setting, where nosocomial infections can be particularly deadly to patients already compromised by a health problem.

nosocomial Infection acquired in a healthcare setting.

 Pathogenic Processes

If an organism has used one of the above methods to protect itself from the body's defenses, it can begin to attach to the host cell and perform all the life functions needed to metabolize, allowing it to multiply and begin killing other host cells. Although this multiplication process causes considerable damage to the host, there are also several other mechanisms by which pathogens can harm the host. Some may produce exotoxins that dissolve in the bloodstream and are transported throughout the system, producing disease as they travel. Exotoxins can be in the form of neurotoxins that interfere with nerve transmissions, enterotoxins that affect the gastrointestinal tract, or cytotoxins that attack the cell and cause damage or death. In some cases the body is capable of producing an antitoxin to block the action of the toxin.

Endotoxins are produced when the bacteria die and the cell wall is lysed, releasing the endotoxin. They can cause fever, chills, and body aches, and in severe cases may result in shock that can lead to death. The bacteria that produce endotoxins can be treated with antibiotics.

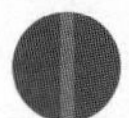 Microbial-Host Relationships

When microorganisms invade a host, there may be varying degrees of harm or benefit. Symbiosis is the name given to the relationship in which two unrelated organisms live together and may benefit each other, cause harm to one or the other, or be harmless to both. An example of this are the normal flora of organisms present in the human body. Disturbing the balance of the flora may result in the overgrowth of one, causing a disease state to develop. There are normal bacterial flora in the

symbiosis Two organisms living together in a close relationship.

normal flora Microscopic organisms adapted to living in the body without causing disease.

intestines. Treatment of a bacterial infection with antibiotics may upset this balance, causing diarrhea. Mutualism is the situation that exists when two organisms live together and both of them benefit from the relationship and depend on it for survival. Synergism describes the relationship in which two organisms work together to produce a desired effect that cannot be produced by either organism alone. In commensalism, one organism benefits from the relationship but the other is not affected either way. Parasitism is a situation in which one organism benefits while causing harm to the host.

mutualism Condition in which two organisms live together and both of them benefit from the relationship and depend on it for survival.

synergism Relationship in which two organisms work together to produce a desired effect that cannot be produced by either organism alone.

commensalism The relationship that exists when two organisms invade a host and one benefits from the relationship but the other is not affected either way.

parasitism Relationship in which one organism benefits while causing harm to the host.

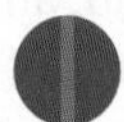

Viruses

Viruses are obligate intracellular parasites. They cannot live on their own and must invade a living cell. They contain either RNA or DNA, but not both. They take over and use the replication processes of the host cell. Viruses are the smallest of the pathogenic microorganisms and are difficult to treat. Infection by a virus often takes place through an exchange of body fluids, ingestion of contaminated food or water, inhalation of respiratory droplets from a diseased individual, or the bite of an infected insect. Viruses can lie dormant in the host until they are reactivated by an immunocompromised host. An example of this is the herpes virus.

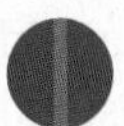

Rickettsiae

Rickettsiae are smaller than bacteria but larger than viruses. They are parasites that live on a host cell, causing disease. They are generally transmitted through the bite of an insect or an animal vector. An example of a disease caused by Rickettsiae transmitted by a tick is Rocky Mountain spotted fever.

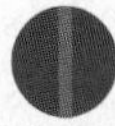

Fungi

Fungi are a group of eukaryotic organisms that include molds and yeasts. Some yeasts that are part of the normal flora in the human body can cause infections known as mycoses when they become overgrown. This proliferation may be due to the use of an antibiotic, which kills the bacteria that normally keep the yeast population in the proper balance. Mycoses are classified according to where they occur. A superficial mycoses affects only the outermost layer of the skin and hair. A cutaneous infection involves the keratin in the skin, hair, and nails, causing inflammation in the skin. Subcutaneous infection involves the soft tissues, muscles, and bones immediately below the skin. A systemic infection goes deep into the tissues and organs of the body. Various antifungal agents are available for treating fungal infections. However, because fungal cells are similar to human cells, these antifungal agents can cause severe reactions in humans. Fungus contamination can be removed from surfaces by cleaning with a fungicide.

Risk Factors for Opportunistic Fungal Infections

Fungal infections are usually the result of exposure to a pathogen at a time when the host's immune system is compromised, allowing the cells to proliferate when they would normally be kept in check by the body's immune system. Factors that increase the risk of opportunistic fungal infections include taking immunosuppressive drugs and undergoing corticosteroid or antibiotic therapy. Disease conditions that contribute to a higher risk for fungal infections include diabetes, certain types of cancer, and diseases that can cause immune deficiencies (e.g., HIV).

Yeasts

As the number of immunocompromised people increases, the incidence of yeast infections is also rising, and an increasing number of yeasts are considered pathogenic. Yeasts are found everywhere—in soil, water, fruits, and vegetables—and some yeasts are considered part of the normal flora of the human body. They are used in the food and beverage industry to ferment sugars when making alcohol or bread. Various *Candida* species of yeasts are part of the natural human flora and are found in the gastrointestinal, rectal, oral, and vaginal mucosa. Overgrowth of these species due to antibiotic treatment or various diseases can result in a number of yeast infections of the skin and nails, and oral and vaginal mucosa. Among the most common of these are vaginal candidiasis and thrush or trench mouth. Immunocompromised patients are prone to more serious systemic infections that can be life threatening and must be treated aggressively.

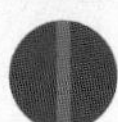

Helminths

Helminths are multicellular animal parasites or worms that are microscopic during certain stages of their life cycle. They can be transmitted through fecal matter or by consumption of uncooked meat, such as pork. They are the largest organisms that are responsible for producing human disease. They may present as roundworms, pinworms, hookworms, trichinella, or flatworms.

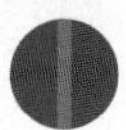

Importance of Microbiology to the Pharmacy Technician

An understanding of the principles of microbiology is essential to the professional pharmacy technician as a foundation for developing excellent aseptic technique. The slightest break in proper technique can create a life-threatening condition for a patient who is already immunocompromised. If the patient survives, they may require weeks or even months of expensive drug therapy, resulting in longer, more expensive hospital stays, increased days of missed work, and lasting ill effects. Even in a retail pharmacy that does not perform IV admixture, the technician has a responsibility to exercise caution when accepting and filling prescriptions to prevent contamination that may be detrimental to the patient or the pharmacy staff. Pharmacy counters should be frequently cleaned with alcohol or some other disinfectant. This is especially true for the intake counter, where patients set children and other personal items. New prescriptions and refill bottles may act as fomites and present an opportunity for transmission of pathogenic organisms. Keep tablet-counting trays and spatulas clean and maintain the counting machines properly. Frequent hand washing is essential and it is wise to keep a box of latex gloves near the intake area to clean spills that may contain body fluids. The professional technician will perform these routine maintenance functions in a discreet manner without causing embarrassment to the patient.

disinfectant Agent used to kill bacteria on inanimate objects.

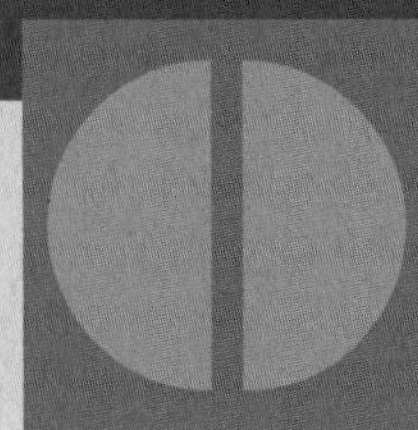

Case Study 19.1

Mark was assigned to spend the day in IV admixture. It was a busy day and he had many IVs to prepare. Mark worked quickly and carefully, trying to keep up with the work. His friend Stan came by and brought a drink to Mark so he could keep working. Stan set the drink on the corner of the table just inside the cleanroom and did not enter the room himself because he was not gowned up. Mark continued to draw fluid from the vial he was working with, but thanked Stan for being thoughtful. After finishing the bag he was working with, Mark went over to the table to get a drink from the cup Stan had left. He was still wearing his latex gloves, so he returned to the IV hood and continued his work. In his haste to complete the work on time, Mark stuck his finger with the needle he was using for IV admixture. It didn't bleed much, so he replaced the needle, wiped his glove with alcohol, and continued with the mixture. As the afternoon continued, it became very warm in the cleanroom. Mark thought it was OK to remove his face mask because there was no one else in the room to talk to. Later, when he was mixing a drug that had

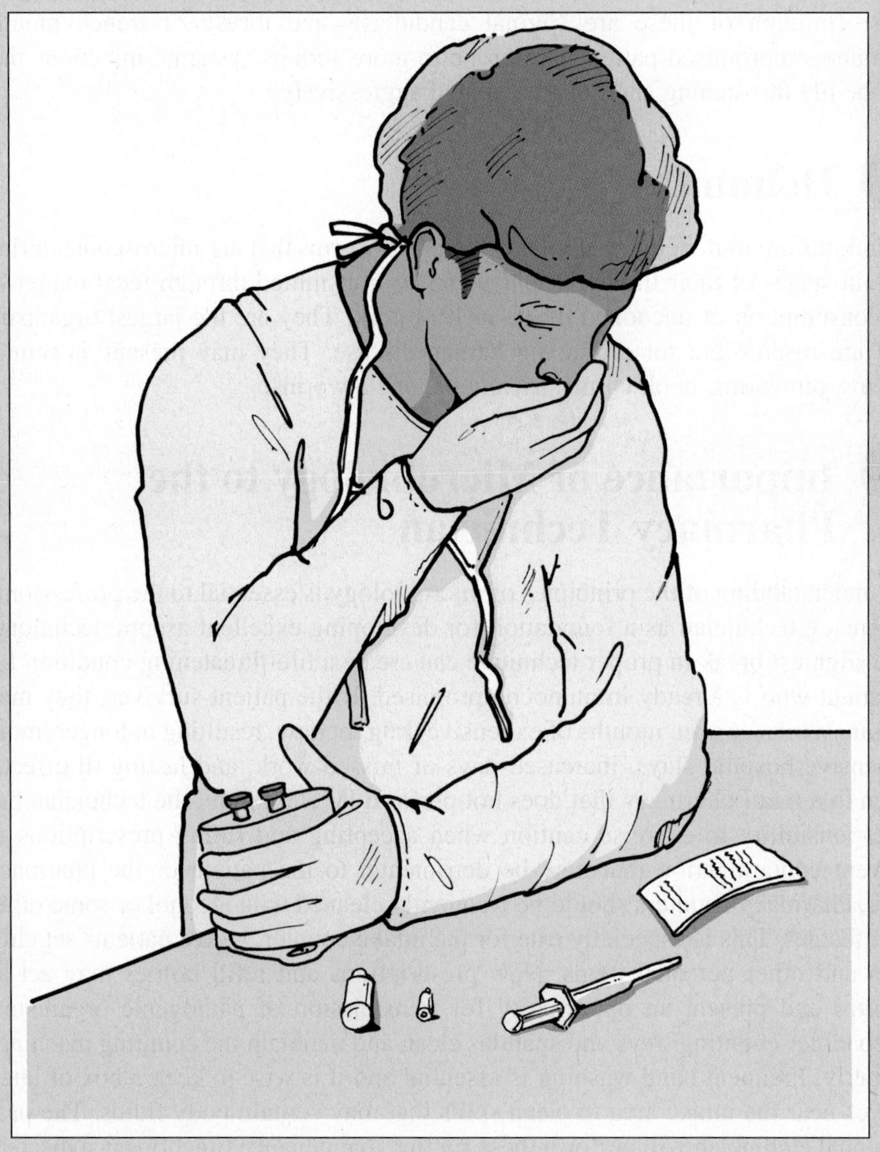

a noxious smell, Mark sneezed. He turned his head away from the hood as he sneezed. Mark knew he didn't have a cold, so he thought there was no harm done. Luckily, he completed all the IV admixtures before the end of his work day.

1. Did Mark use correct aseptic technique as he worked in the cleanroom?
2. Cite some breaches of technique and explain why they may cause a problem.

Chapter Summary

- Microbiology is the study of organisms that can only be seen with a microscope.
- Bacteria may be classified according to morphology growth and motility.
- Bacteria may be classified according to oxygen and nutritional requirements.
- Pathogenicity is the ability of an organism to cause disease or illness in a person.
- Eukaryotes are more complex cells and include plant, animal, and human cells.
- Prokaryotes are less complex cells and include bacteria.
- Fomites can be either living things or inanimate objects that are capable of transmitting pathogens.
- Diseases can be transmitted by direct or indirect contact.
- Pathogenic organisms must find a suitable portal of entry to invade the host.
- Symbiotic human microbe relationships can be either beneficial or harmful to one or both organisms.
- Viruses are obligate parasites that must take over the metabolic processes of the host to multiply and survive.
- Fungi include molds and yeasts that may be part of the normal flora or may cause disease when the normal balance is upset.
- Fungi cause opportunistic infections in immunocompromised patients or those taking certain drugs.
- Helminths are microscopic at certain times during the life cycle and then become animal parasites presenting as various types of worms.
- Avoiding microbial contamination is a prime responsibility of technicians in preparing and dispensing prescription medications.

Review Questions

Multiple Choice

Choose the correct answer to the following statements.

1. Which of the following organisms is the smallest?
   a. bacteria
   b. fungi
   c. viruses
   d. helminths

2. Which of the following bacteria shapes are characterized by a chain formation?
   a. staphylococcus
   b. diplococcus
   c. streptococcus
   d. diplobacilli
3. Which type of bacterial toxin is released only when the cell dies?
   a. exotoxin
   b. endotoxin
   c. pseudotoxin
   d. mortal toxin
4. Which of the following are circular-shaped bacteria?
   a. vibrio
   b. bacillus
   c. cocci
   d. spirochete
5. What is a more common name for helminths?
   a. insects
   b. arthropods
   c. worms
   d. germs

Fill in the Blank

Fill in the blank(s) with the correct word or words to complete the statement.

6. Hairlike processes that cause bacteria to move by wavelike contractions are called ____________.
7. A *Candida* infection seen commonly in the mouths of newborns characterized by white patches is called ____________________.
8. A relationship between two organisms in which one organism is harmed by the presence of the other is called ____________________________.
9. Organisms that are parasites and are much smaller than bacteria but larger than viruses are called ________________________________.
10. A direct pathway for an organism to gain entry into the body is called a ____.

True/False

Mark the following statements True or False

11. _______ Aerobic bacteria must have oxygen to live.

12. _______ Most bacteria prefer direct sunlight for optimal growth.

13. _______ Yeasts are used commercially in the preparation of beer and wine.

14. _______ Helminths are the largest organism known to cause disease in humans.

15. _______ The overall health of the host is a determining factor for the risk of infection.

Matching

Match the terms in column A with the definitions in column B.

Column A	Column B
16. _______ antiseptic	A. Agent used to kill bacteria on inanimate objects.
17. _______ asepsis	B. Agent that kills bacteria.
18. _______ bactericidal	C. Agent that inhibits the growth of bacteria.
19. _______ bacteriostatic	D. The complete absence of microbes.
20. _______ disinfectant	E. Agent used to inhibit growth of microbes on living tissue.

Suggested Readings

Cohen BJ. Memmler's The Human Body in Health and Disease. 10th ed. Baltimore, MD: Lippincott, Williams & Wilkins, 2005.

Engelkirk PG, Burton GRW. Burton's Microbiology for the Health Sciences. 8th ed. Baltimore, MD: Lippincott, Williams & Wilkins, 2006.

Sakai J. Practical Pharmacology for the Pharmacy Technician. Baltimore, MD: Lippincott, Williams & Wilkins, 2008.

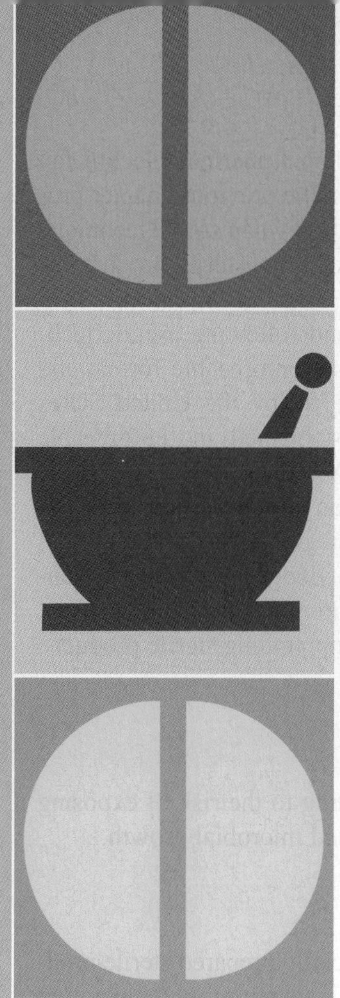

Chapter 20

USP Chapter 797 Guidelines for Compounded Sterile Products

OBJECTIVES

After completing this chapter, the student will be able to:

- Explain the reasons for formalizing 797 requirements.
- Discuss the technician's responsibility to ensure the sterility of compounded sterile products.
- Outline proper hand-washing, gowning, and gloving procedures.
- Establish cleaning procedures for the cleanroom.
- Describe the anteroom requirements and procedures for bringing supplies into the cleanroom.
- Describe the operation of both a horizontal and a vertical laminar airflow (LAF) workbench.
- Differentiate between procedures for using a glovebox and an open workbench.
- Establish a standard operating procedure for performing IV admixture using aseptic technique.

KEY TERMS

- anteroom
- aseptic technique
- barrier isolator
- cleanroom
- ISO Class 5
- ISO Class 8
- laminar airflow (LAF) workbench
- zone of turbulence

aseptic technique Procedure for mixing sterile compounded products with a complete absence of viable microorganisms.

Among the most important responsibilities of a professional pharmacy technician is compounding sterile products using aseptic technique. The previous chapter provided an introduction to the incredible risk of contamination when sterile technique is compromised, and the serious risk to the patient when a nonsterile product enters the bloodstream.

Guidelines for maintaining a sterile environment and following aseptic technique were published years ago, but they were not in an enforceable format and were often ignored. With the publication of Chapter 797 by the United States Pharmacopeia (USP), the guidelines became firmly established and enforceable rules. Many hospital systems have reconfigured their IV admixture areas to bring them into compliance with Chapter 797. The technician should be aware of the types of modifications required, and can often be an integral part of the remodeling team. More importantly, the technician must be knowledgeable about the standards for maintaining a sterile environment and the requirements for hand washing, gowning, and gloving, and the proper technique for compounding sterile products.

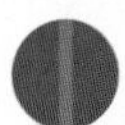

Risk Levels

Requirements for compounding conditions vary according to the risk of exposing patients to inaccurate ingredients, pathogens, or increased microbial growth.

Low Risk Level

Low-risk-level products are compounded from commercially prepared sterile products using commercial sterile devices. The products are stored at room temperature and are completely administered to the patient within 28 hours after preparation.

The compounding procedures should involve only a few basic aseptic manipulations using no more than three products in a closed transfer system and should be performed in a ISO Class 5 (Class 100) laminar airflow (LAF) workbench. An ISO Class 8 cleanroom is recommended. The compounder is required to scrub his or her hands, nails, wrists, and forearms with a brush, warm water, and an appropriate antimicrobial skin cleanser for at least 30 seconds. Makeup, jewelry, false nails, and nail polish are not allowed in the cleanroom. Protective clothing must include gowns, masks, hair covers, shoe covers, and gloves.

A triple-check system of validating that the correct medications and amounts have been mixed should be standard procedure. The compounding area should have an ante area, but this may be just a line to demarcate the cleanroom area. All compounding personnel are required to participate in a yearly media fill procedure to ensure proper technique.

ISO Class 5 International Organization for Standardization Class 5 environment, in which a maximum of 100 particles 0.5 microns in size will be present for every cubic foot of air space.

laminar airflow (LAF) workbench A workbench that meets the ISO Class 5 standard.

ISO Class 8 International Organization of Standardization Class 8 cleanroom environment, in which a maximum of 100,000 particles 0.5 microns in size will be present for every cubic foot of air.

cleanroom An enclosed room with smooth walls, floors, and ceilings that are resistant to damage from sanitizing agents; the air quality meets ISO Class 8 standards.

Medium Risk Level

Medium-risk-level compounded products involve more complex manipulations or the addition of multiple ingredients, such as in a total parenteral nutrition (TPN) mixture, or the preparation of multiple IV bags for the same patient. Also included are products that will be stored at room temperature and administered to the patient more than 28 hours after preparation without the addition of an antibacterial.

All safety precautions for low-risk-level products must be in place for these compounds and the compounding area must be in an ISO Class 7 (Class 10,000) cleanroom with an anteroom area. The annual media fill testing should be a more rigorous test of complex aseptic manipulations performed under stressful conditions to ensure the competency of the compounder.

High Risk Level

High-risk-level compounded sterile products involve the use of nonsterile ingredients or nonsterile devices, or compounds in which the sterile or nonsterile ingredients are exposed to air quality less than Class 5. All of the safety procedures for low- and medium-risk-level products should be in place, but in addition the compounding must take place at ISO Class 8 level with a separate anteroom area. The annual media fill testing of personnel should involve the most challenging manipulations and difficult conditions using nonsterile media.

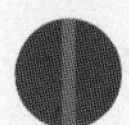

Cleanroom and Anteroom

The cleanroom should be a controlled area separate from the rest of the pharmacy activities. Traffic flow in the sterile area must be minimized to prevent contamination, and boxes, or any item that may generate particulate matter, must be kept at least 3 feet away from the compounding area in the anteroom or ante area. There should be no drains or sinks in the cleanroom. The cleanroom or buffer area must be an ISO Class 8 (Class 100,000). Necessary furniture and fixtures may be present but should be limited. Walls and furniture should be solid surfaces that can be cleaned with liquid disinfectants without being damaged.

anteroom A room adjacent to but separate from the cleanroom where handwashing, gowning, and gloving take place, and where supplies are sanitized before being brought into the cleanroom.

In facilities that compound only low- and medium-risk products, a well-marked ante area may suffice, although a separate anteroom is preferred. In a facility that compounds high-risk sterile products, a physically separate anteroom is required. There are modular cleanroom systems and soft-wall cleanrooms that can be put in place relatively quickly for $20,000 to $30,000. These may satisfy the requirements for lower-volume operations. Refer back to Figure 13.2 for diagrams of a cleanroom and anteroom.

Sanitizing the Cleanroom

All work surfaces in the cleanroom should be cleaned with a detergent and sanitizing solution each day. Flooring should also be cleaned daily with an appropriate sanitizing solution and cleaning tools that are nonshedding and are used only in the cleanroom to avoiding bringing contamination into the room. Walls and ceilings should be cleaned at least monthly with cleaning tools that are either disposable or are sanitized in an appropriate manner. Supply shelves should be cleaned weekly. Trash containers should be lined with plastic bags and the trash should be collected on a regular schedule by trained custodial people using minimal agitation to prevent particulate matter from being released into the air.

Sanitizing the Anteroom

The floors in the anteroom should be cleaned daily as an extension of the daily cleaning of the cleanroom floors, and the walls and ceilings should be cleaned weekly. Supplies should be removed from boxes and cartons in the anteroom and cleaned with a sanitizing agent before they are transferred to the cleanroom.

barrier isolator A sealed laminar flow hood that is supplied with air through a HEPA filter, maintaining a Class 5 ISO environment. It allows the compounder to access the work area through glove openings and maintain sterility without the need for a cleanroom or gowning.

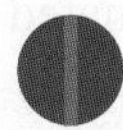

Compounding Equipment

Compounding of sterile products is performed using aseptic technique in an LAF hood or a barrier isolator. Class II LAF hoods contain a HEPA filter that blocks 99.97% of the particulate matter (3 microns or larger) contained in the air entering

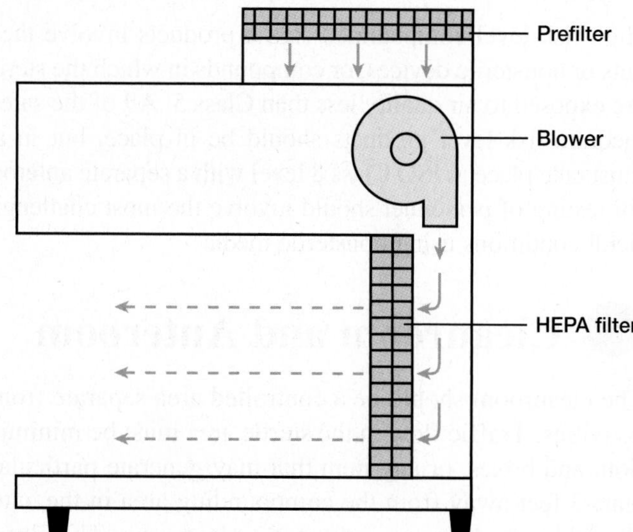

Figure 20.1 Horizontal flow hood. (Reprinted with permission from Thompson JE. A Practical Guide to Contemporary Pharmacy Practice. 2nd ed. Baltimore, MD: Lippincott, Williams & Wilkins, 2004.)

and leaving the hood. This protects the personnel as well as the compounded products. Horizontal airflow hoods direct the filtered air in a horizontal direction from a HEPA filter toward the compounder. See Figure 20.1 for a diagram of a horizontal flow hood.

Vertical flow hoods (sometimes called biologic safety cabinets) direct the HEPA-filtered air in a downward direction through a prefilter and back up through a second HEPA filter before releasing it. The vertical flow hood also has a shield on the front to prevent hazardous materials from reaching the compounder. A vertical flow hood is used to compound chemotherapy drugs and other agents that may be harmful to the compounder. See Figure 20.2 for a drawing of a vertical flow hood.

Barrier isolators (often called gloveboxes) were originally used in nuclear medicine to reduce the hazards of radioactive agents, and in the mixing of hazardous substances for chemotherapy. Some healthcare organizations are now using this technology to satisfy the requirements of Chapter 797 without the expense of constructing a cleanroom. An isolator provides a controlled environment with an air-handling system of blowers and filters, and a system of air locks, gloves, and sleeves that allows for the transfer of materials in and out of the system without contaminating the internal environment by the external air. Openings in the isolator, called glove ports, allow the compounder to perform admixture manipulations without the need for personal garb such as gowns, masks, and hair and shoe covers. Air locks provide a seal between the internal and external environments and serve as an anteroom for the transfer of materials. Refer back to Figure 13.7 for a picture of a barrier isolator.

Automated compounding devices are available for both large-volume and small-volume components of an IV admixture. They are especially useful for mixing TPNs and other complicated preparations. It is vitally important for automated compounders to be accurately programmed and calibrated to ensure the accuracy of the final preparation.

Many IV solutions require refrigeration, and refrigerators (whether ordinary consumer products or commercial refrigerators) must have a thermometer for a

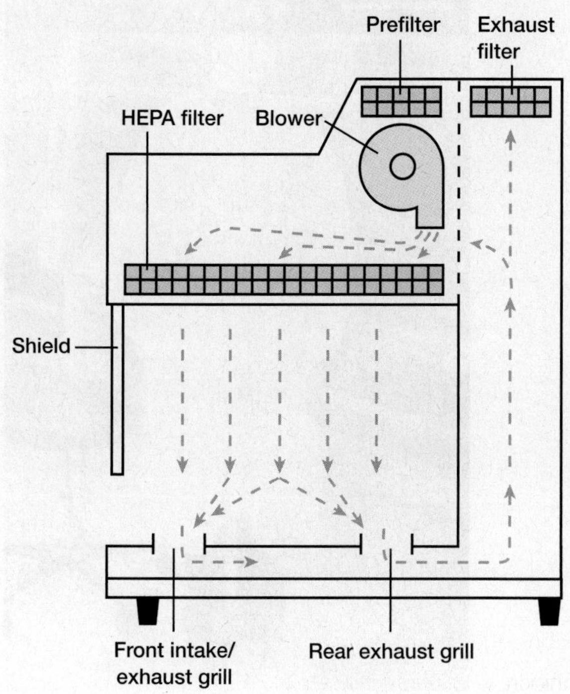

Figure 20.2 Vertical flow hood. (Reprinted with permission from Thompson JE. A Practical Guide to Contemporary Pharmacy Practice. 2nd ed. Baltimore, MD: Lippincott, Williams & Wilkins, 2004.)

daily documentation of the temperature. The refrigerator must not be in a Class 5 cleanroom but may provide access to the cleanroom by two-sided pass-through doors. Some sterile preparations require freezing temperatures (−20°C to −10°C) and the same monitoring documentation requirements are required for freezers.

Computer terminals for record keeping should not be kept in the cleanroom because they interfere with air quality; however, they can be kept in the anteroom. Shelves for storage should be kept to a minimum in the cleanroom. Shelves, tables, and chairs should be made of stainless steel for ease of cleaning and have wheels so they can be easily moved for floor cleaning. Carts for transferring supplies into the controlled area and delivery out of the controlled area should be made of stainless steel and have swivel wheels and brakes.

If laminar flow hoods do not run continuously, they should be turned on at least 30 minutes before any compounding is begun to ensure proper airflow. The work surface, sidewalls, and front edge of the workbench should be sprayed with a suitable disinfectant. The back wall with the HEPA filter should not be sprayed. The work surface should be cleaned by wiping it from side to side with towels made from a nonshedding material, working from back to front. The compounder should be in full gown and glove garb before entering the cleanroom to begin the cleaning process.

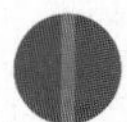 Gowning and Gloving by Compounders

Technicians assigned to compound IV admixtures should remove all jewelry, nail polish, scented cosmetics or those likely to flake, and any outer sweaters or laboratory jackets before entering the cleanroom. False nails should not be worn, and nails should be trimmed and clean. Overall good grooming and cleanliness

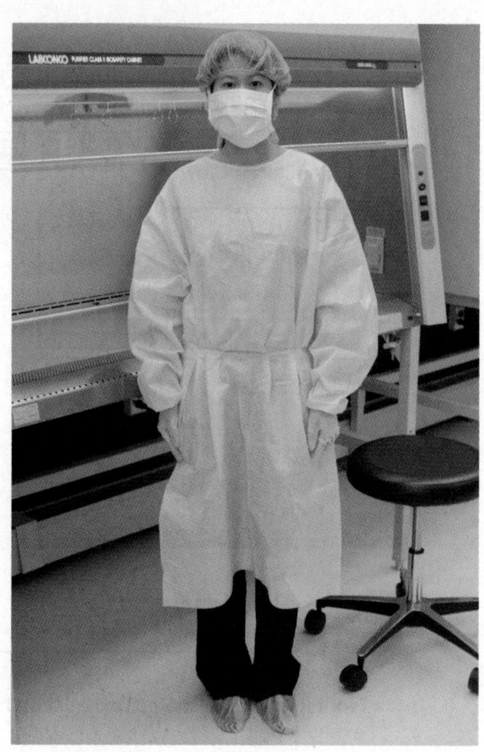

Figure 20.3 Gowned and gloved technician.

are essential, and all hair (on both the head and face) must be covered. A technician suffering from any infectious disease or a skin condition that might cause shedding should be excluded from compounding sterile products until the situation resolves.

Each facility will decide on the type of hand cleanser (whether plain soap or an antimicrobial product) that best suits its needs. Compounders should be sure to perform the following cleanroom procedures:

Scrub hands vigorously, paying attention to all surfaces of the fingers and nails, and scrub arms up to the elbows for 15 seconds. Rinse hands and arms, dry with a disposable towel, and use the towel to turn off the faucet before disposing of it. Apply a hair cover (and beard cover, if needed). Adjust the face mask to cover your nose, and put shoe covers on shoes. Put on the gown and then the gloves. Wearing gloves does not eliminate the need for proper hand washing, and the gloves should be periodically sprayed with a sanitizing solution if worn for a long period of time. On leaving the cleanroom, discard hair cover, mask, shoe covers, and gloves, and replace them with new ones if reentering the area. The gown may be hung inside-out at the entrance and re-used if reentering the same day. See Figure 20.3 for a picture of a properly garbed pharmacy technician about to enter the cleanroom.

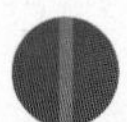 Aseptic Technique

After being properly garbed and the LAF hood has been cleaned, sanitize the IV admixture supplies in the anteroom and transfer them into the cleanroom with the use of stainless steel carts if this has not already been done. Assemble all materials needed for the sterile preparation and examine them before placing them in the

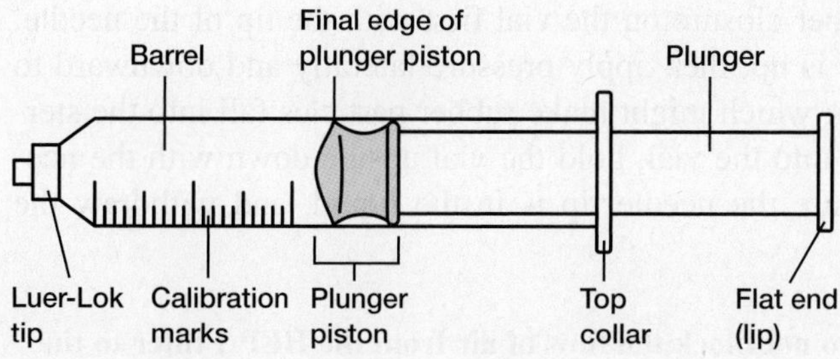

Figure 20.4 Syringe with parts labeled. (Reprinted with permission from Thompson JE. A Practical Guide to Contemporary Pharmacy Practice. 2nd ed. Baltimore, MD: Lippincott, Williams & Wilkins, 2004.)

laminar flow hood. Vials and ampules should not have cracks or particles in the solution. Remove the outer wrappers from plastic IV bags before placing them in the hood. The injection port of the bag should face the HEPA filter when placed in the hood.

Choose syringe sizes according to the amount of fluid to be drawn out of the vial to increase accuracy. The syringe volume should be slightly more than the amount of fluid needed. Check the syringe package for any tears or leaks that may compromise sterility. Open the sterile syringe pack in the hood and discard the wrapper outside the sterile area of the hood. Needles are labeled according to the length of the needle and the gauge that describes the diameter of the opening or bore of the needle. Needles are sterile and lubricated to assist in entering the vial. The package should be opened in the hood and the wrapper placed outside the sterile area. Many needles and syringes have Luer-Lok tips that require a quarter turn to tighten the needle to the syringe. The protective cap should be removed from the syringe and the protective cap should remain on the needle to prevent a needle stick when the needle is applied to the syringe. See Figure 20.4 for a diagram of a syringe with parts labeled. See Figure 20.5 for a diagram of a needle with parts labeled.

Injectable medications are often packaged in sterile vials with a rubber closure covered by a plastic or metal cap. The cap should be removed in the hood and the rubber stopper should be swabbed with a disposable alcohol swab twice in the same direction using a clean part of the swab each time. Spray bottles of alcohol are often used, but there is a risk of contamination from resistant spores when a nonsterile bottle is used repeatedly. The vials and syringes should be placed in the hood so that nothing impedes the flow of air from the HEPA filter to all parts of the object. Each object placed in the hood will create a zone of turbulence that will interfere with the flow of air around the object. For this reason, all items used in aseptic manipulations inside the hood must be placed at least 6 inches from the sides and front of the workbench. Begin the process of adding a liquid from a vial to an IV bag by removing the cap from the needle.

zone of turbulence A disturbance of the airflow pattern created behind an object placed in the laminar airflow hood.

TIP

The needle must be at least ⅜ inch long to penetrate the injection port and the inner diaphragm of the IV bag.

Pull the plunger of the syringe back to fill it with an amount of air equal to the volume of fluid to be extracted from the vial, unless the liquid is a drug that will

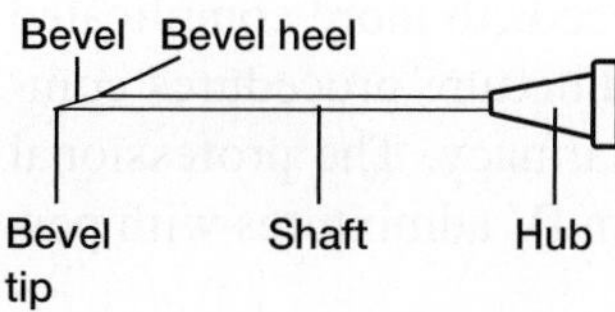

Figure 20.5 Needle with parts labeled. (Reprinted with permission from Thompson JE. A Practical Guide to Contemporary Pharmacy Practice. 2nd ed. Baltimore, MD: Lippincott, Williams & Wilkins, 2004.)

produce gas. Pierce the rubber closure on the vial first with the tip of the needle, making sure the bevel edge is up, then apply pressure laterally and downward to prevent coring of the rubber, which might make rubber particles fall into the sterile solution. Release the air into the vial, hold the vial upside down with the needle still inserted, making sure the needle tip is in the liquid, and withdraw the required amount of fluid.

CAUTION **Be certain that your hands do not block the flow of air from the HEPA filter to the needle.**

Return the vial to its place and remove any air bubbles from the syringe by tapping the side of the syringe to move the air bubble to the surface and slightly depressing the plunger to force the bubble out. Recheck the syringe to ensure that the volume is correct and withdraw more fluid if needed. Grasp the injection port on the IV bag, again making certain that you do not block the airflow from the HEPA filter. Insert the needle through the rubber tip and the inside diaphragm, and push the plunger to release the fluid into the bag.

Place the syringe and needle into a sharps container unless your facility has a policy about leaving the syringe for the pharmacist to check. Visually check the IV bag for any discoloration or particles in the fluid. Apply the proper labels and auxiliary labels and leave with the paperwork in the checking area for the pharmacist.

When the drug to be added is supplied in an ampule, any fluid in the top of the ampule should be moved to the bottom. Accomplish this by tapping on the top of the ampule or gently swirling the ampule until the liquid is all in the bottom section. Place an alcohol swab around the neck and hold the top of the ampul between the thumb and index finger of one hand, while holding the bottom with the thumb and index finger of the other hand. Applying pressure with the thumbs, snap the top of the ampul in one motion. Withdraw the medication using either a filter needle or a filter straw to avoid adding glass particles to the IV bag. Hold the ampul at an angle and insert the filter needle or straw to withdraw the correct amount of fluid. Be aware of the position of hands and the airflow from the HEPA filter so as not to compromise sterility. Replace the filter straw or filter needle with a regular needle before injecting the solution into the injection port of the IV bag.

If the drug to be added is a powder for reconstitution, first add the correct amount of sterile diluent to the vial using aseptic technique.

CAUTION **Be sure to release an amount of air equal to the volume of diluent being added to prevent positive pressure from developing inside the vial.**

Gently rotate the vial and visually check to see that all particles are dissolved. Withdraw the correct amount of the sterile preparation and inject it into the injection port of the IV bag.

Dispose of the syringe in a sharps container according to protocol. Inspect the IV bag for any discoloration or precipitates and apply a seal to the injection port. Place the bag in the appropriate checking area and apply the correct labels.

These basic skills and techniques should be practiced in the laboratory until proficiency is demonstrated before the technician proceeds to more complicated procedures. The next three chapters will expand on admixture procedures commonly performed in an inpatient or home infusion pharmacy. The professional technician will take pride in his or her ability to perform IV admixtures with perfect aseptic technique.

Case Study 20.1

John arrived at work early in the morning at the home infusion pharmacy and discovered there was an order for furosemide 40 mg to be administered by IV infusion that needed to be sent out right away. He decided to mix the compound right away so it would be ready for the pharmacist to check when she arrived. He flipped the switch to turn the laminar flow workbench on and gathered the needed materials. He put on a gown, washed his hands thoroughly, and placed the supplies carefully in the hood. Because the furosemide was packaged in an ampul, John remembered to obtain a filter needle to remove any glass particle that might result from breaking the ampul. He attached the filter needle to the syringe and snapped the tip off the ampul by holding it with his thumbs and index fingers and applying pressure with his thumbs. The glass scraped his finger as the lid came off, but there wasn't much bleeding, so he continued. Using the filter needle and syringe, John withdrew the furosemide from the vial and carefully injected it into the injection port of the piggyback bag. He removed the

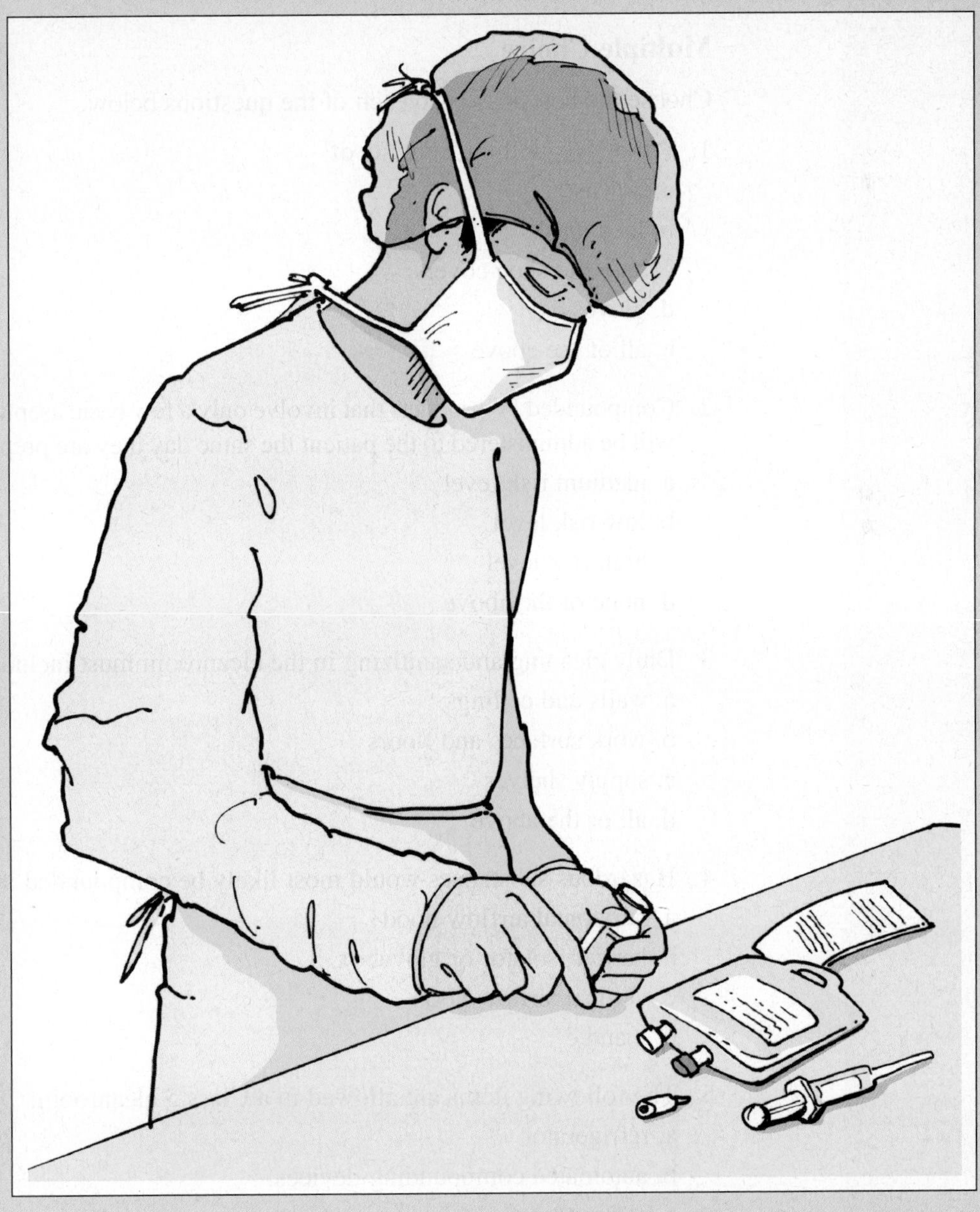

bag from the hood and placed it in the checking area, where he attached the appropriate labels. As he finished, the pharmacist arrived and came over to check the medication. John felt proud that he was able to complete the admixture in a timely manner so it could be sent out to the patient. The pharmacist checked the bag, initialed the paper work, and sent the bag out for delivery.

Did John follow all the 797 guidelines for compounding a sterile product?

How many errors did you notice that would constitute a break in sterile technique?

Review Questions

Multiple Choice

Choose the best answer to each of the questions below.

1. Protective clothing consists of
   a. gowns
   b. face masks
   c. hair and shoe covers
   d. gloves
   e. all of the above

2. Compounded IV products that involve only a few basic aseptic manipulations and will be administered to the patient the same day they are prepared are considered:
   a. medium risk level
   b. low risk level
   c. high risk level
   d. none of the above

3. Daily cleaning and sanitizing in the cleanroom must include:
   a. walls and ceilings
   b. work surfaces and floors
   c. supply shelves
   d. all of the above

4. Hazardous substances would most likely be compounded in a:
   a. horizontal airflow hood
   b. barrier isolator or glovebox
   c. vertical airflow hood
   d. b and c

5. The following items are allowed in a Class 5 cleanroom:
   a. refrigerator
   b. automated compounding devices
   c. computer terminals
   d. cardboard boxes of supplies

Fill in the Blank

Fill in the blank(s) with the correct word(s).

6. If the laminar flow hood does not run continuously, it should be turned on at least ____________________ before compounding is begun.
7. Supplies from the anteroom can be transferred into the cleanroom with the use of ____________________ after being removed from boxes and sanitized.
8. The injection port on an IV bag placed in the hood should face (toward/away from) the HEPA filter.
9. Each object placed in the hood will create a ____________________ that will interfere with the airflow around the object.
10. All items used in aseptic manipulations inside the hood must be at least ____________ from the sides and front of the hood.

True/False

Mark the following statements True or False.

11. _______ When piercing the rubber closure on a sterile vial in the hood, you should make sure the bevel edge of the needle is facing down.
12. _______ When using a filter needle to withdraw fluid from an ampul, you should change the needle before injecting the fluid into a bag.
13. _______ In an ISO Class 5 environment, a maximum of 100 particles sized 0.5 microns or larger can be present for every cubic foot of air.
14. _______ Careful hand washing is not required if gloves are worn during compounding of IV admixtures.
15. _______ A ¼-inch needle is the best length to use for injecting a liquid into the injection port of an IV bag.

Matching

Match the terms with the definitions.

16. _____ zone of turbulence
17. _____ aseptic technique
18. _____ cleanroom
19. _____ barrier isolator
20. _____ anteroom

A. A self-contained glovebox maintaining an ISO Class 5 environment without the need for gowning or a cleanroom.

B. A room adjacent to but separate from the cleanroom where gowning and gloving take place.

C. A disturbance of the airflow pattern created behind an object placed in the hood.

D. A method of manipulating sterile products so that they remain sterile.

E. An enclosed room with smooth walls and ceilings that are resistant to damage from sanitizing agents; the air quality meets ISO Class 8 standards.

LEARNING ACTIVITY

Develop a step-by-step standard operating procedure for making a medium-risk-level IV admixture using a horizontal LAF hood in a cleanroom with a separate anteroom. Include methods for transferring supplies from the warehouse to the anteroom, sanitizing them, and transferring them to the cleanroom. Also include procedures for hand washing, gowning, gloving, and placing supplies in the hood. Include the steps for reconstituting a sterile powder and adding the reconstituted liquid to an IV bag using aseptic technique and checks for quality assurance. Conclude with labeling and placing the product and paperwork in the appropriate area for the final check by the pharmacist. Use diagrams when needed for clarity.

Chapter 21

Large- and Small-Volume Parenterals

OBJECTIVES

After completing this chapter, the student will be able to:

- Define parenteral products and explain the reasons for using them.
- Discuss the disadvantages of parenteral routes of administration.
- Differentiate between large- and small-volume parenterals.
- Explain the handling and use of each type of parenteral container.
- Outline factors involved in determining beyond-use dating.
- List labeling requirements for compounded parenteral products.
- Outline storage requirements for compounded parenteral products.
- Describe media fill processes for compounder validation.

KEY TERMS

- batch preparation
- large-volume parenteral (LVP)
- small-volume parenteral (SVP)
- media fill process

A working knowledge of the types of parenteral administrations and supplies involved in the various forms of administration is vital to the technician receiving and evaluating orders in the IV room. This chapter will discuss the various parenteral routes of administration with emphasis on large- and small-volume parenterals and their uses, advantages, and disadvantages. Labeling requirements, including auxiliary labels and factors involved in beyond-use dating, are covered. Quality-assurance issues and compounder-validation processes are explained.

Parenteral products are intended to be administered by injection through the skin, bypassing two of the body's natural defenses against bacterial invasion: the skin and the gastrointestinal tract. For this reason, it is critical to ensure that the correct drug, in the correct dose, is administered in a product that is entirely free of bacterial contamination. The USP recently issued firm, enforceable guidelines for compounding and administering compounded sterile products, but it still remains the responsibility of each healthcare facility, each pharmacist, and each pharmacy technician to ensure that proper procedure is followed during IV admixture. These guidelines (USP Chapter 797) were discussed in Chapter 19, and technicians should review them on a regular basis to stay current.

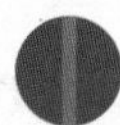

Routes of Administration for Parenteral Products

There are various routes of administration that involve an injection through the skin and require a sterile product. It is important to know the type of syringe and needle required, and the volume of solution that can be injected by each method. Refer to Figure 21.1 for a depiction of the various routes of administration. Intradermal (ID) injections are administered just below the surface of the skin and can range in volume from 0.02 mL to 0.5 mL. They are given with a 1-mL syringe (often called a tuberculin syringe) using a 3/8- to 5/8-inch needle with a 25- to 28-gauge bore. Subcutaneous (SQ or SC) injections are administered in the fat tissue just beneath the skin. This route is most commonly used for insulin injections and can be used for volumes up to 1 mL, so either a 1-mL or 3-mL syringe is used. Insulin syringes are calibrated in units and are available in 30-, 50-, and 100-unit

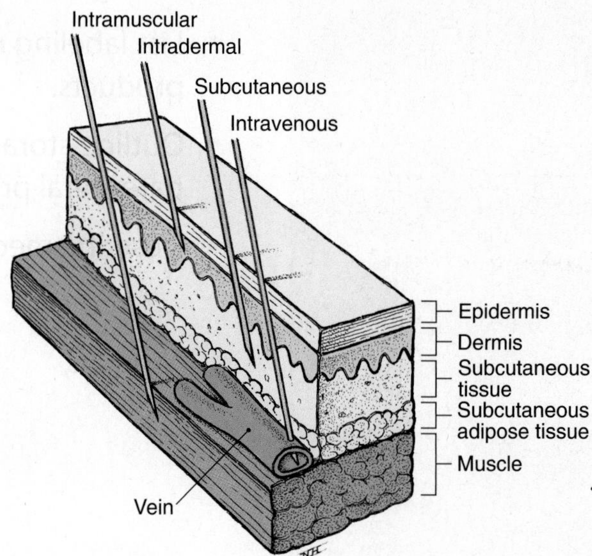

Figure 21.1 Parenteral routes of administration. (Reprinted with permission from Stedman's Medical Dictionary. 27th ed. Baltimore, MD: Lippincott, Williams & Wilkins, 2000.)

sizes; they come with ultrafine needles of 30 to 32 gauge to eliminate the discomfort of daily injections, and short, ultrafine needles that are meant to cause the least discomfort. If a drug for SQ administration is sent to the floor with a Luer cap so the nurse can choose the needle, a slight overfill should be added to the syringe to facilitate priming the syringe. Intramuscular (IM) injections are given into the muscle mass of the arm or buttocks; up to 2 mL can be given in the arm of an adult, and up to 5 mL can be injected into the muscle of the buttocks. For children up to 3 years of age, the maximum volume that can be injected into the muscle is 1 mL. Syringe sizes for IM injections range in size from 1 to 5 mL, and needles range from 20 to 22 gauge and ½ to 1½ inches long. Intravenous (IV) administration includes continuous infusion, intermittent infusion, bolus injections, and IV push. For continuous infusion, a drug is added to a large-volume parenteral (LVP) and allowed to slowly drip into the vein. Intermittent infusion is accomplished by adding the drug to a small-volume parenteral (SVP) bag and infusing it over a set time period at regularly spaced intervals. In an emergency situation, a bolus or IV push dose is usually administered by placing the drug solution in a syringe and injecting it directly into a vein.

large-volume parenteral (LVP) A single-dose injection containing more than 100 mL of solution for intravenous use (i.e., bypassing the gastrointestinal tract).

small-volume parenteral (SVP) A single-dose injection containing 100 mL or less of solution for intravenous use (i.e., bypassing the gastrointestinal tract); also called a minibag or piggyback.

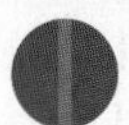

Advantages of Parenteral Products

Parenteral products are used frequently in a hospital setting and are becoming more commonly used for patients recovering at home because they are a convenient way to administer medication to patients who are unwilling or unable to take medications by mouth. They are also useful for giving an immediate dose in an emergency or for administering a given amount of a drug over a period of time with minimal supervision. Patients who need to take drugs for a long period of time may be well served by the use of an implantable pump. In some cases a drug may be injected directly into an organ or a muscle, and often a drug may have to be dosed parenterally because it will be inactivated by passage through the gastrointestinal tract.

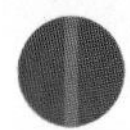

Disadvantages of Parenteral Products

Parenteral products can be extremely expensive because of the time needed to prepare and deliver them to the patient. They must be prepared using specialized equipment in a sterile environment that is costly to maintain. Personnel involved in compounding sterile products require specialized training and must undergo continual validation processes to document their consistent skill levels. An error involving a wrong dose or an incorrect drug may result in serious complications or even death, because when a product is injected it is difficult or impossible to remove and can cause complications very quickly. Contaminating the product by introducing a pathogen as a result of a break in sterile technique can have serious or deadly consequences for an already compromised patient. This risk increases with products sent out of the pharmacy to a home where storage and handling may not be ideal.

Large-Volume Parenterals

IV infusion bags containing more than 100 mL of solution are considered to be large-volume parenterals (LVPs). LVPs are also packaged in glass bottles with or without an air vent tube. Glass containers are generally reserved for drugs that are incompatible with plastic, because plastic bags have clear advantages over glass.

Plastic bags are easier to store because they are compact, and they are easier to dispose of when empty. They also do not break as easily as glass and they weigh less, making it easier to transport them. LVPs are available in plastic bags containing 250 mL, 500 mL, or 1000 mL of solution. The bag comes packaged inside an outer plastic shield that should be removed before the bag is placed in the hood or labeled before it is sent to the floor. Because of the large volume of the solutions, these bags do not include a bacteriostatic agent. LVP fluids are generally used to correct fluid and electrolyte balances that may occur as a result of excessive diarrhea or an illness that causes the patient to restrict fluid intake. They may also be used as a vehicle for administering other drugs.

Each LVP bag has two ports that are nearly the same length at the same end of the bag. The administration port is covered by a plastic cover that must be removed and has a diaphragm about ½ inch inside the port that must be punctured for the solution to pour out of the bag. The other port is covered by a rubber tip through which medications can be added. It also has a plastic diaphragm that must be punctured for solutions to enter the bag. The spike of the administration set is inserted into the administration port, puncturing the diaphragm, and the solution is able to flow out of the bag into the administration set and be delivered to the patient.

Common commercially available LVP solutions include sodium chloride (available as normal saline 0.9%, ½ normal 0.45%, and ¼ normal 0.225%) and dextrose (dextrose 5% in water [D5W] and dextrose 10% in water [D10W]) solutions. Ringer's solution and lactated Ringer's solution are also commonly used. There are many combinations of normal saline and dextrose available in various strengths, so it is important to carefully check any LVP bags being sent to the floor to be certain they contain the correct solution. In the past, potassium chloride (KCl) was often added to an LVP in the pharmacy when ordered by the physician, but because of concerns about medication errors involving KCl, manufacturers now offer commercially prepared LVP bags with various strengths of KCl already added. Be certain that you send a bag with KCl as an additive only if it was ordered by the physician.

Small-Volume Parenterals

Plastic IV bags containing 25, 50, or 100 mL are called small-volume parenterals (SVPs), minibags, or piggybacks. They are often used to add a drug to the therapy of a patient who is receiving fluids through an LVP. The LVP can either be stopped while the SVP bag is administered or the bag can be piggybacked on the LVP for intermittent therapy with a drug. See Figure 21.2 for a picture of an SVP. SVPs are sometimes piggybacked on an LVP, particularly when a patient needs to receive an antibiotic two or three times a day and is on continuous IV fluids. Other forms of SVPs include ampuls, prefilled syringes, and single- and multiple-dose vials containing liquid solutions or lyophilized powder for reconstitution. Some manufacturers offer commercially available, ready-to-mix systems consisting of a minibag and a drug vial attached with a special adapter that can facilitate mixing just prior to administration. Figure 21.3 shows an ADD-Vantage® (Abbott Laboratories) ready-to-mix bag. This type of system reduces waste because the solution can be mixed just prior to administration. It cuts down on medication errors because the medication bottle stays attached to the bag for double-checking; however, such systems are more expensive and occasionally the bag fails to activate properly, resulting in the potential for an inaccurate dose.

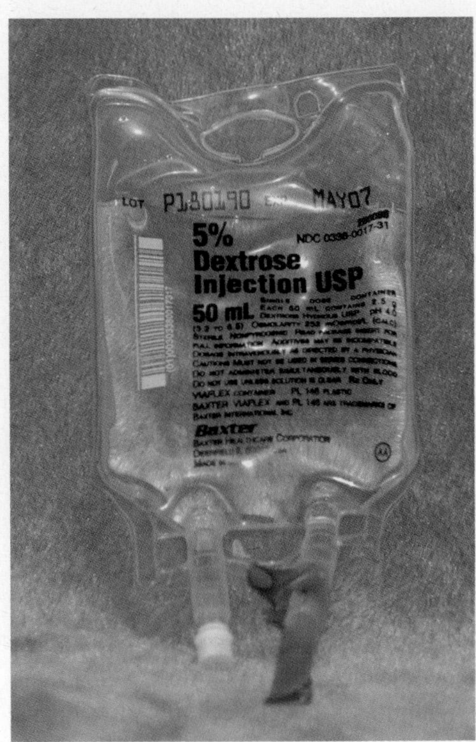

Figure 21.2 Small-volume parenteral (SVP). (Reprinted with permission from Lacher BE. Pharmaceutical Calculations for the Pharmacy Technician. Baltimore, MD: Lippincott, Williams & Wilkins, 2008.)

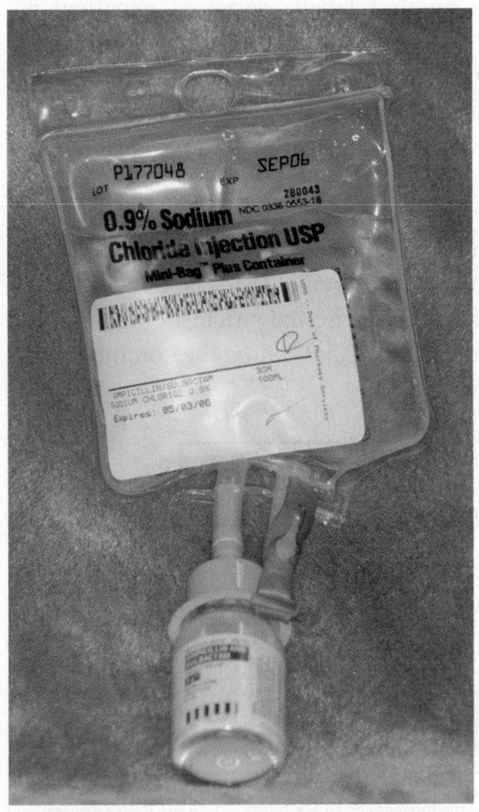

Figure 21.3 The ADD-Vantage® system by Abbott Laboratories. (Reprinted with permission from Lacher BE. Pharmaceutical Calculations for the Pharmacy Technician. Baltimore, MD: Lippincott, Williams & Wilkins, 2008.)

Labeling Requirements for Compounded Parenterals

Correct labeling of compounded sterile products is essential for medication safety. USP Chapter 797 has established firm guidelines regarding information that is required to be on the label of a compounded sterile product. The generic name and concentration or amount of each ingredient used in compounding the product should be listed along with the total volume of the product. The route, time, and frequency of administration must be clearly stated. An accurate beyond-use date must be listed along with any auxiliary labels detailing storage requirements and any other cautionary statements needed to ensure safe handling of a particular drug. Sterile products compounded in an institutional setting will have a label with the name of the institution and will include the name, hospital number, and room number of the patient. The date and time the medication was compounded, and the initials of the compounder and the checking pharmacist should also be included. See Figure 21.4 for an example of a label for a compounded sterile product.

Compounded sterile products that will be sent to a patient's home have some additional requirements. The label must include the name, address, and phone number of the pharmacy; the prescription number; the prescribing physician's name; and the number of refills, if any. The directions must be clear and complete in terms that can be understood by the patient or caregiver, including explicit manipulations or additions of other ingredients, equipment needed (e.g., pumps or tubing), route of administration, and flow rate. Generally, homecare patients receive at least one initial visit by a nurse or pharmacy personnel to ensure that they have the proper training to store and administer the product.

Auxiliary labels, especially brightly colored labels, serve as excellent reminders about information pertaining to the sterile product. Storage information may include a label to "Store in the Refrigerator" or "Protect from Light." There may be a warning to not shake the product, or information about the route of administration. There should be some consistency about the auxiliary labels applied to each product so that the nursing staff or home caregiver can become accustomed to seeing the same information each time.

batch preparation A large number of sterile products prepared by a single compounder at the same time.

Batch preparation products can be made up in advance and stored in the refrigerator or freezer for later use, and have specific requirements for labeling. Most of these products are considered Risk Level 3 and require the strictest compounding technique to ensure sterility. Each item must have a label stating the common name

℞#113 Control # 000000-1 Bottle #1
Patient Name: Brett Favrite Rm. No. 430
Medical Record #: 120579
Additives:
Heparin Sodium 15,000 units

IN: 0.9% Sodium Chloride 500 mL
minutes
hours/start time
40 mL/hr 0.67 mL/min
40 drops/min (60 drops/mL)
1830 00/00/00 date/time prep/Prep by JET
1830 00/02/00 infuse before/Chk'd by BJF

Auxiliary Labels: Keep in the refrigerator do not freeze, 24-28 hrs if no refrigeration

Figure 21.4 Label for a compounded sterile product. (Reprinted with permission from Thompson JE. A Practical Guide to Contemporary Pharmacy Practice. 2nd ed. Baltimore, MD: Lippincott, Williams & Wilkins, 2004.)

by which the preparation is known, in addition to the name and amount of each drug, including any additives or preservatives and the name and strength of any diluents. The total volume in the bag or syringe and the concentration should be listed along with the route of administration, lot number, date of compounding, beyond-use date and time, and the initials of the compounder and checking pharmacist. Any storage information can be included in either the regular label or an auxiliary label.

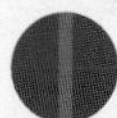

Beyond-Use Dating

An accurate beyond-use date is vital to the safe administration of compounded sterile products. This date should predict as accurately as possible the last date and time when the product will contain 90% of the active ingredients listed on the label in a form that will be bioavailable and free of microbial contamination when stored under the required conditions. A number of factors should be considered when establishing a beyond-use date for a sterile compounded product. The solubility of the ingredients added to the solution and their stability over a period of time must be considered. Variation from the optimum storage temperature (for example, as a result of being subjected to a lower temperature because of refrigeration or, in some cases, freezing) may lower the stability of a drug. Exposure to light will affect the stability of some products, and the type of container should also be considered. Reference books, such as Trissel's *Handbook of Injectable Drugs*, should be consulted for stability and compatibility issues. Lastly, the potential for growth of bacteria in the solution over a period of time under various conditions should be considered.

Preparation Method 21.1
Using Aseptic Technique to Compound a Sterile Product

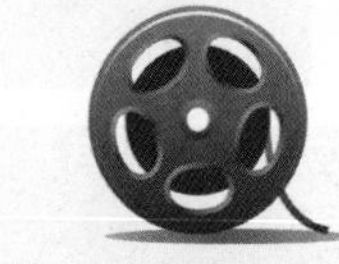

See the student CD and website for a video of this procedure.

Date/Time 05-03-06 Medication Orders

Lasix 40mg / D5W 100ml

Infuse over 30 minutes once daily

M Amado MD

Medical Orders

Patient Information
Sandra Smithson 45 yo female

Pharmacy Copy

(Reprinted with permission from Mohr ME. Lab Experiences for the Pharmacy Technician. Philadelphia: Lippincott Williams & Wilkins, 2006.)

1. Clean the laminar airflow hood with alcohol. (See Fig. 21.5A.)
2. Assemble materials in the hood. (See Fig. 21.5B.)
3. Clean the ampul and minibag port with alcohol. (See Fig. 21.5C.)
4. Open the ampul by snapping off the top. (See Fig. 21.5D.)
5. Attach a filter straw to the syringe and withdraw 4 mL of fluid. (See Fig. 21.5E.)
6. Remove the filter straw and attach a sterile needle to the syringe. (See Fig. 21.5F.)
7. Inject the drug (in this case, Lasix) into the minibag port. (See Fig. 21.5 G.)
8. Rotate the bag to evenly distribute the fluid, and visually inspect for particulate matter. (See Fig. 21.5H.)
9. Apply a seal to the port.
10. Apply the label, expiration date, and auxiliary labels.
11. Leave the product and paper work for the final check by the pharmacist.
12. Discard trash and clean the hood if there are any spills.

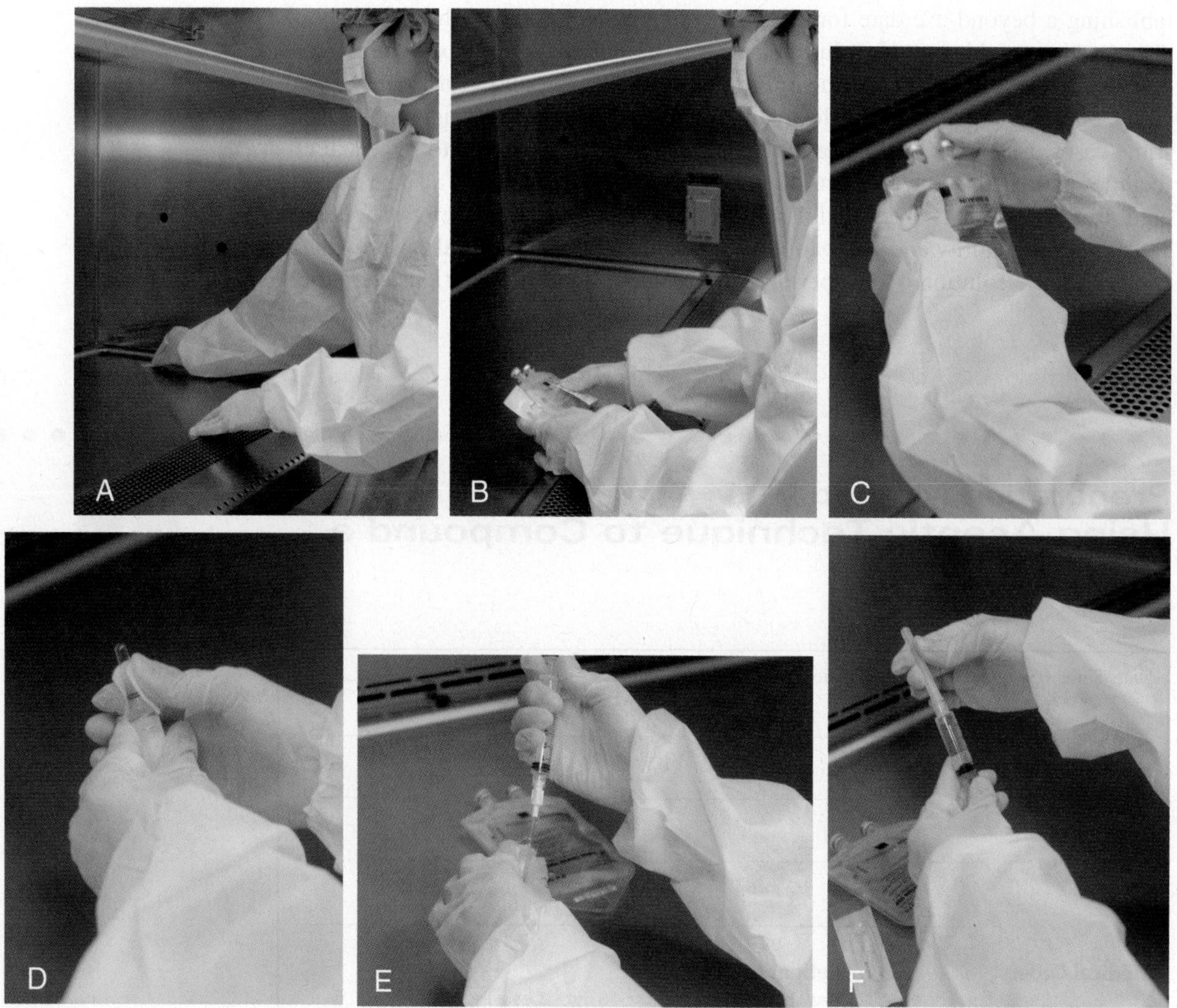

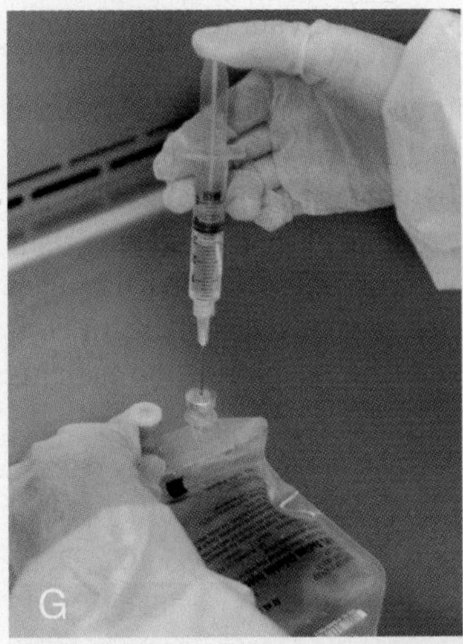

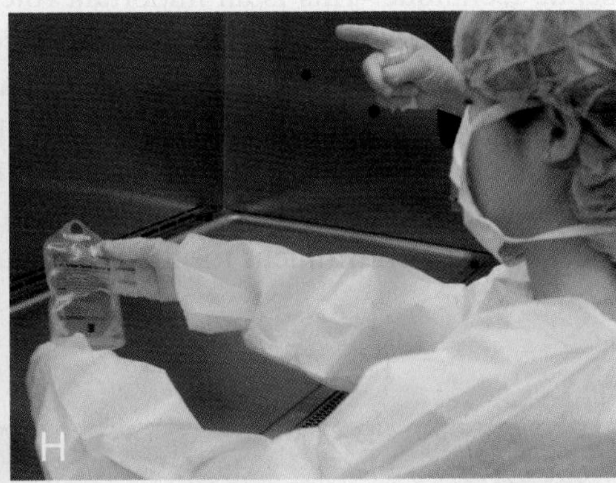

Figure 21.5 Steps for using aseptic technique to compound a sterile product.

Media Fill Processes for Compounder Validation

USP Chapter 797 regulations require that each person involved in compounding sterile products must meet training and testing requirements before being allowed to compound a sterile product for a patient, and must do so again on a regular basis after the initial training. For personnel involved in preparing only low- and medium-risk-level preparations, the training and testing for revalidation must be performed once a year. Personnel who compound high-risk-level compounds must be revalidated every 6 months. An important component of the revalidation involves a media fill process using a soy culture medium that is capable of supporting the growth of microorganisms that would be likely contaminants during the compounding process. There are several media fill kits available commercially, but they do not necessarily include materials for all of the sterile manipulations normally performed in a pharmacy. Each pharmacy should base its media fill process on the types and risk levels of the compounded products produced in that pharmacy. The sterile manipulations performed by each compounder during his or her validation test should be comparable with the most involved preparation that would be prepared in that compounding pharmacy, and should be performed under the most stressful conditions that would be encountered in that work area.

media fill process
Required on an annual basis for compounding personnel. A simulated product is prepared by the compounder with the use of a culture medium, such as soy broth, to perform manipulations using aseptic technique. The product is then incubated and checked after a predetermined amount of time for growth contamination.

All media testing should take place in an ISO Class 5 environment with the compounder gowned and gloved and following protocol for aseptic technique. A low-risk-level media fill test would involve transferring four aliquots of a sterile solution into each of three vials of soybean culture medium, sealing them with sterile closures, and incubating the mixture for 14 days. They should be read daily for microbial contamination, but must be read on day 7 and again on day 14. If no evidence of contamination is found, the compounder has passed the validation test. The number of test vials and aseptic transfer manipulations will increase as the risk level of the compounded products increases, so that the validation process will be a true test of the aseptic technique of the compounder for the types of sterile compounds produced in that pharmacy.

Professional technicians take pride in their ability to compound sterile products using aseptic technique. This is an important role that affords technicians the opportunity to assist the pharmacist in providing excellent pharmaceutical care to patients. By observing the validation processes of the technicians and observing their daily work ethic, the pharmacist can form a mutual trust relationship with each technician that creates an atmosphere of respect in the workplace. This team concept provides a set of checks and balances that impacts the health of the patients and creates a sense of fulfillment for the technicians.

Case Study 21.1

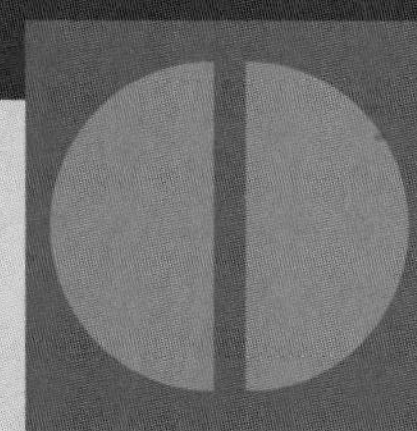

Southwest Memorial Hospital is a small rural hospital with a low patient census, and usually requires only 10 to 20 compounded sterile products a day. One technician is assigned to the IV room each morning. Janet has been scheduled as the IV technician today, and she gathers the daily IV orders from the printer and prepares to enter the IV room. Before the advent of USP Chapter 797, the IV hood was located along a wall in the open area of the pharmacy. Recently, the IV area has been sectioned with walls and a demarcated area to serve as a buffer area. The compounding at Southwest is all low-risk level.

Janet gathers all the supplies, removes extraneous wrappers and boxes, and sanitizes the materials before placing them on the cart to transport them into the cleanroom. She then begins the process of hand washing, gowning, and gloving. Janet removes all of her jewelry and meticulously washes her hands, making sure to scrub her nails, between each finger, and up to her elbows. She gowns appropriately, pushes the cart into the cleanroom, turns on the hood, and cleans it with alcohol before placing the supplies for the first round of admixtures in the hood. As Janet puts on the gloves, she concentrates on her sterile technique and the process for each admixture. She takes a great deal of professional pride in her ability to compound sterile products.

By lunchtime, Janet has completed all of the admixtures, carefully labeled them, and placed them in the checking area for the final check by the pharmacist. Janet disposes of the wrappers from the supplies used, cleans the IV hood, and removes and disposes of her gloves, mask, and hair and shoe covers. She removes her gown, hangs it on a hook on the door of the cleanroom, and checks out for a well-deserved lunch.

Shortly after Janet leaves the pharmacy, a stat order for an IV antibiotic for infusion prepared in a 100-mL piggyback bag is received in the pharmacy. The remaining technicians all look at each other and then become very busy in another area. No one wants to go to the trouble of gowning up for one IV. Finally, the supervisor taps Samantha on the shoulder and she begrudgingly begins to gather the supplies for the mixture. As she washes her hands, Samantha grumbles under her breath: "Why does she always pick on me? My project was just as important as the other technicians'. I'm not the IV technician and I'm not going to spend a lot of time gowning up for just one IV bag."

Samantha washes her hands quickly, not bothering to remove her watch and rings. She grabs a gown and tosses the supplies into the hood. Her training in aseptic technique ensures that she uses proper technique when she reconstitutes the antibiotic powder and adds the correct amount to the 100-mL bag of D5W. She applies the correct labels and lets the pharmacist know that the "stat order" is ready to be checked. The pharmacist checks the IV bag and Samantha's calculations, and sends the bag to the floor.

The patient was an elderly gentleman who was well known and loved by everyone in the area. Samantha hadn't paid any attention to his name, but it turned out she knew him also. He had developed a severe kidney infection, and despite therapy with a potent antibiotic and constant caring attention from nurses and doctors, he passed away during the night.

When Samantha returned to work the next morning, she heard that the patient had passed away during the night. She was saddened along with her coworkers because he had been a loving, caring individual who was always ready to lend a hand

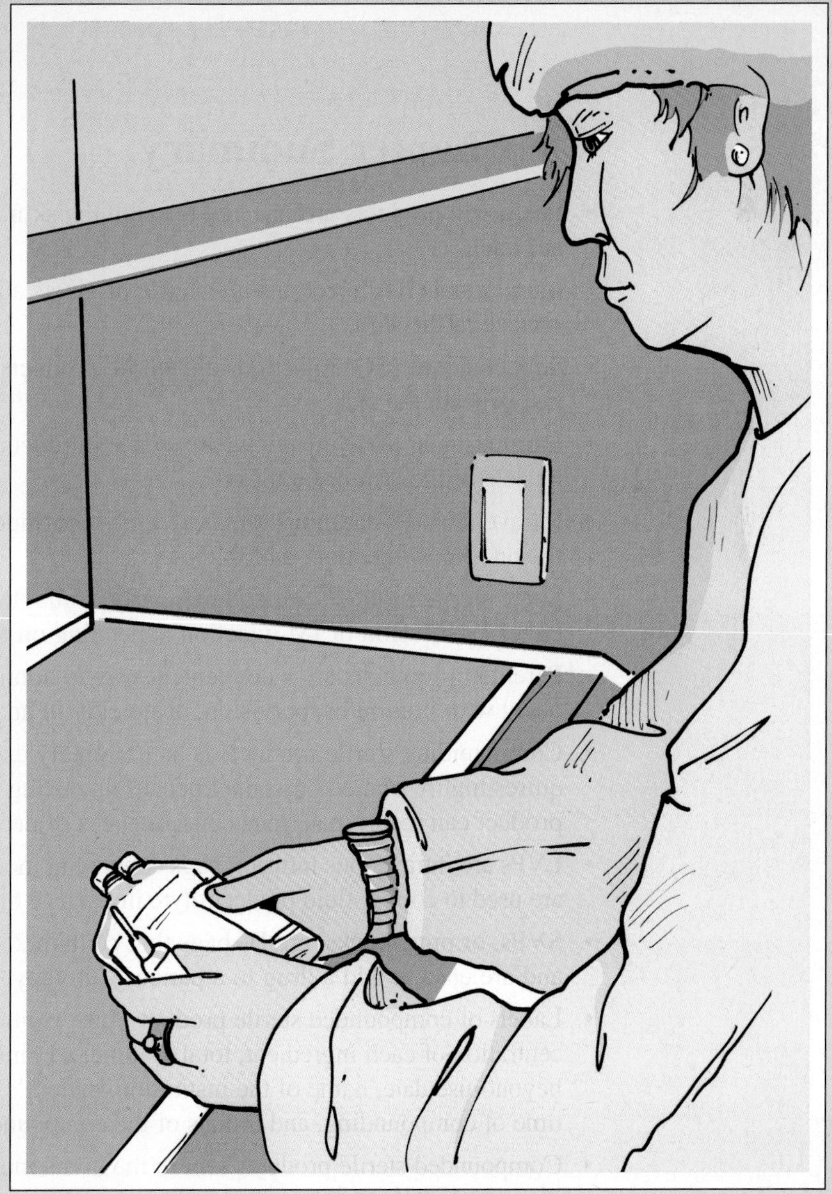

or a smile to someone in need. Later in the day, Samantha began to have some nagging thoughts: "Did I do everything I could to prepare his medication properly? Was my haphazard hand washing and not wearing a mask enough of a break in technique to introduce microbial contamination into the bag? Could I be responsible for the death of this generous, loving man?"

1. Do you think Samantha caused this man's death?
2. Does the fact that it was a stat order and was administered immediately after it was mixed increase or reduce the risk of microbial growth in the solution?
3. Did Samantha do something illegal or unethical?
4. Because Samantha is a very competent technician who allowed her discontent to affect her work ethic, how should she deal with her feelings of guilt and prevent this from happening again?

Chapter Summary

- Parenteral products are injected through the skin and bypass the gastrointestinal tract.
- Intradermal (ID) injections are sterile products administered just below the surface of the skin.
- Subcutaneous (SQ) injections are sterile products administered in the fat tissue just beneath the skin.
- Intramuscular (IM) injections are sterile products administered into a large muscle of the arm or buttocks.
- Intravenous (IV) administration includes continuous infusion, intermittent infusion, bolus injection, and IV push.
- Some sterile products are commercially available in a vial that can be used for either IV infusion or IM injection depending on the preparation method used.
- Parenteral products are a convenient way to administer medications continuously with minimal supervision, or quickly in an emergency.
- Compounding sterile products is an extremely expensive procedure that requires highly trained personnel because a dosing error or contamination of the product can result in serious consequences or death.
- LVPs are intravenous infusion bags containing more than 100 mL of solution that are used to correct fluid or electrolyte imbalance or as a diluent for other drugs.
- SVPs, or piggybacks, are IV bags that contain 25, 50, or 100 mL of solution and are used to add a drug to a patient's therapy.
- Labels of compounded sterile products must contain the generic name and concentration of each ingredient, total volume, administration route and directions, beyond-use date, name of the institution, patient's name and number, date and time of compounding, and initials of the compounder and checking pharmacist.
- Compounded sterile products sent to the home must also include the name, address, and phone number of the pharmacy; the prescribing physician's name; the prescription number; and clear directions that can be understood by a lay person.

- Auxiliary labels provide warnings or reminders for storage requirements.
- Beyond-use dating is based on factors such as the stability of the compound, compatibilities of ingredients, storage requirements, and risk of microbial contamination.
- Validation processes for compounders of sterile products include yearly education, skills examinations, and media fills to verify that the compounder is using correct aseptic technique.

Review Questions

Multiple Choice

Choose the most correct answer to the following.

1. Parenteral products bypass the
   a. liver
   b. gastrointestinal tract
   c. bloodstream
   d. muscles

2. Intramuscular injections into the buttocks of an adult can contain a volume of solution up to
   a. 1 mL
   b. 10 mL
   c. 20 mL
   d. none of the above

3. All of the following would be considered LVPs except
   a. a 1-liter IV bag
   b. a 500-mL IV bag
   c. a 100-mL bag
   d. all of the above are LVPs

4. Small-volume parenterals are also called
   a. minibags
   b. SVPs
   c. piggybacks
   d. all of the above

5. Which of the following affect the beyond-use date of a compounded sterile product?
   a. potential for growth of bacteria
   b. storage requirements
   c. stability of the solution
   d. all of the above

Fill in the Blank

Fill in the blank(s) with the correct word(s).

6. Injecting sterile solutions into a soybean culture medium using aseptic technique is a ______________________________ process designed to validate the technician's use of aseptic technique to prevent microbial ____________________ in sterile compounded products.

7. All media testing should take place in an ISO ________________ environment.

8. LVPs are generally used to replenish ________________, correct ____________________________ and provide a __________________ for an addition to the patient's drug therapy.

9. The two ports at the end of an IV bag are called the injection port and the ____________________________ port.

10. A half-normal sodium chloride solution in an IV bag contains ___________% sodium chloride.

True/False

Mark the following statements True or False.

11. ______ D10W is dextrose 1% in sterile water.

12. ______ When an SVP is added to the IV therapy of a patient receiving a continuous infusion of IV fluids, the LVP must be stopped before the SVP is started.

13. ______ When using an ADD-Vantage® ready-to-mix IV preparation, the powder in the vial must be reconstituted before it is mixed with the diluent.

14. ______ Insulin injections are given subcutaneously.

15. ______ LVPs do not contain a bacteriostatic agent.

Matching

Match the terms in column A with the definitions in column B.

Column A	Column B
16. _____ LVP	A. A large number of sterile products prepared by a single compounder at the same time.
17. _____ media fill process	B. SVPs containing 100 mL or less.
18. _____ batch preparations	C. Products that are injected through the skin and bypass the gastrointestinal tract.
19. _____ piggybacks	D. Adding sterile products to a soy culture medium using aseptic technique and incubating the mixture to verify that the compounder is using aseptic technique.
20. _____ parenterals	E. Single-dose infusions containing more than 100 mL of solution for intravenous use.

LEARNING ACTIVITY

Using the scenario presented in Case Study 21.1, complete the following:

1. Develop a policy that would facilitate the mixing of IV preparations that arrive in the pharmacy when the assigned IV technician is unavailable.
2. Discuss ways to develop a team approach to the responsibilities in the pharmacy setting.
3. Plan ways to deal with the emotions involved in losing a patient, and the feelings of guilt that may accompany an error regardless of whether it causes harm to the patient.

Suggested Reading

Trissel LA. Handbook of Injectable Drugs. 14th ed. Bethesda, MD: American Society of Health-System Professionals, 2007.

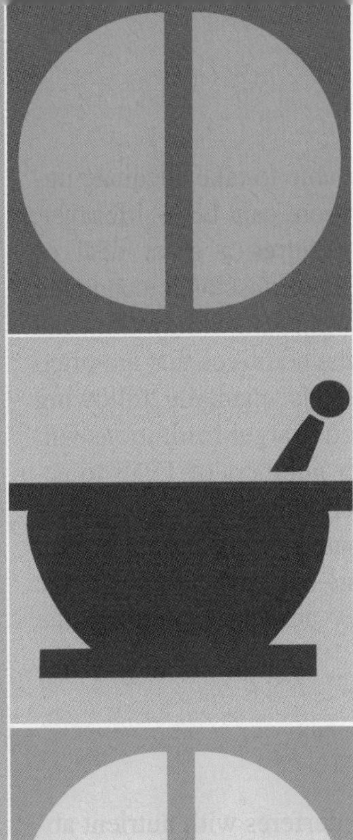

Chapter **22**

Total Parenteral Nutrition

OBJECTIVES

After completing this chapter, the student will be able to:

- List types of patients who require total parenteral nutrition (TPN).
- Outline the basic types of ingredients in TPN.
- Discuss the advantages of having standard TPN formulas.
- Describe the use of automated compounders for compounding TPNs.
- List quality-assurance initiatives required by USP Chapter 797.

KEY TERMS

- electrolytes
- fat emulsion
- partial parenteral nutrition
- peripheral parenteral nutrition
- protein (amino acids)
- total fluid volume
- total nutrient admixture (TNA)
- total parenteral nutrition (TPN)
- trace elements

There are a number of reasons why a patient may not be able to take adequate nutrition by mouth. For these patients, parenteral nutrition can be a lifesaver. Compounding these medium-risk-level formulations requires a great deal of knowledge and expertise on the part of the technician. The professional technician will strive to gain a basic knowledge of nutritional requirements and how they can be met with a basic formula of fluids and nutrients, and the additives that are often used. Some smaller institutions may still compound TPNs manually following aseptic technique in a cleanroom with a laminar flow hood. Larger institutions will use automated compounders to facilitate preparing larger numbers of TPNs to accommodate patients' needs. The professional technician should have a basic understanding of the procedures for both manual and automated preparations of total parenteral nutrition (TPN). This chapter will present some background knowledge to prepare technicians for hands-on practice before they attempt to perform the media fill validation process.

total parenteral nutrition (TPN) Intravenous therapy designed to provide nutrition for patients who cannot or will not take in adequate nourishment by mouth.

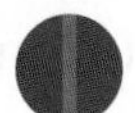

Uses of TPN

Patients who are malnourished or have a condition that interferes with nutrient absorption from the gastrointestinal tract are candidates for TPN. This would include patients who have had severe nausea and vomiting for more than a week. Also, patients with anorexia nervosa who restrict their oral intake and become malnourished may need parenteral therapy to restore their nutritional balance. Patients who have had bowel surgery or a severe bowel disease, skin lesions, or severe burns, and those with various types of cancer affecting the gastrointestinal tract would also be candidates for parenteral nutrition therapy. See Figure 22.1 for an illustration of the routes of oral, enteral, and parenteral nutrition.

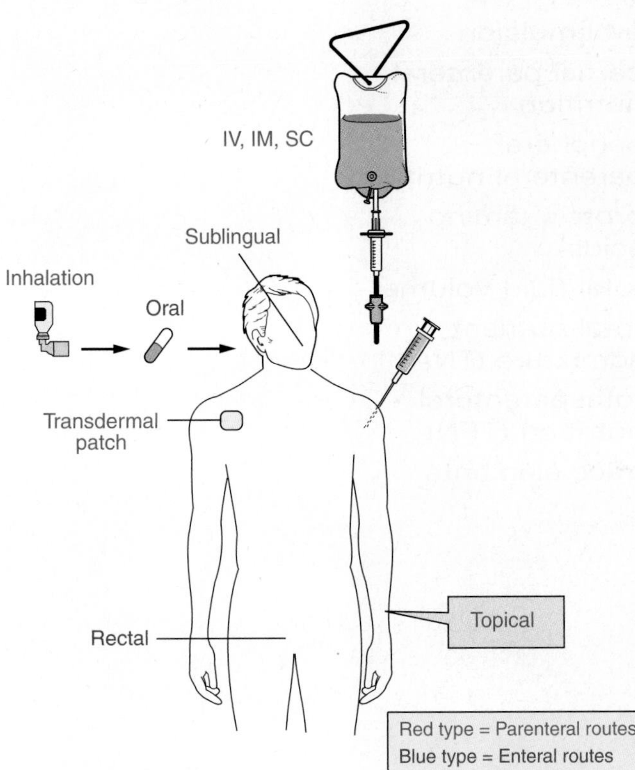

Figure 22.1 Oral, enteral, and parenteral routes of administration. (Reprinted with permission from Sakai J. Pharmacology for the Pharmacy Technician. Baltimore, MD: Lippincott Williams & Wilkins, 2009.)

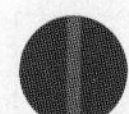 Base Components of a TPN

Dextrose is the main source of calories in a TPN and is a relatively inexpensive form of carbohydrates. The patient's daily requirement is calculated by the physician, using the patient's weight. A concentrated dextrose solution is used in TPNs to avoid exceeding the daily fluid requirements of the patient. Dextrose preparations ranging from 5% to 70% are commercially available. Usually a concentration between 30% and 70% (depending on the liquid volume of the other components in the formula) is used in a TPN. The final concentration of dextrose varies depending on the caloric needs of the patient and whether the preparation is to be infused through a central vein or a peripheral vein. Infusion through a peripheral vein limits the maximum concentration to only 10% to 12%, although it can be as high as 25% if the solution is infused through a central vein. An important component of the parenteral nutrition formula is protein (amino acids). There are commercially available preparations ranging from 8% to 15% that can be diluted according to the needs of the patient during compounding. A 70-kg adult would require 0.8 to 2 g/kg of body weight depending on his stress level and injuries to the body. Protein is required for tissue synthesis to encourage tissue growth or repair.

protein (amino acids) Parenteral solution required for tissue synthesis and repair.

fat emulsion A lipid emulsion intended to supply extra calories and essential fatty acids.

electrolytes Salts of sodium, potassium, chloride, acetate, phosphate, magnesium, and calcium added to a TPN to correct any deficiencies and help meet daily metabolic needs.

An intravenous fat emulsion provides extra calories as well as essential fatty acids that are needed on a daily basis. Fats usually account for 1% to 4% of the total calories. When adding fats to a TPN formulation, it is important to check the bag for precipitates before adding the fat emulsion because the opaque white color of the fats will make it impossible to visually spot a precipitate. A combination of dextrose, amino acids, electrolytes, and fats in one container is called a "three-in-one" or "all-in-one" solution.

A TPN containing a fat emulsion should always be visually inspected before it is administered to ensure that there has been no separation or coagulation of particles. CAUTION

The amount of electrolytes used in a TPN formulation is calculated according to the daily metabolic needs of the patient, with consideration given to any conditions the patient may have, such as liver disease or heart failure. Sodium, potassium, calcium, magnesium, and phosphorus are the electrolytes that are usually included in a TPN. They are all commercially available in a salt form of the element, such as sodium chloride or potassium phosphate.

There have been reports of precipitates of calcium phosphate forming in TPN formulations that contain both calcium and phosphate. The amounts of these two elements and the order in which they are mixed are critical. The FDA recommends that when calcium and phosphate are added to a mixture, phosphate should be the first electrolyte added and calcium should be the last. CAUTION

Trace elements are commercially available in a number of formulations containing chromium, copper, manganese, selenium, and zinc. It is important to double-check the formula against the amounts ordered for the TPN being prepared to ensure that the correct product is selected.

trace elements Small amounts of elements, such as copper, zinc, chromium, manganese, selenium, iron, and iodine, that are commercially available in combinations for addition to TPNs.

Multiple vitamins come in several forms because the stability of the product may be compromised if all the vitamins are packaged together. They are available as a powder for reconstitution and in mix-o-vial units so they can be mixed together and added to a TPN just before use. When vitamins are added to a TPN, the beyond-use date should reflect the stability of the vitamin formulation. When the

STANDARD CENTRAL LINE FORMULA

Standard ❑ Modified ❑

Amino Acid 4.25% ________%

Dextrose 25% ________%

Rate ________mL/hr

Electrolytes (per liter)

Standard ❑ Modified ❑

Na 35 mEq ________mEq

K 30 mEq ________mEq

Mg 5 mEq ________mEq

Ca 3 mEq ________mEq

P 15 mM ________mM

Acetate: Cl = 1 : 1

Each bag contains the standard amount of multivitamins and trace elements.

Additional Ingredients (per liter)

Standard ❑ Modified ❑

___Cimetidine 900 mg/24 hr OR:_____ mg/24 hr

___Ranitidine 150 mg/24 hr OR:_____ mg/24 hr

___Reg Insulin _____units/L

Other:

____

____

____

STANDARD PERIPHERAL LINE FORMULA

Standard ❑ Modified ❑

Amino Acid 2.75% ________%

Dextrose 10% ________%

Rate ________mL/hr

Electrolytes (per liter)

Standard ❑ Modified ❑

Na 35 mEq ________mEq

K 30 mEq ________mEq

Mg 5 mEq ________mEq

Ca 3 mEq ________mEq

P 15 mM ________mM

Acetate: Cl = 1 : 1 ________

Each bag contains the standard amount of multivitamins and trace elements.

Additional Ingredients (per liter)

____

____

____

____

STANDARD RENAL CENTRAL LINE FORMULA

Standard ❑ Modified ❑

Amino Acid 1.95% ________%

Dextrose 44% ________%

Rate ________mL/hr

Electrolytes (per liter)

Standard ❑ Modified ❑

Na 0 mEq ________mEq

K 0 mEq ________mEq

Mg 0 mEq ________mEq

Ca 0 mEq ________mEq

P 0 mM ________mM

Check if you wish to add the standard amount of trace elements and multivitamins.

Trace Elements ________

Multivitamins ________

Additional Ingredients (per liter)

____

____

____

____

Intravenous Fat 10% 500 mL (1.1 kcal/mL):________________(rate)

Intravenous Fat 20% 500 mL (2 kcal/mL):________________(rate)

Date:________________ MD ________________

NOTE:
Standing physician's orders for line management and patient monitoring of parenteral hyperalimentation will be followed unless initialed here:________

Figure 22.2 Order form for adult parenteral nutrition. (Reprinted with permission from Lacher BE. Pharmaceutical Calculations for the Pharmacy Technician. Baltimore, MD: Lippincott Williams & Wilkins, 2008.)

TPN is delivered to another site, such as a nursing home, to be administered, the vitamin preparation is often sent separately to be mixed by the caregiver just before administration.

total fluid volume The amount of fluid a patient needs to receive from the TPN to satisfy daily fluid requirements (usually about 2500–3000 mL daily for an average adult).

TPNs are also used to maintain a patient's fluid requirements. Although most of the fluid is present in the various components of the TPN, sterile water is often added to complete the fluid requirements. A typical TPN for an adult patient might contain a total volume of 2400 mL to be infused at a rate of 100 mL/hr. The total volume of each component of the TPN is calculated and the amount of water required to bring the total fluid volume to 2400 mL (or the volume ordered by the physician) is added. Figure 22.2 shows an example of the components of a standard TPN.

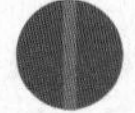

Using a TPN as a Drug Delivery Vehicle

Frequently a drug, such as ranitidine, is added to the TPN mixture, but occasionally the physician may want to include other drugs that are a part of the patient's drug therapy. It is important to ensure that the drug in question will remain stable in the solution for the entire 12- to 24-hour period in which the TPN will be infused. It also must be checked for compatibility with all other agents in the TPN mixture, including any additional drugs being added. The drug being added must also have a steady dose that will not need to be adjusted during the 12 to 24 hours during which the solution will be infused.

Compounding TPN

Smaller pharmacy facilities that require few TPNs will compound them manually. Strict aseptic technique must be followed regardless of the method used. An empty bag may be obtained commercially and filled in the laminar flow hood. The base ingredients are allowed to flow into the bag by gravity. The electrolytes, trace elements, and any other additives are then added by drawing them up in a syringe and using the injection port on the large IV bag to inject them into the bag one at a time.

Parenteral nutrition solutions containing the base ingredients (amino acid solution and dextrose solution) are commercially available in 2000- and 3000-mL bags. Such bags require only the addition of electrolytes, trace elements, multivitamin solutions, and lipids. These ingredients can be added manually using a syringe. The lipid emulsion can either be added to the bag or sent separately to hang as a piggyback on the base solution. When fats are added to a TPN, it is considered a total nutrient admixture (TNA). When a TPN is formulated to only partially supply the daily needs of the patient, it is a partial parenteral nutrition bag (TPN). A TPN administered through a peripheral vein, usually in the arm, is a peripheral parenteral nutrition bag.

total nutrient admixture (TNA) A three-in-one IV solution that includes a lipid emulsion added to the base components.

Manual filling of TPN solutions must be performed using the strictest aseptic technique. It is vitally important to add each additive correctly according to the formula ordered for the individual patient. Quality-assurance methods should be in place for the pharmacist to double-check the amounts of each ingredient added. If there is even one error in the addition of an additive, the formula should be discarded and remade because the error would invalidate the concentrations of everything in the bag. The bag should be visually checked during the compounding process to determine that there are no precipitates. After the lipids are added, it is extremely difficult to see precipitates, but it is important to do a final check to ensure that the addition of the lipids has not resulted in a separation or coagulation of the solution. Needless to say, manual filling of TPN bags is extremely time-consuming, so as the volume of TPN bags needed on a regular basis increases, the pharmacy will begin to consider purchasing an automated compounder.

There are two basic types of automated compounders: macro compounders and micro compounders. The macro compounder has special tubing that is strong enough to pump the large volumes of fluids needed in the base solution into the bag. The specific gravity of the solution can be programmed into the computer, and the machine can calculate the final weight of the bag. The micro compounder uses computer software to calculate the amount of each additive from the specific gravity and the volume needed, and weighs the final product for comparison with the calculated weight. The computer can be programmed for alarms when a line is plugged or maximum safe quantities are reached. An automated compounder does not replace the many checks that must be done by the technician and pharmacist. Refer back to Figure 2.8 for a picture of an automated compounder. The technician must learn the proper way to set up the machine and program the specific gravity, and this process should be checked and verified by the pharmacist. The automated compounder must be placed inside a laminar airflow hood and cleaned according to protocol daily. It may be the technician's responsibility to perform regular maintenance and check the calibration periodically. The pharmacy should have a written policy regarding cleaning and maintenance. The professional technician will be knowledgeable about the policy and make sure it is followed.

It is important to administer parenteral nutrition admixtures within 24 hours of mixing if they have been stored at room temperature. If the TPN has been refrigerated, it should be started within 24 hours of rewarming. Allowing the TPN to be warmed for too long a period of time will encourage the formation of precipitates. The caregiver administering the infusion should check for the presence of precipitates and report any sign of respiratory distress experienced by the patient. TPN preparations without lipids are usually administered with a 0.22-micron filter to filter out precipitates; however, if a lipid emulsion has been added, a 1.2-micron filter should be used to avoid filtering out the fat globules.

Most institutions have developed a standard TPN order form to prevent medication errors resulting from illegible handwriting. All of the base components and the commonly used additives are listed on the form. The ordering physician only needs to write in the amounts of each ingredient. Figure 22.2 shows an example of a standard adult TPN formula that can be modified by the physician to meet the special needs of the patient.

Case Study 22.1

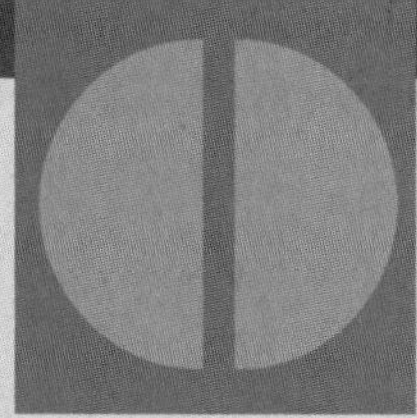

John arrives at work in a small rural hospital and discovers that a patient has been admitted who will need to be started on TPN. While he is waiting for the orders to reach the pharmacy, he turns on the horizontal laminar airflow hood and begins the cleaning process. This pharmacy does not have an automated compounder because it does not often have a patient on a TPN. John begins to gather some of the basic supplies he knows will be needed and places them on the stainless-steel cart in the buffer area. He chooses an empty 3000-mL IV bag because he knows the physician usually writes for a 2400 to 3000-mL total fluid volume. He gathers an amino acid bag, a large-volume bag of dextrose, a lipid emulsion, and a bag of sterile water to complete the fluid requirements. As John is placing these items on the cart, the order is received in the pharmacy. John is experienced at performing the calculations and having them double-checked by the pharmacist before beginning the procedure. The order reads as follows:

Patient Name: James Jones   ID #64352   Room #212   Wt: 85 kg

Infusion Volume 2400 mL   Infusion Rate 100 mL/hr

Protein	120 g
Dextrose	350 g
Lipids	60 g
Additives	
Sodium chloride	60 mEq
Potassium acetate	40 mEq
Magnesium sulfate	10 mEq
Calcium gluconate	10 mEq
Adult multivitamins	1 ampul
Trace elements	3 mL

The concentration of each item available in the pharmacy is as follows:

protein (amino acids)	10%
dextrose	D70W
fat emulsion	20%
sodium chloride	4 mEq/mL
potassium acetate	2 mEq/mL
magnesium sulfate	4 mEq/mL
calcium gluconate	0.45 mEq/mL
potassium chloride	2 mEq/mL
multiple vitamins	10 mL
trace elements	3 mL

1. Using the above concentrations, calculate the volume of each component that will need to be added to the TPN.
2. Calculate the amount of sterile water, if any, that must be added to bring the total volume of the TPN to 2400 mL.

After completing the calculations, John has the pharmacist check his figures and initial the order before he begins to compound the TPN. He finishes adding the supplies and equipment to the cart in the buffer room, sanitizes each item, and begins the hand-washing, gowning, and gloving procedure in preparation for entering the cleanroom.

Chapter Summary

- Patients who are unable or unwilling to take adequate nourishment by mouth or through a feeding tube are candidates for parenteral nutrition.
- The base components of a TPN are dextrose for carbohydrates, amino acids for protein, and a lipid emulsion for fatty acids and calories.
- Sterile water is added to the final formulation of a TPN to bring the fluid volume up to the daily fluid requirement of the patient.
- Electrolytes are added to the base solution in amounts calculated to supply the daily metabolic needs of the patient.
- Trace elements are added to the formulation in amounts calculated to supply the special needs of each patient.
- Multivitamin preparations are commercially available and may either be added at the time of compounding or sent with the bag to be added at the time of administration.
- Small pharmacy facilities may compound TPNs manually by the gravity-fill method.
- Larger facilities use automated compounders to prepare TPNs.
- Automated compounders require diligent cleaning and maintenance, which are frequently the responsibilities of a technician.
- Strict aseptic technique is required whether the TPN is prepared manually or with an automated compounder.
- Proper temperature and length of storage are critical for a TPN.

Review Questions

Multiple Choice

Choose the correct answer for the following statements.

1. When a TPN has been stored in the refrigerator, how soon after rewarming must the infusion be started?
   a. 30 minutes
   b. 1 hour
   c. 24 hours
   d. 6 hours

2. Potential candidates for receiving a TPN include all of the following except:
   a. patients with fluid loss from prolonged diarrhea
   b. patients who have nausea and vomiting for a few days
   c. patients with severe bowel disorders
   d. patients who are severely malnourished

3. The components of the base ingredients in a three-in-one TPN that will provide calories to the patient are:
   a. amino acids
   b. dextrose
   c. lipids
   d. b and c

4. The protein component of the TPN formulation is provided by:
   a. lipid emulsion
   b. trace elements
   c. amino acids
   d. electrolytes

5. An automated compounding device that is used to add the base components to a TPN is called a:
   a. manual compounder
   b. macro compounder
   c. micro compounder
   d. gravity-fill compounder

Fill in the Blank

Fill in the blanks with the correct word or words.

6. When both calcium and phosphate are added to a TPN mixture, _____________ should be the first additive and _____________ should be the last.

7. If the base ingredients and the additives ordered for a TPN formula do not add up to the total volume required for the TPN, a calculated amount of ______________________ should be added.

8. When using the TPN as a drug vehicle for a patient's drug therapy, the ______________ and the ______________ of each drug should be considered.

9. TPN compounding is considered Risk Level ________.

10. An automated compounder must be set up properly by the technician, and the ______________ ______________ of the additives must be correctly programmed into the machine.

True/False

Mark the following statements True or False.

11. ______ If the automated compounding machines are located in a cleanroom, they do not need to be in a laminar flow hood.

12. ______ It is customary for the fat globules in a TPN to separate from the rest of the solution and coagulate.

13. ______ A TPN formulation including a lipid emulsion is usually administered with a 0.22-micron filter to remove any precipitates.

14. ______ Most adult patients need a total volume of 2400 to 3500 mL of fluid daily.

15. ______ A commercial multivitamin preparation is often sent separately with the TPN to be added just before administration because of stability concerns.

Matching

Match the terms in column A with the definitions in column B.

Column A

16. _____ amino acids
17. _____ total nutrient admixture (TNA)
18. _____ total parenteral nutrition (TPN)
19. _____ lipid emulsion
20. _____ peripheral parenteral nutrition

Column B

A. Parenteral nutrition administered through a vein in the arm.
B. Intravenous therapy designed to provide nutrition for patients who are unable to take nourishment by mouth.
C. A fat emulsion intended to supply extra calories and essential fatty acids.
D. A parenteral solution to supply protein needed for tissue synthesis and repair.
E. A three-in-one solution that includes fats with the base components.

LEARNING ACTIVITY

Design a step-by-step procedure to prepare the above formulation by the manual gravity-fill method. Include proper placement of the items in the hood and the mixing procedure. Design a label containing the required information to be placed on the TPN, any storage requirements, and the expiration date.

Suggested Readings

Buchanan CE, Schneider PJ. Compounding Sterile Preparations. 2nd ed. Bethesda, MD: American Society of Health-System Pharmacists, 2005.

Mirtallo JM, Lehman K. Assessment Tools and Guidelines: Parenteral Nutrition Therapy. Pharmacy Practice News Special Edition, 2004.

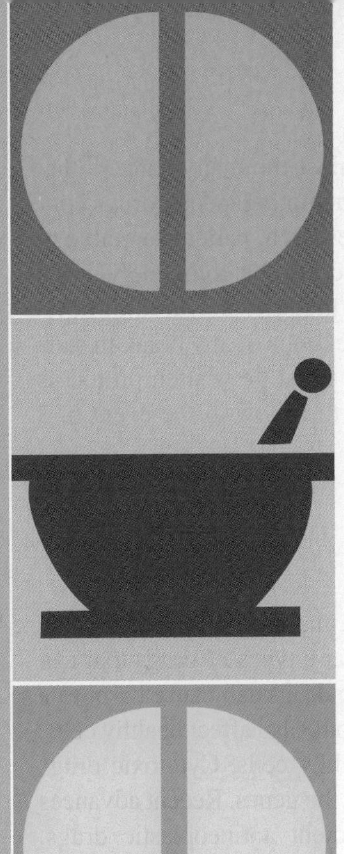

Chapter 23

Compounding Sterile Chemotherapeutic Products

OBJECTIVES

After completing this chapter, the student will be able to:

- List types of chemotherapeutic drugs that may be hazardous.
- Detail precautions to protect the compounder from harm.
- Contrast the aseptic manipulations in a horizontal flow hood with those in a vertical flow hood.
- Identify the components of a hazardous spill kit and describe their use.
- Illustrate labeling and packaging requirements for a sterile chemotherapeutic compound.

KEY TERMS

- antineoplastic drugs
- barrier isolator
- biohazard
- biological safety cabinet (BSC)
- chemo spill kit
- chemotherapeutic drugs
- cytotoxic
- genotoxic agent
- material safety data sheets
- mutagenic
- oncogenic
- personal protective equipment
- teratogenic

chemotherapeutic drugs Drugs used in the treatment of cancer that can destroy normal living cells. Extra precautions are needed to ensure the safety of the compounder.

As the medical profession continues the battle against the many cancers that afflict our patients, the volume of sterile compounded chemotherapeutic drugs continues to increase. As a result of advances in medical research, patients are able to live longer, enjoy a better quality of life, and, in some cases, be completely cured of cancer. The professional technician will understand the serious nature of deviating even slightly from the ordered dose, and the implications of any break in sterile technique when preparing these compounds. There must be written protocols about the safe handling of these drugs and procedures to follow in the event of a hazardous spill or an inadvertent exposure incident.

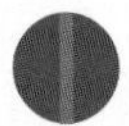

Types of Hazardous Drugs

teratogenic Capable of causing damage to a developing fetus or the reproductive system.

oncogenic Capable of destroying cancer cells.

mutagenic Causing changes in DNA that can increase mutations.

antineoplastic drugs Chemotherapeutic agents that help control or cure cancer.

A few years ago when hazardous drugs were discussed, the term referred to a few drugs used in cancer chemotherapy. Today, there are many types of drugs that can be hazardous in a number of different ways. Teratogenic drugs can cause harm to a developing fetus. Oncogenic drugs kill cancer cells, but may also affect healthy cells. Mutagenic drugs can cause mutations in otherwise healthy cells. Cytotoxic drugs damage cells within the body. Genotoxic drugs can affect the genes. Recent advances have resulted in the development of newer, more potent antineoplastic drugs. Immunosuppressants play a vital role in preventing rejection of transplanted organs. More complex antiviral drugs are constantly being developed to continue the fight against HIV, and biological response modifiers are playing an ever-increasing role in modern drug therapy.

All of these drugs have the potential to create risk for persons who are even minimally exposed to them on a daily basis. Any drug or chemical for which there is sufficient evidence that acute or chronic health hazards may result from exposure is considered a hazardous product and requires special handling procedures. There must be Material Safety Data Sheets (MSDS) available for all hazardous drugs and chemicals in the pharmacy.

Potential for Exposure to Hazardous Drugs

Some procedures performed before, during, and after the compounding of sterile hazardous drug products create an opportunity for exposure through skin contact, inhalation, ingestion, or injection. Understanding the risks and following safety guidelines will help to minimize or even eliminate some of these risks. Manipulations that are routinely performed by pharmacy technicians and require extra thought and precautions include reconstituting powdered or lyophilized drugs and further diluting either the powder or concentrated liquid form of hazardous drugs. Expelling air from syringes filled with hazardous drugs and contacting measurable amounts of drugs present on the outside of drug vials, work surfaces, floors, and the final drug container can create the risk of exposure. Improper handling of unused hazardous drugs or contaminated waste is another area of concern. The technician is also responsible for decontaminating and cleaning the drug preparation area. Finally, the technician should remove and dispose of personal protective equipment (PPE) according to policy after handling hazardous drugs.

personal protective equipment (PPE) Includes gloves, gowns, goggles, respirators, and face shields.

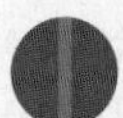

Safe Handling of Hazardous Drugs

Safe handling begins when the hazardous drugs enter the pharmacy. Technicians checking in an order containing hazardous drugs should be wearing proper PPE, including chemotherapy gloves and respiratory masks, to prevent exposure from breakage or drug spills from damaged containers. Hazardous drugs should be clearly labeled as hazardous materials and stored separately from other drugs in closed containers to minimize breakage. The storage area should have adequate ventilation to limit airborne contaminants. Hazardous drugs should not be stored on shelves above eye level, to avoid having the technician reach over his or her head and possibly allowing supplies to fall. Access to areas where hazardous drugs are prepared should be limited to persons who have been trained to participate in hazardous-drug preparation.

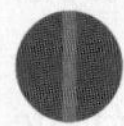

Compounding Sterile Hazardous Preparations

Hazardous sterile products should only be compounded in a Class III biological safety cabinet (BSC) or a barrier isolator. Extensive training is required to acquaint the technician with the extra precautions and the different manner of working in a barrier isolator or a vertical flow BSC. Hand washing, gowning, and gloving are performed the same as for nonhazardous sterile compounding except that the technician should be double-gloved, with one pair of gloves worn under the cuffs of the gown and the second pair worn over the cuffs. When working in the hood for prolonged periods of time, technicians should change their gloves every 30 minutes or whenever they leave the BSC and reenter, or when one of the gloves is torn or contaminated.

biological safety cabinet (BSC) A ventilated cabinet designed to protect the worker, the product, and the environment with a downward HEPA-filtered airflow and a HEPA-filtered exhaust; a vertical flow laminar flow hood used to compound chemotherapeutic agents.

barrier isolator A sealed laminar flow hood that is supplied with air through a HEPA filter, maintaining a ISO Class 5 environment. It allows the compounder to access the work area through glove openings and maintain sterility without the need for a cleanroom or gowning.

After completing the gowning process, complete with a hair shield, shoe covers, and face mask, the operator should sanitize the hood and carefully place only the needed supplies in the hood to avoid blocking the air vents. IV bags can be hung in the hood, keeping in mind that the BSC is a vertical flow hood and the hanging bags must not block the airflow by being placed directly above items placed in the hood. Aseptic manipulations in a vertical flow hood are conducted in a different manner than in a horizontal flow hood because of the different direction of the airflow.

When reconstituting a hazardous drug, it is important to create a slight negative pressure in the vial. The syringe used should be no more than three-quarters full when the solution is drawn up, and the needle should be inserted into the vial and drawn back slightly to create a slight negative pressure. Small amounts of diluent can be transferred to the vial while small amounts of air are removed. With the needle still in the vial, the contents are swirled until mixed. The vial can then be inverted with the needle still in the vial, and the process is reversed as small amounts of the reconstituted solution are withdrawn into the syringe alternately with small amounts of air.

Use the following procedure to fill an IV bag with a hazardous drug: When the correct amount of solution is in the syringe, turn the vial and withdraw a small amount of air into the hub of the needle before removing the needle from the vial. Carefully puncture the injection port of the IV bag, being careful not to puncture the sides. Wipe the IV port and the container, and cover the IV port with a protective shield. Clean the final preparation and remove your outer gloves, being careful to dispose of them as hazardous waste. Put on new gloves to remove the final preparation, label it, add auxiliary labels, and place it in a transport bag. Decontaminate the equipment using the agent prescribed by pharmacy protocols. Use proper procedure for removing your gown, gloves, and other PPE, and dispose of them properly as hazardous waste.

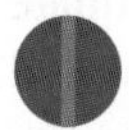 Hazardous Material Spill Kit

chemo spill kit A kit that contains PPE and equipment for cleaning up a hazardous spill; it can be either purchased commercially or assembled by the pharmacy.

Any pharmacy that handles hazardous substances should have a chemo spill kit immediately available. There are several spill kits available commercially, but the required items can also be assembled into a kit by the pharmacy. The kit should contain a complete set of PPE, including a gown, two pairs of gloves, a respirator mask, and a pair of goggles. If the spill takes place inside the hood area, the technician may already be wearing the PPE, but some or all of the items may be contaminated by the spill. If so, they should be removed. If the spill has penetrated the PPE and contacted the skin or any area of the body, the PPE should be removed and disposed of properly and the area flushed with water or an eye flush kit if the eyes have been exposed. After all contaminated areas have been washed with soap and water, the affected person should be taken to the emergency room.

At this point, a second person will need to don the PPE in the chemo spill kit and begin to contain and clean up the spill. The kit should contain a sign stating "CAUTION: Chemo Spill" to warn others to avoid the area and plastic disposal bags labeled "Hazardous Waste." The kit should also contain a scoop and brush for picking up any glass that may have broken, plenty of absorbent towels, and extra chemo hazard labels. Either in the kit or somewhere in the compounding area there should be chemo incident forms for writing up the details of the spill and the actions taken.

Only very experienced technicians with experience mixing compounded sterile products should be chosen for training as hazardous-drug compounders. These technicians must demonstrate an educated understanding of the risks posed to workers and the environment, and an ability to adhere to all policies and procedures. This could potentially become an advanced specialty area for competent technicians.

Case Study 23.1

As Alex was walking by the cleanroom window, he noticed that John seemed very agitated as he worked in the hood. He asked John if he needed any help, and John replied that he had spilled one of the chemo drugs he was working with in the BSC. The vial had broken and torn a small area of his gloves, and some of the solution had contacted his skin. Alex went in the room to assist John as John removed his gown and gloves and disposed of them in the biohazard waste receptacle. Without touching John, Alex turned on the water for John to flush the skin on his hand and called for another technician to accompany John to the emergency room.

biohazard A hazardous biological agent, such as contaminated tissue, blood or body fluids, needles, and syringes, that presents a risk to the health of humans exposed to it.

Detail the steps Alex should take to clean up the spill and decontaminate the area. Include the correct use of each item in the chemo spill kit.

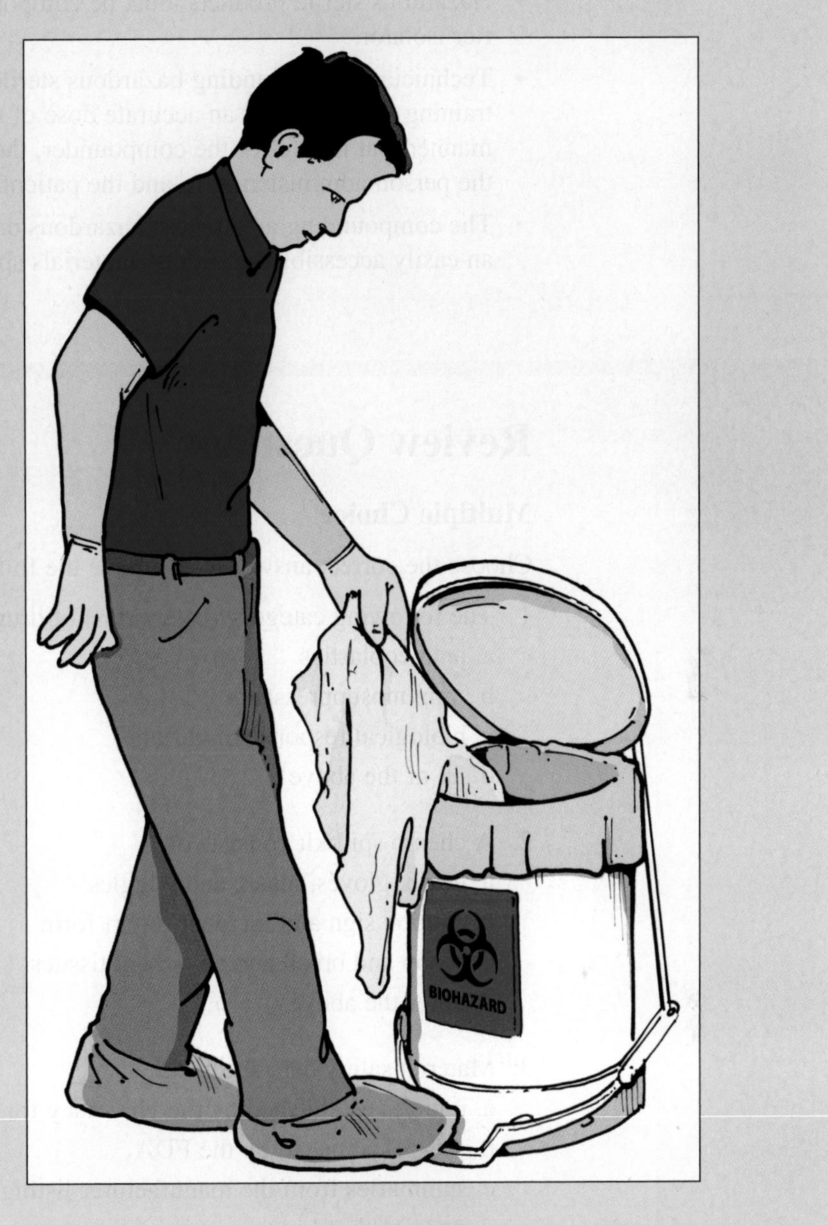

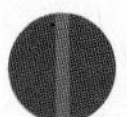

Chapter Summary

- Categories of hazardous drugs have expanded from antineoplastic drugs to include antivirals, immunosuppressants, and biological response modifiers, and the list continues to grow.
- Risks for technicians handling hazardous drugs include spills during reconstitution and dilution, expelling air from syringes, and contact with drugs on vials, work surfaces, or floors.
- Safe handling of hazardous drugs begins when they enter the pharmacy. Technicians checking in the order should be wearing proper PPE.
- Hazardous drugs must be clearly labeled as hazardous and stored separately in well-ventilated areas.

- Hazardous sterile products must be compounded in a Class III BSC or a barrier isolator.
- Technicians compounding hazardous sterile products must have extensive training to ensure that an accurate dose of the correct drug is prepared in a manner that is safe for the compounder, the person delivering the medication, the person administering it, and the patient.
- The compounding area where hazardous drugs are compounded should have an easily accessible hazardous-materials spill kit.

Review Questions

Multiple Choice

Choose the correct answer to complete the following statements.

1. The following category (categories) of drugs may be considered hazardous:
   a. antineoplastics
   b. immunosuppressants
   c. biological response modifiers
   d. all of the above

2. A chemo spill kit consists of
   a. gown, gloves, mask, and goggles
   b. caution sign and incident report form
   c. scoop and brush and absorbent tissues
   d. all of the above

3. Material safety data sheets are
   a. policies established by the pharmacy for safe drug use
   b. rules established by the FDA
   c. summaries from the manufacturer listing the properties and hazards of drugs
   d. none of the above

4. In a BSC the airflow through the HEPA filter is
   a. horizontal, flowing out toward the room
   b. vertical, flowing from the top of the cabinet down
   c. flowing up through the vents on the work surface
   d. none of the above

5. When working in a BSC, technicians should change their gloves
   a. every hour
   b. when leaving the hood to get more supplies
   c. every 30 minutes
   d. b and c

Fill in the Blanks

Fill in the blanks with the correct word(s).

6. Technicians checking in an order containing hazardous substances should be wearing ____________ ____________ ____________.

7. When drawing up a hazardous drug, technicians should use a syringe that is no more than ____________ full.

8. When reconstituting a hazardous substance, it is important to create a slight ____________ pressure in the vial.

9. A hazardous biological substance, such as contaminated blood or body fluids, that poses a risk to human health from exposure is called a ____________.

10. A sealed device with air supplied through a HEPA filter that allows the performance of aseptic manipulations through attached rubber gloves is called a ____________ ____________.

True/False

Mark the following statements True or False.

11. _______ When compounding hazardous drugs, the technician should be double-gloved so that if only the outer glove is torn, the compounding can continue.

12. _______ Damaged boxes containing hazardous substances should not be taken into the pharmacy.

13. _______ IV bags cannot be hung in the BSC when hazardous drugs are being compounded.

14. _______ When completing the compounding of a hazardous substance, the technician should put new gloves on before removing the IV bag from the hood.

15. _______ An IV bag containing a hazardous substance must be put in a specially marked transport bag before it is removed from the pharmacy.

Matching

Match the items in column A with the definitions in column B.

Column A	Column B
16. ______ cytotoxic	A. Capable of destroying cancer cells.
17. ______ oncogenic	B. Capable of damaging DNA.
18. ______ teratogenic	C. Drugs used to treat cancer and other diseases.
19. ______ chemotherapeutic drugs	D. Destructive to cells in the body.
20. ______ genotoxic agent	E. Damaging to a developing fetus.

LEARNING ACTIVITY

Practice setting up vials, IV bags, syringes, and needles in a vertical flow cabinet without interrupting the airflow from the HEPA filter or the air vents. Then practice the aseptic manipulations involved in transferring fluids and discuss how they differ from aseptic manipulations in a horizontal flow hood.

Suggested Readings

Buchanan CE, Schneider PJ. Compounding Sterile Preparations. 2nd ed. Bethesda, MD: American Society of Health-System Pharmacists, 2005.

National Institute for Occupational Safety and Health. Preventing Occupational Exposure to Antineoplastic and Other Hazardous Drugs. http://www.cdc.gov/niosh/docs

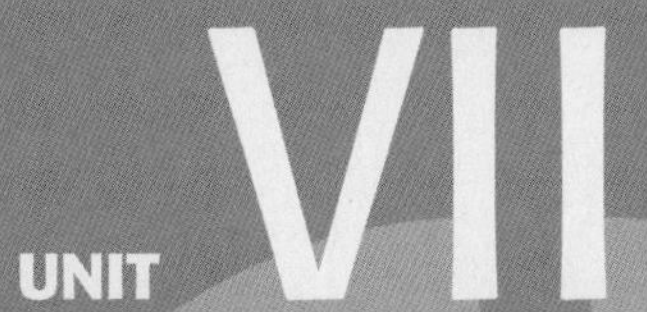

UNIT VII

Professionalism and Career Exploration

Chapter **24**

Professional Organizations and Education

OBJECTIVES

After completing this chapter, the student will be able to:

- List professional organizations that are pertinent to the pharmacy technician profession.
- Outline the importance of each organization to the profession.
- Discuss reasons for technicians to maintain memberships in professional organizations.
- Plan ways to organize a local chapter of an organization.
- Devise ways to work with an organization to enhance the profession.
- Name the two national certification examinations.
- Explain the importance of national certification.
- Discuss reasons for mandatory education standards.
- Detail a plan to keep current through continuing education.

KEY TERMS

- AACP
- AAPT
- ACPE
- ASHP
- APhA
- ExCPT
- NABP
- NACDS
- NPTA
- PTCB
- PTCE
- PTEC

As the profession of pharmacy technician continues to evolve, it is important for all technician professionals to become vested in their profession. There are a number of ways to demonstrate this professional vesting and contribute to the growth and development of the profession and of each technician personally. Pharmacy technicians must nurture a basic education in the standards of practice by following a continuing education plan to ensure that their knowledge remains current. Another mark of a true professional is active membership in a professional organization. This allows technicians to help direct the future course of the profession by creating a unified voice concerning important decisions affecting the profession. This chapter will describe some important organizations and their relevance to pharmacy technicians.

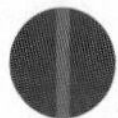

ASHP

ASHP American Society of Health-System Pharmacists.

The ASHP is a national professional organization for pharmacists and pharmacy technicians who work in hospitals and health systems. This organization has served as the accrediting body for pharmacy technician training programs for 20 years and has accredited about 100 programs across the country. Accreditation by the ASHP signifies that a program has met certain standards and a course curriculum is based on the Model Curriculum for Pharmacy Technician Training Programs. The Council on Legal and Public Affairs has adopted a policy position stating that the pharmacy profession should move toward adopting the following model for pharmacy technicians:

- Development of uniform state laws and regulations for pharmacy technicians.
- Mandatory completion of a nationally accredited pharmacy technician education and training program as a prerequisite to taking a national PTCE.
- Mandatory certification by the PTCB or a comparable certification exam approved by the state board of pharmacy (BOP). Practicing technicians with at least 1 year of experience could become eligible to take the certification exam.

PTCE Pharmacy Technician Certification Exam.

PTCB Pharmacy Technician Certification Board.

The ASHP works with the state BOPs and state pharmacy associations to advocate for technician initiatives. Most state associations have a local chapter of the ASHP that encourages technician membership. Technician members of the ASHP who meet certain qualifications are eligible to serve on the Pharmacy Technician Advisory Group or other committees that may be available at the national or state level. The ASHP is actively involved in advancing the technician profession through education and training. There are many opportunities for technicians to speak at ASHP conferences and exhibit poster presentations, in addition to technician networking opportunities.

TIP **The web address for the American Society of Health-System Pharmacists is http://www.ashp.org.**

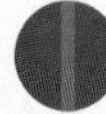

APhA

APhA American Pharmaceutical Association.

The APhA is the oldest and largest professional pharmacy association. It represents 66,000 pharmacists, technicians, students, and others who believe in its mission to advance the profession of pharmacy. Although it does not have a separate section for pharmacy technicians, it offers many advantages to technicians. A journal is offered to all members to help them stay abreast of new developments in the profession, and a Drug Information Center is available to members on the website. Some continuing education programs can be used to fulfill requirements for renewing national certification. An online career center helps with job placement, and the organization has published several books for pharmacy technicians. More importantly, the APhA affords the technician another opportunity to band together with thousands of members to promote initiatives that will move the profession forward.

The APhA's web address is http://www.aphanet.org. **TIP**

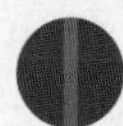

ACPE

The ACPE is the national agency for accrediting pharmacy degree programs and providers of continuing education for pharmacists and pharmacy technicians. In 2003 the ACPE conducted a profession-wide dialogue concerning the need for national standards for pharmacy technician education and training. The profession has yet to reach a consensus on this subject. In January, 2007, the ACPE adopted new standards for differentiating between continuing education requirements for pharmacists and technicians.

ACPE Association for the Credentialing of Pharmacy Education.

As of January 1, 2008, continuing-education programs for pharmacists have a "P" in the program number and will further pharmacist-specific objectives based on initiatives from the Institute of Medicine, the American Association of Colleges of Pharmacy, the National Association of Boards of Pharmacy, and the Joint Commission of Pharmacy Practitioners. Continuing education for pharmacy technicians will address pharmacy technician-specific performance objectives derived from the Pharmacy Technician Certification Board's Practice Analysis, and will have a "T" in the number. If a continuing-education activity is developed to include both pharmacists and technicians, there must be separate objectives for each. The program number will be the same for both, except for the last letter, which will be either a "P" or a "T." This will be important information for technicians when they acquire continuing-education credits to renew their national certification.

The ACPE's web address is http://www.acpe-accredit.org. **TIP**

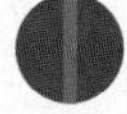

AACP

The AACP is a group of pharmacy school educators who have joined together to improve pharmacy education, be an advocate for professional and interprofessional education, facilitate discussion and networking in the profession, and maintain open communications. The AACP as a group has not been directly involved in pharmacy technician education, but it hopes to work more closely with pharmacy technician educators in the future.

AACP American Association of Colleges of Pharmacy.

The AACP's web address is http://www.aacp.org. **TIP**

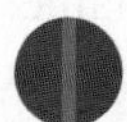

NABP

The NABP is an international organization that was founded to assist the state BOPs in developing and enforcing uniform standards to provide safe medications to the public. The NABP is not directly involved with pharmacy technicians, but it has been supportive of standardized technician education and training.

NABP National Association of Boards of Pharmacy.

 NACDS

NACDS National Association of Chain Drug Stores.

The NACDS was founded to represent the leading retail chain pharmacies and their suppliers. It has nearly 200 member companies and represents nearly 37,000 retail community pharmacies. They represent the views and policy positions of the chain drug industry and promote the role of retail community pharmacies in the health-care system. Retail chain pharmacies employ a tremendous number of pharmacy technicians with varying levels of education and training. In some states, education and training standards have been mandated by the state BOP. Often a chain pharmacy will implement a company training program and encourage its technicians to pass the national certification exam within a prescribed time period after beginning employment. Technicians in the retail community chain setting play a vital role in dispensing medications to the public. Although they are supervised by a pharmacist, these technicians are often in a position to discover a possible drug interaction that a pharmacist might not notice. The technician is the ambassador of the pharmacy who greets the customers and establishes a relationship with them. The patient will often confide a health issue to a technician and not "bother" the pharmacist. An educated technician will be alert for any signs of a problem and alert the pharmacist that patient counseling may be needed. Quality education and training are a must for these very important members of the pharmacy profession.

TIP **The NACDS's web address is http://www.nacds.org.**

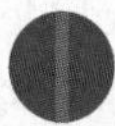 ExCPT

ExCPT Exam for the Certification of Pharmacy Technicians.

The ExCPT is a national exam that is recognized by the NACDS and is used to determine whether a minimum knowledge base has been achieved by pharmacy technicians who assist pharmacists in retail pharmacy outlets. It is offered by the Institute for the Certification of Pharmacy Technicians (ICPT) and is accepted by some state BOPs. Be sure to check with your state's pharmacy board to verify which certification exam is accepted.

TIP **The web address for the ExCPT is http://www.nationaltechexam.org.**

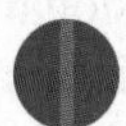 PTCB

The PTCB began offering the PTCE in 1995 and since its inception has certified over 262,000 pharmacy technicians. The exam has proven to be psychometrically sound and legally defensible as an indicator that a technician possesses the basic knowledge to function as a pharmacy technician in the various work environments of the pharmacy profession. Passing the exam confers on the technician the right to use the credential CPhT (Certified Pharmacy Technician) after his or her name. This is a nationally recognized credential by members of the pharmacy profession and many state BOPs. After certification, the certificate must be renewed every 2 years. A total of 20 hours of continuing education is required, at least 1 hour of which must concern pharmacy law. The PTCB exam has recently become available in a computerized format offered at testing sites across the country during several testing windows to provide more convenient access to technicians. The PTCB has several volunteer committees that afford technicians the opportunity to become involved in this very important organization. Each year a group of volunteers are chosen to assist in writing questions for the exam. More information and an application for this important work may be found on the website.

The web address for the PTCB is http://www.ptcb.org. TIP

PTEC

The PTEC began in 1989 when a networking conference was organized for technician educators. It has since evolved into a national organization that provides information and support to pharmacy technician educators across the country. The mission of the PTEC is to assist the profession of pharmacy in preparing high-quality, well-trained personnel through education and practical training. PTEC also promotes the profession of pharmacy through professional activities and dissemination of information and knowledge to members, pharmacy organizations, and other specialists and professions. The organization has an e-group for member communications about technician issues and conducts a yearly conference for networking with other technician educators.

PTEC Pharmacy Technician Education Council.

The web address for the PTEC is http://www.rxptec.org. TIP

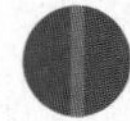

AAPT

The AAPT was the first pharmacy technician association. The association began in 1979 with a group of volunteer technicians dedicated to providing leadership and representing the interests of its members. It promotes safe, efficacious, cost-effective dispensing and use of medications, provides continuing-education programs for technicians, and promotes pharmacy technicians as an integral part of the patient-care team. The AAPT conducts an annual convention each year to provide continuing education and networking opportunities for its members.

AAPT American Association of Pharmacy Technicians.

The web address for the AAPT is http://www.pharmacytechnician.com. TIP

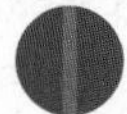

NPTA

The NPTA is the largest pharmacy technician association and is dedicated to advancing the value of pharmacy technicians and the vital roles they play in pharmaceutical care. The organization was founded in 1999 and believes that individuals should be required to complete a standardized education and training program, pass a competency exam, and register with the state BOP to practice as a pharmacy technician. The NPTA is composed of pharmacy technicians from diverse practice settings, and offers many opportunities for technicians to get involved on a volunteer basis to advance their profession. Numerous continuing-education and certification programs are offered in various locations around the country.

NPTA National Pharmacy Technician Association.

The web address of the NPTA is http://www.pharmacytechnician.org. TIP

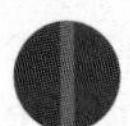

State BOPs

Each state has a state BOP—Board of Pharmacy—that is the regulating body for the pharmacy profession. The state board establishes policy, and issues or suspends licenses for pharmacists, technicians, and pharmacy practice settings in the state. BOP inspectors perform annual inspections of retail and hospital pharmacies to ensure that regulations are being followed. Technicians should know how to contact the state board to report a concern about a pharmacy issue.

TIP **To contact the state BOP in your state using the Internet, put "board of pharmacy" into the web browser followed by a semicolon and the name of the state.**

State pharmacy associations exist to provide support and continuing education to pharmacists and technicians in each state and to advance the profession of pharmacy. The state associations generally work closely with legislators to introduce bills that pertain to the practice of pharmacy. Most state associations have a pharmacy technician section organized by and for pharmacy technicians to provide networking opportunities and continuing education, and to have a voice in the legislative process. There are a number of opportunities for technicians to become involved in volunteer activities.

If the state association in your state does not have a technician section, you should establish one. To accomplish this, contact several other technicians who are interested in becoming involved in such an association. Meet to decide what role you would like to see technicians play in the state association. Learn the mission and bylaws of the state association, and develop mission and policy statements that are within the parameters of those of the state association. Request permission to be put on the agenda of a board meeting of the association and present your proposal for a technician section. Once permission has been granted, be prepared to assume a leadership role in recruiting members and organizing activities. Assuming an active role in the state pharmacy association will give technicians access to continuing-education offerings, information about new legislation that affects their profession, and a voice in the direction the profession will take in their state.

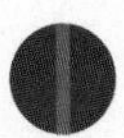

Chapter Summary

One of the marks of a professional is active membership in one or more professional organizations to remain current in professional knowledge, enhance the image of the profession, and have a voice in the future of the profession. Visit the web addresses of the organizations in this chapter and decide where your talents can best be used. Decide to be a leader in your profession. The rewards are great.

- Being vested in the pharmacy technician profession means having a basic education in the standards of practice, staying current with continuing education, and maintaining active membership in one or more professional organizations.
- The ASHP is the accrediting body for pharmacy technician education and training programs.
- The APhA is the largest and oldest professional pharmacy organization, with 66,000 pharmacist, student, and technician members. It offers continuing education, job placement assistance, and networking opportunities to members.
- The ACPE accredits pharmacy degree programs and continuing education for both pharmacists and technicians.

- The AACP is a group of pharmacy school educators who work to improve pharmacy education.
- The NABP assists state BOPs in establishing policy.
- The NACDS represents the chain pharmacies that employ thousands of pharmacy technicians. These pharmacy technicians should have a voice in the organization.
- The PTCB offers the PTCE in a computer-based format. Technicians who pass the exam may use the designation CPhT after their name.
- The PTEC is a national organization of pharmacy technician educators who are dedicated to preparing well-educated and well-trained pharmacy technicians to assist pharmacists.
- The AAPT was the first pharmacy technician organization. Its members are strictly volunteers and work to promote safe, efficacious, and cost-saving medications.
- The NPTA is the largest pharmacy technician organization. It provides a forum for technician networking, supports continuing education, and promotes mandatory standardized education for technicians.
- State BOPs are the regulating bodies for the practice of pharmacy in each state.
- State pharmacy associations provide support and continuing education for pharmacists and technicians, and work with legislators to introduce bills that are fair and effective for the practice of pharmacy.

Review Questions

Multiple Choice

Choose the correct answer to the following:

1. A mark of a professional technician is:
   a. continuing education
   b. basic education and training
   c. active membership in a professional organization
   d. all of the above

2. The oldest and largest professional pharmacy organization is the:
   a. ASHP
   b. APhA
   c. NACDS
   d. AACP

3. The organization that accredits pharmacy technician education and training programs is the:
   a. ACPE
   b. NPTA
   c. NACDS
   d. ASHP

4. The organization that is responsible for accrediting continuing-education programs for pharmacists and pharmacy technicians is the:
   a. AACP
   b. ACPE
   c. ASHP
   d. state BOP

5. Pharmacy policy in each state is regulated by the:
   a. FDA
   b. state pharmacy association
   c. state BOP
   d. NABP

Fill in the Blank

Fill in the blank with the correct word or words to complete the statement.

6. The first professional pharmacy technician association that was organized and is still run by volunteer technicians is the ______________.

7. The largest professional pharmacy technician organization is the ______________.

8. The oldest and most nationally recognized PTCE is the ______________.

9. The professional organization developed specifically for educators of pharmacy technicians is called ______________.

10. A recently developed pharmacy technician exam accepted by some state BOPs is called ______________.

True/False

Mark the following statements True or False.

11. _______ As of January 2008, continuing-education programs for pharmacists and technicians must have separate objectives.

12. _______ The questions on the PTCE exam are all written by pharmacists.

13. _______ Mandatory standardized education will enhance the professional status of pharmacy technicians.

14. _______ Technicians can renew their PTCB certification every 2 years by just paying the fee.

15. _______ State pharmacy associations often work with legislators to introduce and support laws pertaining to pharmacy.

Matching

Match the abbreviations in column A with the terms in column B.

Column A	Column B
16. ______ ASHP	A. National Pharmacy Technician Association.
17. ______ APhA	B. Pharmacy Technician Certification Board.
18. ______ NPTA	C. American Society of Health-System Pharmacists.
19. ______ AAPT	D. American Pharmacists Association.
20. ______ PTCB	E. American Association of Pharmacy Technicians.

LEARNING ACTIVITY

The Academy of Pharmacy Technicians, a section of the Indiana Pharmacists Alliance, is an active group of technicians from many different practice settings around the state. Among their many activities, they planned and implemented a project to offer a service to the community. They decided to participate in the "Vial of Life" program. This involves distributing prescription vials containing a refrigerator magnet with the Vial of Life symbol, and a Vial of Life form for patients to fill in their medical history and their current medications. The medical form is placed in the vial, the vial is placed on the top shelf in the right side of the refrigerator door, and the refrigerator magnet is placed on the front of the refrigerator to alert medical personnel who may be called to the house in an emergency that information is available. To facilitate distribution of the vials, the technicians solicited a donation of vials from a local pharmacy chain and spent a day placing the magnets and the medical forms in the vials. They set up a booth at a senior citizens fair that was being held in the city and distributed thousands of vials to grateful senior citizens.

1. Develop a service project that could be carried out by your pharmacy technician class.
2. Map out details and organize members of the class to participate in carrying it out. After the project is complete, do an evaluation and make recommendations for improvements to the process.

Chapter **25**

Expanding Horizons for Technicians

OBJECTIVES

After completing this chapter, the student will be able to:

- List specialty areas for experienced technicians.
- Explore other positions using the knowledge and skills of technicians.
- Develop a career ladder for technicians.
- Construct a professional resume including knowledge and skills.
- Search for professional opportunities.

As the pharmacy technician profession progresses, many specialty areas are beginning to evolve. Eventually these specialty areas will require extra education and training, and be validated by a specialty certification exam. There will always be a need for competent pharmacy technicians who are cross-trained in many areas and play a vital role in community and health-system pharmacies. Although this will provide a rewarding career as a pharmacy professional, some pharmacy technicians will develop special interests and seek further knowledge in a specialty area. As other healthcare professionals discover the technical skills possessed by pharmacy technicians, they will begin to seek competent technicians to perform in positions outside of the pharmacy. Begin early to construct a career ladder for your ideal position and keep an ongoing resume listing the many skills you possess to be prepared when opportunities arise.

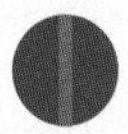

Pharmacy Technician Specialty Areas

As was mentioned earlier, nuclear pharmacy is one area where extensive education programs are offered by several universities across the country to provide a certification for pharmacy technicians. Nuclear pharmacy involves the compounding and dispensing of radioactive materials for use in nuclear medicine procedures. In November 2002, the Academy of Pharmacy Practice and Management issued guidelines for nuclear pharmacy technician training programs. In addition to all the skills required of a certified pharmacy technician, nuclear technicians must also have a working knowledge of radiopharmaceutical terms, and abbreviations and symbols used in compounding radiopharmaceuticals. They must also be capable of performing the mathematical calculations required for the dosage and solution preparation of radiopharmaceuticals, and understand the record-keeping and safety requirements for radioactive materials. There are several nuclear pharmacy technician courses available, including some offered by the nuclear medicine department of a college of pharmacy, and at least one online course that requires the student to be working in a nuclear practice setting under the guidance of a preceptor pharmacist.

TIP **The web address for the Academy of Pharmacy and Management guidelines for nuclear pharmacy technician training programs is http://www.nuclearpharmacy.uams.edu/tech.**

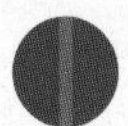

Pharmacy Technician Oncology Specialist

As more cancer-specialty hospitals and outpatient centers are being built in major cities across the nation, many pharmacists are attaining specialty certification in oncology to better serve their patients. In addition to their experience working in a pharmacy dispensing oncology medications, these pharmacists have spent a great deal of time studying the treatments, dosages, side effects, and drug interactions of oncology medications, and have passed a rigorous exam. These pharmacists are often assisted in their work by professional pharmacy technicians who have adapted to their practice setting by conscientious on-the-job training. In the future, this would be an excellent area for developing a certification training program for pharmacy technicians who would then be prepared to sit for a certification exam that would validate their knowledge in this very important specialty.

Pharmacy Technician HIV-AIDS Specialist

At one time AIDS was considered to be a terminal illness. There were few antivirals on the market and the virus quickly developed resistance to the available drugs. With so many lives at stake, drug manufacturers stepped up research efforts and the FDA even allowed a fast track for approval of AIDS drugs. HIV pharmacotherapy has become very complex and patients are living long and functional lives as a result of new drug regimens. Specialty pharmacies are being developed to meet the special needs of HIV-positive patients and those with full-blown AIDS. These patients face many challenges in their lives as they deal with the psychological, emotional, and financial issues brought on by their disease. A caring technician with special knowledge of AIDS drugs and the concerns of AIDS patients could be a valuable asset to a pharmacist dedicated to serving these patients. A certificate program to prepare technicians to work in this specialty could be a stepping-stone toward a rewarding career.

Stepping-Stones for Technicians

As the healthcare industry becomes more cognizant of the knowledge and skills possessed by a professional pharmacy technician, opportunities for advancement in other areas of healthcare will be abundant. A position as a nutrition and dietetics technician would be a natural stepping-stone for a pharmacy technician. This could involve managing the enteral formula room—ordering, preparing, and delivering enteral formulas to the patient floors. Or it could involve working in the Newborn Intensive Care Unit (NICU), using the nurse's documentation of the infant's "ins and outs" to calculate the amount of formula needed for the following day.

Traditionally, state board of pharmacy (BOP) inspectors have been retired police officers trained to enforce the law. Although such training would be important in situations involving a flagrant violation of the law that could result in an arrest, some of the finer points of pharmacy law may be overlooked. An educated, well-trained pharmacy technician professional with a strong foundation in the state pharmacy practice act would be well-equipped to perform inspections and report infractions to the board.

A pharmacy technician with knowledge and interest in inventory management can advance through the pharmacy warehouse system as a pharmacy warehouse technician supervisor. This progression could open the door to a position in a chain pharmacy warehouse, or an entire hospital system, as a buyer or manager.

A pharmacy technician with an interest in computer technology might begin by assisting with computer issues in the pharmacy. Many hospital systems will offer reimbursement for tuition, especially if the courses are job-related. With continued experience and knowledge, the technician could become the computer expert for the pharmacy system. This position could lead to a position with information services for an entire hospital system or a large retail chain.

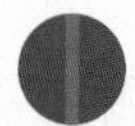

Developing a Career Ladder

These are but a few of the opportunities available for a professional pharmacy technician. It is important to be proactive in planning your career path. Becoming a certified pharmacy technician is the major first step to success. This may lead to a position that becomes a fulfilling career for many years. But if you know that you want to advance beyond an entry-level position, you should begin planning a career ladder immediately. Decide on a time frame to reach your ultimate goal. Whether it is 5 years or 10 years away, planning should begin as soon as possible. Perhaps you hope to become a pharmacist. The education and training you receive as a pharmacy technician will give you great insight into the day-to-day responsibilities of this profession. Begin planning your career ladder immediately. See Figure 25.1 below to view several of the many possible career ladders available. Begin with your present position, a student in a pharmacy technician program. Your next steps will be to complete the program, pass the national certification exam, interview for a position, and be hired for the position of your choice. Research the various pharmacy schools and visit several schools. Using your research, decide whether this is still a feasible option. Can you meet all the qualifications? Can you find financing? Can you devote 6 years to your education? If the answers to these questions are all affirmative, then it is time to apply for and take the Pharmacy College Aptitude Test (PCAT) and begin the application process for pharmacy school.

Perhaps your ultimate career goal does not require further education. Planning the steps to reach your goal is still important because it gives you the opportunity

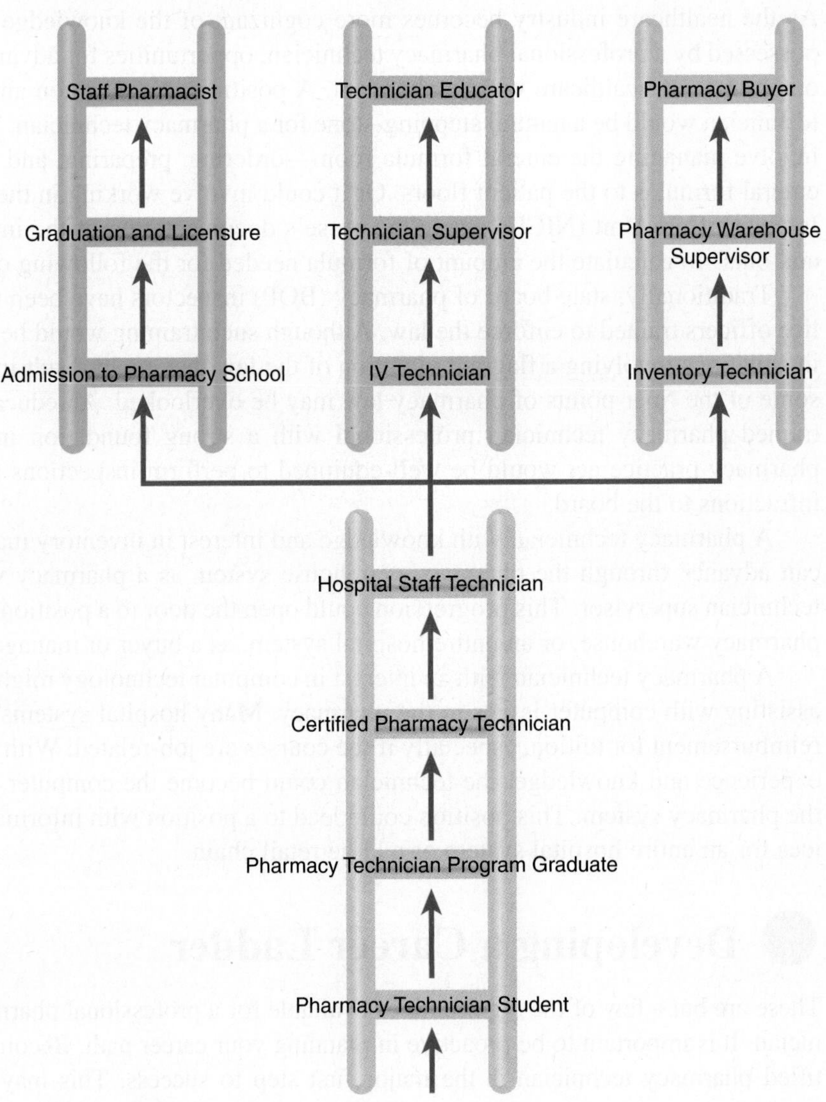

Figure 25.1 Three possible career ladders that can be followed by the pharmacy technician student.

to chart a course and check periodically to see how far you've come and how far you still have to go until you reach your ultimate goal. Don't be discouraged if your career path takes unexpected turns along the way; one of those turns may actually point you in a direction you hadn't anticipated and lead to an unexpected position that may be very exciting. The important thing is to continue to grow in knowledge and experience, and to demonstrate professionalism and dependability. Be a problem solver, avoid gossip and negativity, and search for ways to make yourself indispensable to the organization. If, after a reasonable amount of time, this hasn't resulted in any advancement in your career, it may be time to look outside the organization for other opportunities.

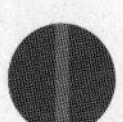

Search for Career Opportunities

Search the Internet for openings that use your skills and knowledge base. An important benefit of active membership in a professional organization is the opportunity to network with other professional technicians. Attending meetings and developing camaraderie with professional colleagues and gaining their respect for your knowledge and skills will often open the door to new opportunities. The most effective way to gain an interview for a new position in an organization is to receive a recommendation from a person who is employed by that organization and knows you well. Among the active members of a state pharmacy technician association there will be technicians from many different practice settings in the pharmacy arena. There will be discussions about new positions that will become available before the positions are posted for the general public. You may have a chance to explore the feasibility of applying for the position, and then interview and be hired before others discover the opening.

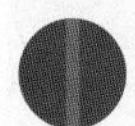

Resume Construction

As you complete your education, you should begin constructing your resume. This is an extremely important document because it must represent you well enough to make the hiring manager want to meet with you for an interview. There are a number of software programs and templates that provide guidance in formatting a professional resume. Be sure to follow one of them as you construct your document. The objective on your resume can be adapted to apply to the particular position you are seeking. Your educational listings should include any formal instruction you have completed, degrees awarded, and certificates of completion for continuing-education courses that enhance your skills. When listing your experience, detail briefly the responsibilities of each position you have held. Where applicable, use verbs such as "developed," "managed," "supervised," "directed," and "trained" to accurately describe the job skills you have demonstrated. Your resume should not be a stagnant piece of paper that is resurrected from your computer files only when you are searching for a new position. Rather, it should be a living, growing document that is updated regularly as new skills and responsibilities are mastered. This will assure that each new skill is documented and will allow you to be prepared for any unexpected opportunity that may arise. Before listing a person's name as a reference, you should contact that person to request permission to include him or her as a reference. Choose your references carefully, listing professional people who know and appreciate your work. An unfavorable reference can destroy your chance for a new position.

Once you have been hired into a position, put your heart and soul into fulfilling your responsibilities to the best of your ability. Even if it is an entry-level position and you aspire to a higher position, the best way to advance is to excel in every way to be envisioned as a professional. Some characteristics of such a professional are shown in Figure 25.2.

Pride in performing each duty with precision

Responsibility for arriving at work on time each day

Objectivity when asked to change processes and procedures

Forming excellent work habits that will continue throughout your professional career

Exceeding expectations in each task undertaken

Skills kept current through continuing education

Superseding basic requirements in performing each task

Integrity when making decisions

Opportunities for service

Neat and clean professional attire

Attitude always positive

Live by the laws and ethics of your pharmacy practice act

Figure 25.2 Characteristics of a professional.

Case Study 25.1

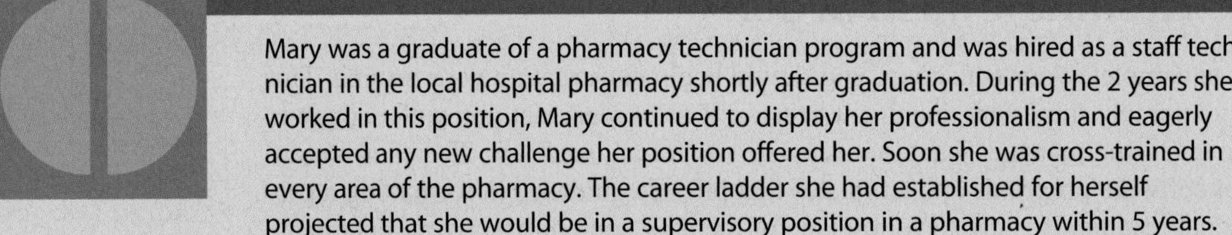

Mary was a graduate of a pharmacy technician program and was hired as a staff technician in the local hospital pharmacy shortly after graduation. During the 2 years she worked in this position, Mary continued to display her professionalism and eagerly accepted any new challenge her position offered her. Soon she was cross-trained in every area of the pharmacy. The career ladder she had established for herself projected that she would be in a supervisory position in a pharmacy within 5 years.

Although Mary was relatively content with her position, she decided to do an Internet search to see what else might be available. Mary really enjoyed IV admixture, so when she discovered a position available in a home infusion pharmacy, she decided to apply. Mary had continually updated her resume as she gained new experiences and acquired new skills, so she just needed to adapt the objective to more specifically coincide with the new position and add her current references. When an interview was scheduled, Mary dressed in her most professional attire and arrived on time. She greeted the interviewer with a friendly smile and explained her satisfaction with her current position and the desire to explore a new challenge. When Mary was offered the new position, she accepted, gave 2 weeks' notice to her current employer, and thanked each person in her practice setting for a wonderful learning experience.

Mary approached her new position with the same enthusiasm and desire to learn as before. Before long, she was performing all the duties of her new position with precision, and her pleasant personality was noticed by all. Mary was offered a position in customer service because of her ability to communicate with others and her precision in preparing orders for patients. She would now be the first person the patient would speak with when ordering IV medications and supplies. This was a great promotion and was very fulfilling for Mary because she loved to have contact with the patients and assist them with their needs. Mary so enjoyed this position that she discontinued searching for other opportunities and thought she might stay there forever.

She joined the state pharmacy technician association and began to attend meetings. With her experience and leadership abilities, she was soon elected as a board member. At one of the board meetings, a fellow board member who was a technician supervisor at a nearby hospital informed Mary that a position had opened up for another technician supervisor in the hospital system. Again, Mary had continued to update her resume, so it needed only minor adjustments. Mary donned her professional interview attire and her professional attitude, and arrived on time for the interview. Her fellow board member had already spoken with the interviewer to reference Mary's outstanding background. Mary was offered the position and realized that she had attained her 5-year career goal by accepting a supervisory position in a large hospital system.

1. Using the above information, diagram a career ladder for Mary.
2. What important professional attributes did she use to reach her goal?

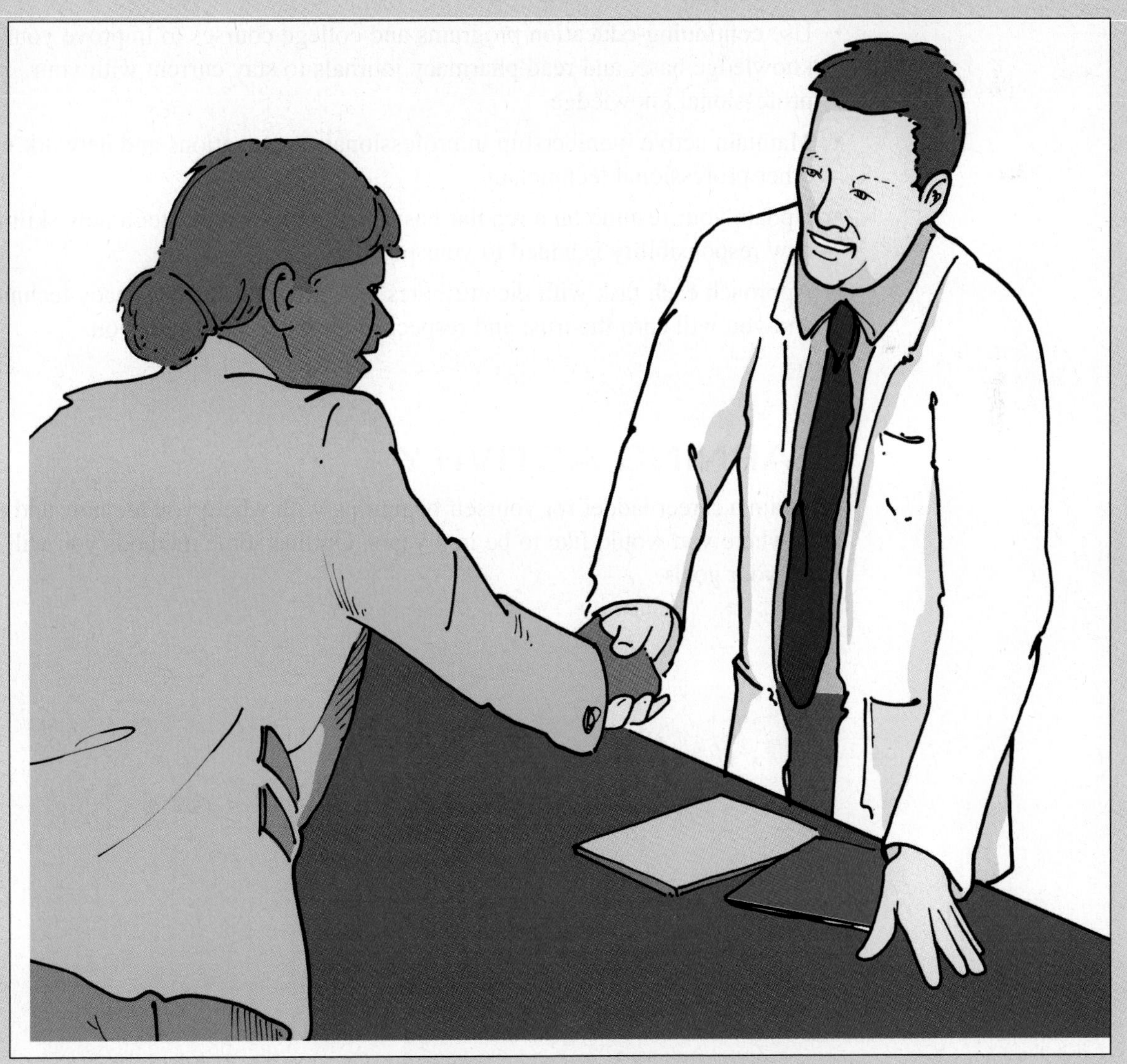

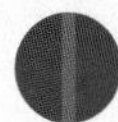

Chapter Summary

- The future of the pharmacy technician profession will involve certification programs for various specialty areas.
- Nuclear pharmacy technician is a specialty certification program already in existence.
- Pharmacy technician oncology specialist and pharmacy technician HIV-AIDS specialist are two specialty areas that could evolve into certification programs.
- There are a number of allied-health areas that could use the knowledge and skills possessed by a pharmacy technician.
- Develop a career ladder, with the first step indicating your present position and the last step indicating your ultimate goal. Then plot the steps that will be needed to reach that goal.
- Steps and goals on the career ladder will change from time to time as a result of life experiences.
- Unless you have found Utopia, the search for new opportunities should be ongoing.
- Use continuing-education programs and college courses to improve your knowledge base, and read pharmacy journals to stay current with your professional knowledge.
- Maintain active membership in professional organizations and network with other professional technicians.
- Update your resume on a regular basis whenever you master a new skill or a new responsibility is added to your position.
- Approach each task with the attributes of a professional pharmacy technician and you will earn the trust and respect of all those who meet you.

LEARNING ACTIVITY

Diagram a career ladder for yourself beginning with where you are now and ending with where you would like to be in 5 years. Outline some methods you will use to reach your goals.

Appendix A • Calculation Formulas and Tables

Percent Weight in Volume

The percent weight in volume of a solute in a liquid is the number of grams of the solute in 100 mL of solution. A 5% solution would have 5 g of solute in 100 mL of solution. To determine how many grams of solute would be needed for 50 mL of a 5% solution, set up the following proportion: 5 g/100 mL = x g/50 mL; cross multiply; 250 = 100x; x = 2.5 g of solute in 50 mL of solution.

Percent Volume in Volume

The percent volume in volume is the number of milliliters of active ingredient in 100 mL of solution. A 5% volume in volume solution would have 5 mL of active ingredient in 100 mL of solution. To determine how many milliliters of active ingredient would be needed for 50 mL of a 5% solution, set up the following proportion: 5 mL/100 mL = x mL/50 mL; cross multiply; x = 2.5 mL of active ingredient in 50 mL of a 5% solution.

Percent Weight in Weight

The percent weight in weight is the number of grams of active ingredient in 100 g of total weight of the product. A 5% weight in weight mixture would have 5 g of active ingredient in 100 g of mixture. To determine how many grams of active ingredient would be needed for 50 g of a 5% mixture, set up the following proportion: 5 g/100 g = x g/50 g; cross multiply; x = 2.5 g of active ingredient.

Solution Strength

A 1:1000 solution of an active ingredient contains 1 g of active ingredient in 1000 mL of solution.

Alligation

Note: This example is reprinted with permission from Lacher BE. Pharmaceutical Calculations for the Pharmacy Technician. Baltimore, MD: Lippincott Williams & Wilkins, 2008.

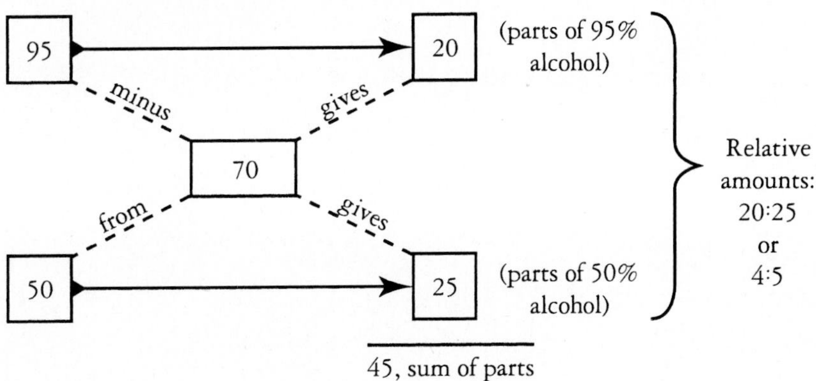

In what proportion should alcohols of 95% and 50% strengths be mixed to make 70% alcohol? The difference between the *strength of the stronger component* (95%) and the *desired strength* (70%) indicates the *number of parts of the weaker* to be used (25 parts), and the difference between the *desired strength* (70%) and the *strength of the weaker component* (50%) indicates the *number of parts of the stronger* to be used (20 parts).

Pediatric Formulas

Young's Rule

Age/Age + 12 × adult dose = pediatric dose

Fried's Rule

Age (in months) × adult dose/150 = infant dose

Clark's Rule

Weight (pounds) × adult dose/150 = pediatric dose

Cowling's Rule

Age at next birthday (in years) × adult dose/24 = pediatric dose

Dose calculation based on weight

mg/kg/day

1 kg = 2.2 lb

IV flow rates

Drop factor = number of drops the IV set will deliver per milliliter

Volume per milliliter × drop factor/time in minutes = flow rate in drops per minute

Body Surface Area

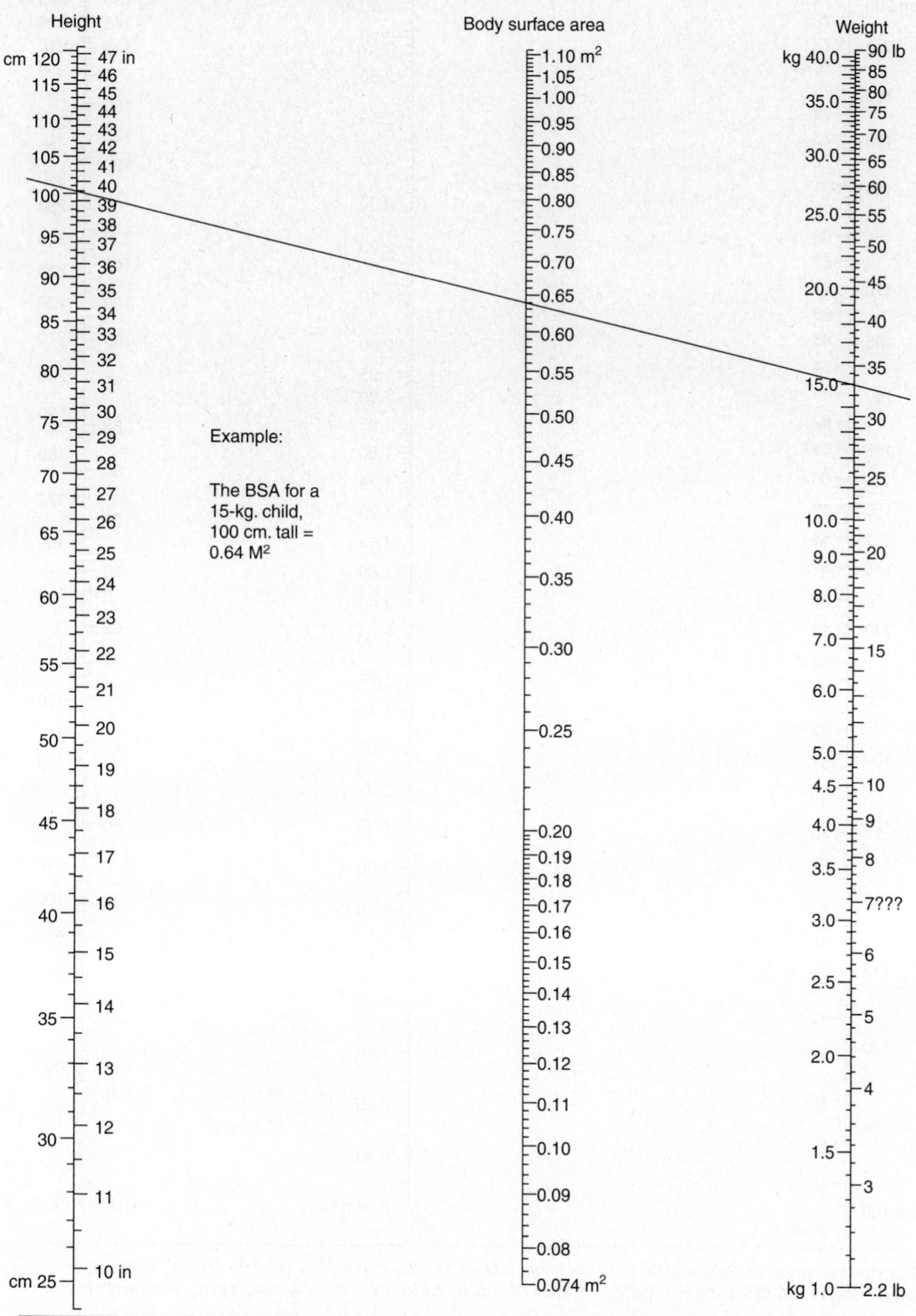

From the formula of Du Bots and Du Bots, *Arch Intern Med.*, 17, 863 (1916): $S = W^{0.425} \times H^{0.725} \times \cdot 71.84$, or $\log S = \log W \times 0.425 + \log H \times 0.725 + 1.8564$ (S = body surface in cm², W = weight in kg, H = height in cm).

Figure A.1 Body surface area of children. From Diem K, Lentner C, Geigy JR. Scientific Tables. 7th ed. Basel, Switzerland: JR Geigy, 1970:538.

Nomogram for Determination of Body Surface Area From Height and Weight

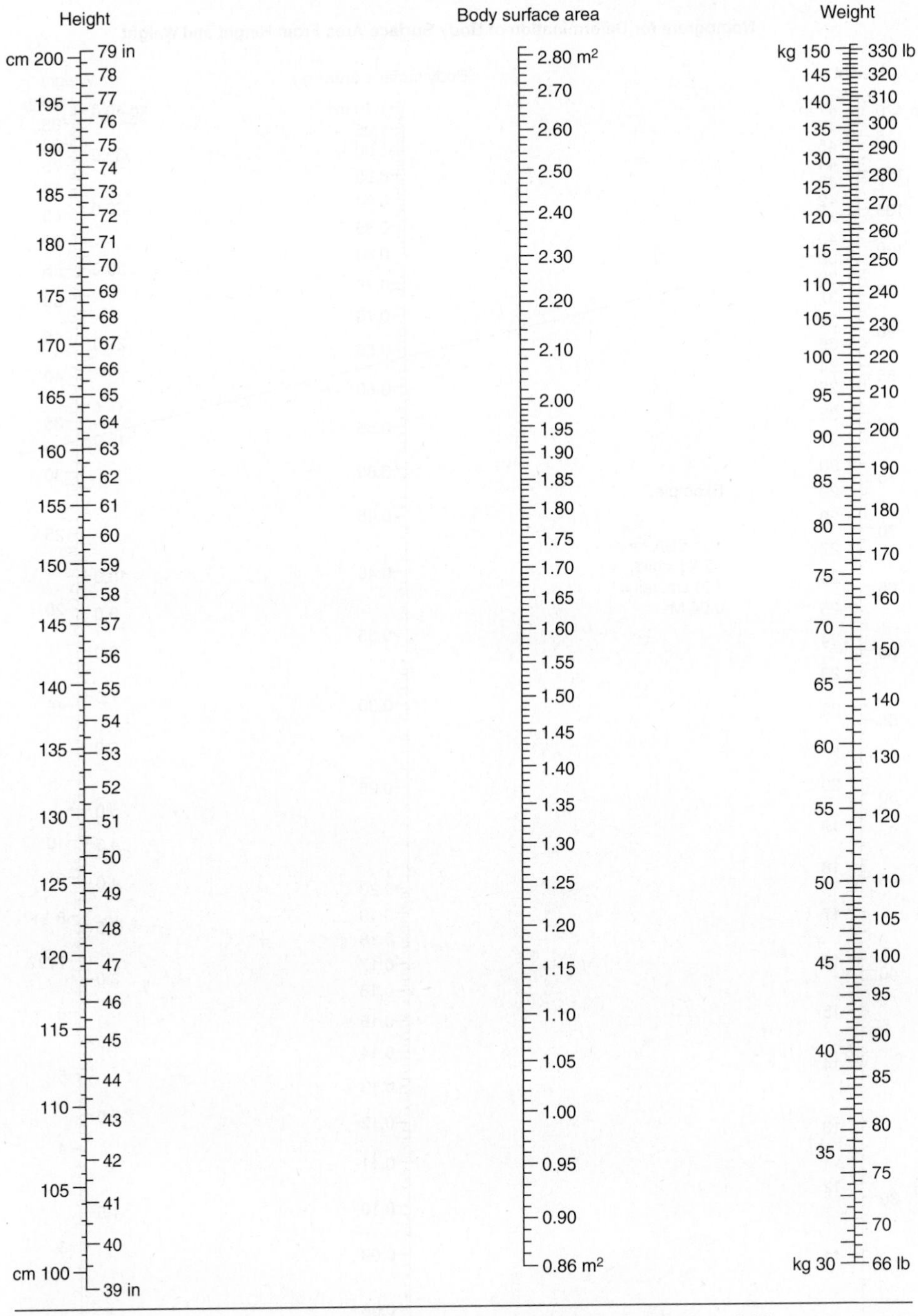

From the formula of Du Bots and Du Bots, *Arch Intern Med.*, 17, 863 (1916): $S = W^{0.425} \times H^{0.725} \times \cdot 71.84$, or $\log S = \log W \times 0.425 + \log H \times 0.725 + 1.8564$ (S = body surface in cm², W = weight in kg, H = height in cm).

Figure A.2 Body surface area of adults. From Diem K, Lentner C, Geigy JR. Scientific Tables. 7th ed. Basel, Switzerland: JR Geigy, 1970:538.

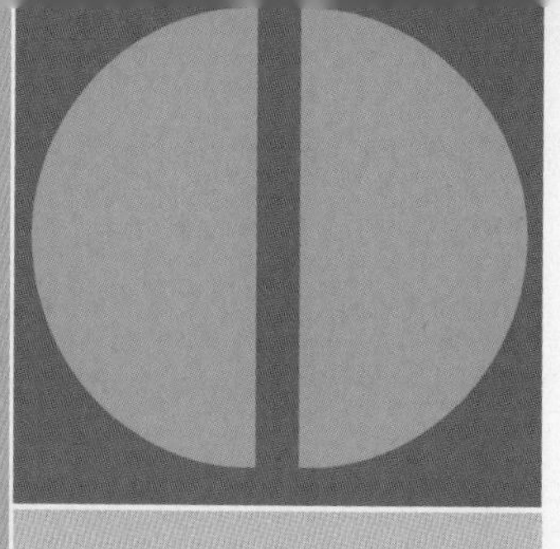

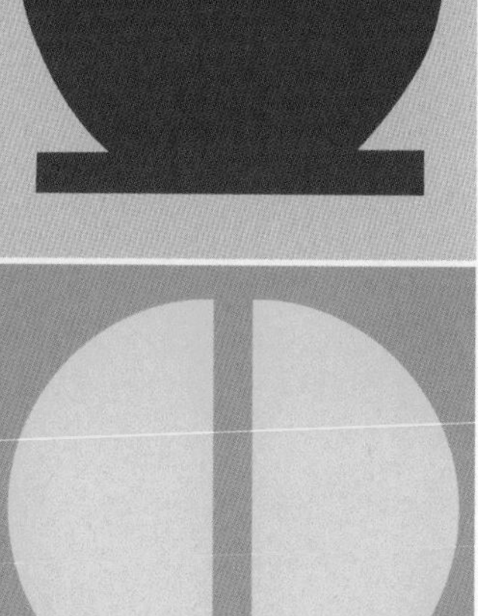

Appendix B • Abbreviation Watch List

Abbreviation	Correction
AD, AS, AU	write out "right ear," "left ear," or "each ear"
OD, OS, OU	use "right eye," "left eye," or "each eye"
Cc	use "mL"
HS	use "bedtime"
QD	use "daily"
QOD	use "every other day"
QHS	use "nightly"
QOD	use "every other day"
TIW	use "three times weekly"
U or u	use "unit"

Each institution should add error-prone abbreviations to its institutional watch list.

Trailing zeros should not be placed after a decimal point for doses expressed in whole numbers.

A leading zero should always be used before a decimal point when the dose is less than a whole unit.

Do not place a period after the abbreviation mL or mg, because it may be mistaken for a 1.

Use commas for dosing units at or above 1,000, or use the words to avoid errors.

Appendix C • **High-Alert Medications**

Electrolytes

- Magnesium sulfate injection
- Potassium acetate injection
- Potassium chloride injection concentrate
- Potassium phosphate injection
- Sodium chloride (concentrations greater than 0.9%)

All hazardous drugs

All anticoagulants

- Heparin
- Enoxaparin
- Fondaparinux
- Warfarin

All insulins

Narcotics/sedatives

- Diazepam
- Fentanyl
- Hydromorphone
- Lorazepam
- Meperidine
- Midazolam
- Morphine
- Propofol

Glossary

AACP: American Association of Colleges of Pharmacy.

AAPT: American Association of Pharmacy Technicians.

Abbreviated New Drug Application (ANDA): Must be filed by a generic company before it markets its generic version of a brand-name drug to prove its bioequivalence to the brand-name drug.

absorption: The process by which a drug enters the bloodstream.

absorption bases: Bases that can absorb water.

ACE inhibitors: Class of antihypertensive drugs that may be chosen for therapeutic substitution.

ACPE: Association for the Credentialing of Pharmacy Education.

actual acquisition cost (AAC): The actual price that is paid for a drug after all discounts and shipping costs have been applied.

adsorbent: An anti-diarrheal product that promotes fluid and electrolyte absorption by the intestine to prevent dehydration and electrolyte imbalance.

adulterated drugs: Drugs that contain any unclean substance, are prepared in unsanitary conditions or containers, or differ in strength, quality, or purity from the official drug standards.

aerobe: Microorganism that requires oxygen.

affective behaviors: An important aspect of professionalism; they convey attitude, cooperation, and initiative apart from knowledge and skills.

alcoholic solution: A solution in which alcohol is used as the vehicle.

aliquot: Calculations required when the quantity of drug required for a compound is less than the minimum amount that can be weighed on a Class A prescription balance. An aliquot is produced by adding a diluent to a weighable amount of the drug and weighing the part of the mixture that contains the correct amount of the desired drug.

altruism: True concern for the well-being of the patient.

American Pharmaceutical Association (APhA): Founded in 1852 to provide for more uniform standards of education.

American Society of Health-System Pharmacists (ASHP): Founded in 1942 to establish minimum standards for pharmaceutical services in hospitals.

anaerobe: Microorganism that lives without oxygen.

analgesic: A substance that provides pain relief.

anesthetic: Chemical agent used to numb an area to pain.

angina: Chest pain caused by reduced blood flow in the coronary arteries.

anhydrous absorption bases: Ointment bases that do not contain water but can absorb significant amounts of water and moderate amounts of alcoholic solutions.

anteroom: A room adjacent to but separate from the cleanroom where hand-washing, gowning, and gloving take place, and where supplies are sanitized before being brought into the cleanroom.

antibacterial: Agent used to inhibit the growth of bacteria.

antifungal: Agent used to treat fungal infections.

anti-inflammatory: A substance that reduces inflammation caused by an allergic reaction, irritation, or disorder (such as arthritis).

antineoplastic drugs: Chemotherapeutic agents that help control or cure cancer.

antipruritic: A drug or chemical that reduces itching.

antipyretic: A substance that lowers fever.

antiseptic: Agent used to inhibit the growth of microbes on living tissue.

antitussive: A substance that inhibits or reduces the cough reflex.

APhA: American Pharmaceutical Association.

apothecaries: Name given to early dispensers of medicines and their shops in Great Britain.

Apothecaries Act of 1815: Separated the apothecaries from the grocers and established the apothecaries as professionals who were required to be licensed.

approved abbreviations and symbols: Each institution should develop a list of abbreviations and symbols that are standardized as acceptable for use and a list of unacceptable abbreviations.

asepsis: The complete absence of microbes.

aseptic conditions: Conditions in which there is a complete absence of living pathogenic organisms.

aseptic technique: Procedure for mixing sterile compounded products with a complete absence of viable microorganisms.

ASHP: American Society of Health-System Pharmacists.

average inventory: A figure calculated by adding a beginning inventory and an ending inventory for the desired period of time and dividing that sum by two.

average wholesale price (AWP): The calculated national average price that a retail pharmacy might pay for a given package size of a drug.

bactericidal: Agent that kills bacteria.

bacteriostatic: Agent that inhibits the growth or development of bacteria.

barrier isolator: A sealed laminar flow hood that is supplied with air through a HEPA filter, maintaining a ISO Class 5 environment. It allows the compounder to access the work area through glove openings and maintain sterility without the need for a cleanroom or gowning.

batch preparation: A large number of sterile products prepared by a single compounder at the same time.

beakers: Glass receptacles that are suitable for mixing liquid preparations but not for accurately measuring volume.

binary fission: Manner of cell division of prokaryotes.

binders: Materials added to a tablet formulation to hold the powders together.

bingo card: A heat-sealed card with rows of blister packs designed to hold a 30-day supply of medication.

bioavailability: The ability of a drug to exert its therapeutic effect on the body.

biohazard: A hazardous biological agent, such as contaminated tissue, blood or body fluids, needles, and syringes, that presents a risk to the health of humans exposed to it.

biohazard spill: The spill of a chemotherapeutic drug that is capable of causing damage to living cells through contact or inhalation.

biological safety cabinet (BSC): A ventilated cabinet designed to protect the worker, the product, and the environment with a downward HEPA-filtered airflow and a HEPA-filtered exhaust; a vertical flow laminar flow hood used to compound chemotherapeutic agents.

black box warning: Warning included by the manufacturer at the beginning of the package insert concerning a serious adverse effect.

bolus dose: A large initial dose given to quickly bring the blood level of a drug up to a therapeutic level.

bowl of Hygeia: Bowl with a snake coiled around it, often depicted as a symbol of pharmacy. Hygeia was the Greek goddess of health.

brand name: The trade name given to a drug by the manufacturer for marketing purposes.

breach of duty: Not providing a reasonable amount of care in performing a duty that is expected of a technician.

broth test: Another name for a media fill procedure used to assess the aseptic technique of a technician performing IV admixture. Fluid is withdrawn from one container and injected into another, then incubated for a period of time and checked for microbial growth.

buccal tablets: Tablets designed to be placed in the cheek so that the drug can be absorbed through the oral mucosa.

burden of proof: The person filing the complaint must prove that the defendant committed a violation.

calibrate: To test the accuracy of a balance by comparing it with known weights.

capsule body: The bottom part of the capsule shell that contains the solid ingredients.

capsule filling machine: A device that holds the capsule body while it is being filled with powdered ingredients before it is capped.

capsule lid: The top part of a two-piece gelatin capsule that fits over the capsule body.

chain pharmacy: A group of pharmacies, usually owned by a corporation, that have the same name and policies.

chemical name: Official name of a drug that describes the exact chemical formula of the drug.

chemo spill kit: A kit that contains PPE and equipment for cleaning up a hazardous spill; it can be either purchased commercially or assembled by the pharmacy.

chemotherapeutic agent: A drug used to treat diseases such as cancer.

chemotherapeutic drugs: Drugs used in the treatment of cancer that can destroy normal living cells. Extra precautions are needed to ensure the safety of the compounder.

child-resistant cap: Special safety caps required on prescription vials by the Poison Prevention Packaging Act to reduce poisoning in children.

cleanroom: An enclosed room with smooth walls, floors, and ceilings that are resistant to damage from sanitizing agents; the air quality meets ISO Class 8 standards.

clinic pharmacy: A pharmacy in an outpatient clinic building to serve the patients of physicians located in the clinic.

clinical coordinator: The faculty member who manages the laboratory skills and on-site experience of students in a pharmacy technician education and training program.

code of ethics: A list of principles formulated to guide members of a profession in making decisions about matters that are not firmly established by laws.

commensalism: The relationship that exists when two organisms invade a host and one benefits from the relationship but the other is not affected either way.

comminution: The process of reducing particle size.

competence: Possessing the education and skills to perform the tasks of the profession.

compliance: Medication compliance requires that the patient take their medication exactly as directed.

compressed tablets: Tablets that are produced by a tablet press exerting great pressure on powders and shaped by punches and dies of various sizes.

computerized inventory management: A system that records all purchases and dispensing of items and produces a purchase order when items reach a certain minimum level.

computerized physician order entry (CPOE): A plan to use technology to eliminate handwriting errors by having physicians enter orders directly into the computer.

confidentiality: Accessing only the patient information that is required for the specific task being performed and extending the information only to those who have a genuine need to know.

conical graduates: Graduates with volumetric markings for measuring liquids. The sides of the graduate flare out from the bottom to the top.

consent: Final step in the process of informed consent, in which the patient makes a final decision to participate in a trial.

consequential ethics: Emphasizes the end result. (Does the end result justify the means?)

continuous infusion: Administering a drug by placing it in solution in an IV bag and allowing the solution to slowly enter a vein over a prescribed period of time.

controlled-release tablets: Tablets that have been formulated to release a drug slowly over a predetermined period of time.

contributory negligence: An action or inaction on the part of the patient or a family member that caused or increased the risk of harm.

Controlled Substances Act: Legislation by Congress to regulate the sale of habit-forming and addictive drugs.

convalescent supplies: Medical needs such as catheters, braces, band-aids, slings, etc.

co-pay: The amount of money that patients are required to pay at the pharmacy, which is determined by their insurance plan.

counter-prescribing: Common practice in which patients describe their symptoms and the pharmacist prescribes an over-the-counter drug without consulting a physician.

cream: Semisolid dosage forms containing one or more drug substances dissolved or dispersed in a water-removable base.

cross-sensitivity: Some medications have similar structures to another medication and may cause an allergic reaction in a patient who is allergic to either medication.

cylindrical graduates: Graduates that have volumetric markings and parallel sides from top to bottom.

cytotoxic: A compound that is destructive to cells within the body.

damages: Harm (physical or emotional) caused to the patient by the technician's failure to perform a duty.

DEA form 222: The form required to order Schedule II drugs from a wholesaler.

DEA number: Number issued by the Drug Enforcement Administration to authorize the prescribing and dispensing of controlled drugs.

decongestant: A drug that reduces swelling in the nasal passages and sinus cavity.

deductible: The amount that patients are required to pay before their insurance begins to cover medical expenses.

defendant: The person against whom a legal complaint has been brought.

demulcent: Agent used topically to soothe irritated tissue in the mouth or throat.

density factor: The weight of a substance that will displace a given amount of the base.

dereliction of duty: Failure to perform an expected duty.

diluents: Usually inert powders added to a drug to increase the volume.

direct cause: A determination of whether the action or inaction of the technician was the reason for the harm.

disclosure: Providing the patient with all of the pertinent information needed to make a decision.

disinfectant: Agent used to kill bacteria on inanimate objects.

disintegrates: Compounds added to a tablet formulation to ensure that the tablet will break apart and be available for absorption into the system.

dispersion: Uniform distribution of each ingredient in a powder mixture; a way of defining how the active ingredient is mixed throughout the base.

displacement: Uses the density factor to determine the amount of base that will be needed to compound a given quantity of product when the density factor is more or less than one.

double-blind study: An investigational drug study in which neither the patient nor the physician knows whether the patient is receiving the study drug or a placebo. Only the pharmacy knows.

duplicate therapy interaction: An interaction alert indicating two drugs with the same indication for the same patient.

Drug Abuse Control Amendments: Amendments enacted in 1965 to deal with abuse of stimulants, depressants, and hallucinogens.

drug–disease interaction: Interaction created by the addition of a drug that will cause a problem with a disease or condition of the patient.

drug–drug interaction: An adverse event that may occur as the result of two incompatible drugs being used together.

drug duplication: Computer alert to signal the data entry of a drug that is already in the patient's profile.

drug recalls: Official notices (warnings) issued by the manufacturer or the FDA that a drug must be removed from the shelf and returned to the manufacturer. They are classified according to the seriousness of the problem.

duplicate therapy interaction: Two drugs used for the same indication prescribed simultaneously.

durable medical equipment (DME): Reusable medical equipment, such as crutches or wheelchairs.

Durham-Humphrey Amendment: Law mandating that certain drugs require a prescription written by a licensed practitioner.

duty: A responsibility that is expected of a technician.

Ebers papyrus: Document discovered in ancient Egypt that contained a list of herbs and drugs used to improve health. It is considered the precursor to the pharmacopeia of today.

effervescent tablets: Tablets that are compounded with an effervescent salt that releases a gas when placed in water, causing the medication to dissolve rapidly.

electrolytes: Salts of sodium, potassium, chloride, acetate, phosphate, magnesium, and calcium added to a TPN to correct any deficiencies and help meet daily metabolic needs.

electrolyte imbalance: A debilitating condition that occurs due to a loss of electrolytes resulting from diarrhea or poor nutrition.

electronic balance: A single pan balance with internal weights and a digital readout display.

elixir: A hydroalcoholic solution that contains one or more dissolved drugs and is sweetened and flavored for oral use.

emergency drug kits (EDKs): Kits that are kept stocked with drugs that may be needed in an emergency situation. They are kept readily available in strategic locations.

emollient: A chemical used to soften and lubricate the skin.

endotoxins: Toxic substances released when a bacterial cell dies and the cell wall is lysed.

enteral feedings: Measured liquid nutritional supplements that can be inserted into a stomach tube or consumed orally by patients who need additional nourishment because they are unable or unwilling to consume adequate amounts of food.

enteric-coated tablets: Tablets formulated to pass through the stomach unchanged and dissolve in the intestine.

E-prescribing: Using an electronic health record system that checks formulary compliance of the patient's health plan and performs a drug utilization review (DUR) at the point of prescribing, with computer messages that allow the physician to correct issues before the prescription is transmitted to the pharmacy.

errors of commission: Errors resulting from something that was done that should not have been done.

errors of omission: Errors that occur as the result of something that should have been done but was not done.

ethical: Following a set of principles or values when making moral decisions that affect the care of patients in the community where the practice exists.

eukaryotes: Complex cells, including fungi and all plant and animal cells.

eutectic mixture: Two or more chemicals that change from a solid form to a liquid when mixed together.

excipients: Ingredients added to a drug in a solid dosage form to create an acceptable tablet or capsule.

ExCPT: Exam for the Certification of Pharmacy Technicians.

exempt narcotics: Controlled drugs that can be sold in limited quantities without a prescription.

exotoxins: Enzymes secreted by bacteria that can damage the host cell.

expectorant: A substance that helps to thin mucus so it can be coughed up.

expiration date: Date established by the manufacturer of a drug after which the potency of the drug is no longer guaranteed.

expired drugs: Drugs that have passed the date printed on the bottle indicating the manufacturer's guarantee of safety and potency. They must be removed from the shelf according to the protocols of the pharmacy.

extemporaneous compound: A medication compounded in the pharmacy pursuant to a prescriber's order for a given patient.

facultative anaerobes: Organisms that can function with or without oxygen.

fast-dissolving tablets: Tablets designed to liquefy on the tongue within one minute.

fat emulsion: A lipid emulsion intended to supply extra calories and essential fatty acids.

Federal Food, Drug and Cosmetic Act: Act passed by Congress in 1938 requiring new drugs to be proven safe before marketing. It also extended controls to cosmetics and therapeutic devices.

film-coated tablets: Tablets covered with a thin layer of polymer designed to dissolve at the desired place in the gastrointestinal tract.

filter paper: Porous paper intended to be placed in a funnel to remove unwanted substances from a liquid preparation.

flagella: Hairlike appendages on bacteria that create movement.

flocculated suspending agent: A viscosity-increasing agent that forms a controlled lacework-like structure of particles that cause the suspension to settle slowly at rest but readily disperse the particles when shaken.

fluid (total fluid volume): The total amount of fluid that the patient needs to receive from the TPN to satisfy daily fluid requirements (usually about 2500–3500 mL daily for an average adult).

fomites: Living or inanimate objects containing pools of bacteria.

Food and Drug Administration (FDA): The regulating body established by Congress to enforce rules regarding the sale of food and drugs.

Food and Drugs Act: Original act passed by Congress in 1906 to prohibit misbranded and adulterated foods and drugs to be sold across state lines.

formulary system: A system in which a committee establishes a list of drugs approved for use by an institution.

four D's of negligence: Duty, dereliction of duty, damages, and direct cause.

fungicide: Agent that destroys fungus.

Galen: Early Greek physician who practiced in Rome and created a system of therapy, based on humors of the body, that influenced the practice of medicine for decades.

gels: Ointment bases that are semisolid systems of organic or inorganic particles penetrated by a liquid; also called jellies.

generic name: Specific name given to a drug by the United States Adopted Names (USAN) Council; official name of a drug listed in the USP along with the standards that must be met to make it official regardless of the manufacturer.

genotoxic agent: An agent capable of damaging DNA.

geometric dilution: The process of mixing two solid chemicals together by taking equal parts of each in small amounts, mixing them thoroughly, and continuing to add small, equal parts of each until both are thoroughly mixed.

germ theory: Major breakthrough in modern medicine originated by Pasteur after he grew anthrax bacilli in the laboratory and theorized that some diseases are caused by bacteria.

glycerite: A solution in which one of the vehicles is glycerin; such solutions are usually thick and oily in nature and sometimes used in the ear.

good manufacturing practices (GMP): Regulations that set minimum standards to be followed by the manufacturing industry for human and veterinarian drugs. Standards should also be observed for extemporaneous compounds.

Gram staining: Laboratory procedure used to identify bacteria.

granules: Powders that have been wetted and broken into coarse particles to increase stability.

Health Insurance Portability and Accountability Act (HIPAA): Federal law passed in April 2003 to set standards for the healthcare industry for sharing and transmitting health information.

Hippocrates: Ancient Greek physician considered to be the father of medicine.

Hippocratic oath: Code of ethics still recited by physicians today, attributed to the teachings of Hippocrates outlining the responsibilities of the physician to the patient.

hospital protocols: Policies established by a hospital to standardize procedures in different departments.

humoral system: A system set forth by Galen to establish a treatment plan based on the assumption that disease is caused by an imbalance of one or more of the four humors of the body (blood, black bile, yellow bile, and phlegm).

humors of the body: Blood, black bile, yellow bile, and phlegm.

hydroalcoholic solution: A solution in which both alcohol and water are used as vehicles; the ratio of alcohol to water may vary greatly.

hydrocarbon bases: Oil-based bases used to soothe and protect the skin.

hypercalcemia: A condition of excess calcium in the bloodstream, possibly from overconsumption of chewable antacid tablets containing calcium.

implant: A drug or device temporarily placed under the skin to release a medication at a controlled rate.

independent retail pharmacy: A pharmacy owned by one or more individuals who make all the management and buying decisions.

indication: Condition for which a drug has been approved by the FDA.

informed consent: Consent given by the patient after being provided with adequate information about the positive and negative effects of a medication or treatment.

inhalers: Aerosolized medications containing medications to treat asthma.

inhalation: Administration route used to deliver medications to the lungs by breathing them in through the mouth.

inpatient prescription: A medication order written by a prescriber for a patient who is in an institution; the order is intended to be dispensed by the hospital pharmacy and administered to the patient by a healthcare professional.

institutional review board: A group of professionals and a lay person who monitor protocols during a new drug investigation.

insurance formularies: Each insurance plan establishes a list of covered drugs and will not pay for any drug that is not on the list.

insurance information: A series of plan numbers, group numbers, and member ID numbers that when entered into the computer database will identify patients and their benefits.

interaction override: An interaction indicated by the pharmacy software during the prescription-filling process that requires the pharmacist's judgment to override or ignore the interaction and continue filling the prescription.

interaction severity level: *Drug Interaction Facts* categorizes interactions according to their severity level by listing the probability that the reaction will occur and the degree of harm it may cause the patient.

intra-arterial administration: An injection into an artery.

intra-articular administration: An injection into a joint.

intracardiac administration: An injection directly into the heart.

intradermal injection: An injection between the layers of the skin.

intramuscular (IM) administration: An injection into a large muscle.

intraperitoneal administration: An injection into the abdominal cavity.

intrapleural administration: An injection into the pleural sac surrounding the lungs.

intravenous administration: An injection or infusion into a vein.

intravenous medication: A medication that is prepared under aseptic conditions and formulated to be injected or infused into the veins of a patient.

inventory: All of the items a pharmacy has available for sale.

inventory budget: The total amount of money allocated for the purchase of items to be sold by the pharmacy.

inventory control: Management of the products that are bought and sold, and the resulting profit and loss.

inventory management: An organized method of controlling inventory to optimize profitability while serving the needs of patients.

investigational drug: A drug for which the manufacturer has submitted a New Drug Application to the Federal Drug Administration and received approval to begin trials in humans.

Investigational New Drug Application (INDA): Application that must be filed before a new drug is approved for human testing.

invoice: Document that accompanies each order and lists the items sent, the quantity, the cost of each item, the total invoice cost, and the terms of payment.

ISO Class 5: International Organization for Standardization Class 5 environment, in which a maximum of 100 particles 0.5 microns in size will be present for every cubic foot of air space.

ISO Class 8: International Organization of Standardization Class 8 cleanroom environment, in which a maximum of 100,000 particles 0.5 microns in size will be present for every cubic foot of air.

isotonic: A medication having an equal pressure as the area of application.

IV admixture: Process of preparing intravenous fluids using aseptic technique.

Kefauver-Harris Amendment: Amendment passed in 1962 that requires manufacturers to prove the effectiveness of products before marketing them.

laminar airflow (LAF) workbench: A workbench that meets the ISO Class 5 standard.

laminar flow hood: A workbench that provides an environment of air filtered through a high-efficiency particulate air (HEPA) filter to facilitate aseptic work conditions.

large-volume parenteral (LVP): A single-dose injection containing more than 100 mL of solution for intravenous use (i.e., bypassing the gastrointestinal tract).

laws: Regulations enacted by the federal or local government to guide the actions of people; violations are punishable by fines or prison.

lead technician: The technician assigned to establish technician schedules, track attendance, and assist with technician concerns as a liaison between the management and the technicians.

levigating agent: A substance added to slightly wet powdered ingredients.

levigate: To reduce the particle size of a chemical by triturating or spatulating it with a small amount of liquid in which it is not soluble.

levigation: The process of reducing the particle size of a chemical by triturating or spatulating it with a small amount of liquid in which it is not soluble.

license number: The identifying number from the license of the prescriber. Most insurance numbers require this number for insurance coverage.

log book: A book used to document compounding ingredients and techniques, or the repackaging of bulk products into single-dose packaging.

Louis Pasteur: French scientist who developed the germ theory to explain infectious diseases.

lozenge molds: Manufactured devices for measuring and dispensing lozenge formulations.

lubricant: Agent that softens the skin and reduces friction when a suppository is inserted.

lubricants: Topical compounds that are intended to soothe and moisturize dry irritated skin.

malpractice: A form of professional negligence, a careless mistake, breach of confidentiality, or an error in judgment.

material safety data sheets: Summaries from the manufacturer listing the properties and hazards of a drug, and ways to prevent exposure.

media fill process: Required on an annual basis for compounding personnel. A simulated product is prepared by the compounder with the use of a culture medium, such as soy broth, to perform manipulations using aseptic technique. The product is then incubated and checked after a predetermined amount of time for growth contamination.

medical ethics: A set of principles to guide the provision of healthcare by professionals.

medication administration record (MAR): Form used by the nursing staff to document the administration of medication to the patient. The forms are often prepared by a pharmacy.

medication error: Any variation from the correct patient, medication, dosage form, route of administration, or time of administration.

medication order: Any drug ordered by a qualified prescriber, but usually considered to be an inpatient order.

medication reconciliation: Process of evaluating the list of drugs a patient is taking against any admission or discharge orders to check for interactions or duplications.

Medwatch: A federal program for reporting medication errors and adverse events.

meniscus: The curved margin formed at the top of a liquid being measured in a graduate. The measurement should be taken at the bottom of the curve.

merchandise facing: The process of bringing all merchandise on a shelf to the front edge of the shelf in an orderly manner.

microaerophiles: Organisms that need only 5% oxygen to survive.

microbiology: The study of microscopic organisms.

microorganisms: Minute living bodies that are visible only with the aid of a microscope.

min/max system: An ordering system based on establishing the minimum and maximum levels for each item carried.

misbranded: Labeling error or difference between the label information and the actual product.

miscible: Liquids that can be mixed without separating into two layers.

model curriculum for pharmacy technician training: Comprehensive set of guidelines for effective pharmacy technician education in a formal program.

modem connection: Pharmacies under contract to an insurance company may establish a dial-up or wireless Internet connection through a modem to communicate via computer with an insurance provider to verify coverage of prescriptions.

moral standards: Personal beliefs based on cultural, environmental, and religious beliefs.

morphology: The size, shape, and arrangement of bacteria.

mortars: Pharmacy receptacles used for mixing, triturating, or pulverizing substances.

mucilage: A mixture used to hold powders together when compounding lozenges.

mutagenic: Causing changes in DNA that can increase mutations.

mutualism: Condition in which two organisms live together and both of them benefit from the relationship and depend on it for survival.

NABP: National Association of Boards of Pharmacy.

NACDS: National Association of Chain Drug Stores.

national provider identifier (NPI): A standard unique identifying number assigned to healthcare providers to facilitate transmission of health information in accordance with HIPAA regulations. Each pharmacy that is involved in providing Medicare and Medicaid services is required to apply for this number.

NDC number: Identifying number given to each prescription drug before it is marketed.

network pharmacies: Pharmacies that have contracted with an insurance company to accept its insurance.

New Drug Application (NDA): An application that must be filed by a company before marketing a new drug.

nonconsequential ethics: A set of principles based on the rightness or wrongness of each action performed regardless of the outcome.

noncovered drugs and devices: Any drug or device that is not listed on the formulary established by the insurance company.

normal flora: Microscopic organisms adapted to living in the body without causing disease.

nosocomial: Infection acquired in a healthcare setting.

NPTA: National Pharmacy Technician Association.

nutrient (total nutrient admixture): A three-in-one solution that includes the lipid emulsion added into the base components.

obligate aerobes: Organisms that require an atmosphere with oxygen to survive.

obligate anaerobes: Organisms that require an atmosphere with no oxygen to survive.

occlusive: Covered in a manner that does not allow penetration by air or moisture.

ointments: Semisolid formulations containing one or more active ingredients intended to be applied to skin or mucous membrane.

ointment mill: A device used to process ointments to ensure their smooth consistency.

ointment pad: A pad of papers used to spatulate ointments in lieu of a glass ointment slab.

oleaginous: A base in which the oil is the external phase; usually greasy and non-washable.

Omnibus Budget Reduction Act of 1990 (OBRA '90): Mandates that patient counseling be performed by the pharmacist for each prescription dispensed.

oncogenic: Capable of destroying cancer cells.

on-line adjudication: Process of submitting an insurance claim for a prescription through a computer modem and receiving a response indicating the amount of coverage.

oral syringe: A syringe intended to administer oral liquids; also used as a measuring device in compounding.

order verification sheet: An order container with controlled drugs will be secured and have a form requiring the signature of the pharmacist to verify that the correct drugs were delivered.

Orphan Drug Act: Federal Act to subsidize manufacturers for marketing drugs, needed for rare conditions, that would not otherwise be profitable.

outpatient prescription: A medication ordered by a prescriber on a prescription blank intended to be dispensed in a pharmacy outside the hospital, with instructions for the patient to take the doses at home.

ovals: Another name for amber prescription bottles with volumetric markings.

O/W emulsion: Emulsion in which the oil is the internal phase and the water is the external phase.

package insert: Informational sheet required to be included by the manufacturer in drug packaging intended for health professionals.

paradigm shift: A change in the format or basic design of a model. The model of a pharmacy technician is undergoing a paradigm shift from a clerk or assistant to a pharmacy professional.

parasitism: Relationship in which one organism benefits while causing harm to the host.

parenteral dose forms: Injectable doses of medications to be delivered subcutaneously, intramuscularly, or intravenously.

partial parenteral nutrition: Parenteral nutrition that is formulated to supply some of a patient's daily nutritional needs.

paste: An ointment base to which a sizeable amount of powder has been added.

patent medicines: Medicines for which a patent has been applied and received, allowing marketing to the general public and restricting duplication by another person or company.

patent protection: After receiving FDA approval for a new drug, the manufacturer is granted a patent that gives it the exclusive right to market the drug for a number of years.

pathogens: Microbes capable of causing disease.

patient authorization: Written consent to share health information, signed by the patient, if possible with specific instructions about the content of the material shared.

patient package insert (PPI): Patient information sheet that is required to be given to the patient for certain drugs before the first dose is taken.

patient profile: Computer file that lists a patient's medication history, including allergies, diagnoses, age, weight, and all medications ordered.

peak flow meters: Devices used in the management of asthma to determine a patient's optimum expiration volume and establish a danger zone to indicate when the patient needs to seek help.

percutaneous absorption: Systemic diffusion through the lining of the skin as with a transdermal patch.

peripheral parenteral nutrition: Parenteral nutrition administered through a peripheral vein, usually in the arm.

personal protective equipment (PPE): Includes gloves, gowns, goggles, respirators, and face shields.

pestles: Devices used with mortars to mix, triturate, or pulverize substances being compounded.

pharmacopeia: Term used to denote an official listing of drugs.

pharmaceutical elegance: A term used to describe a compounded formulation that is expertly made and packaged to present a pleasing appearance.

Pharmacy and Therapeutics (P&T) Committee: A group of health professionals who are chosen to research drugs and make decisions about which drugs to include in the formulary of an institution.

pharmacy benefit manager (PBM): An individual or company that has contracted with an insurance company to manage formulary guidelines for the insurance company.

Pharmacy Practice Act: Legal document passed by the legislature of each state to outline laws governing the practice of pharmacy in that state.

Pharmacy technicians: Well-trained, educated professionals who have complied with the requirements of the Pharmacy Practice Act of the state in which they practice and are qualified to assist the pharmacist in providing pharmaceutical care to patients.

pipettes: Thin hollow tubes used for volumetric measuring; they may be either single-volume or calibrated to measure more than one amount.

plaintiff: The party bringing a complaint against a defendant.

pneumatic tube system: A system of tubes connecting the units of a hospital with the pharmacy so that certain medications can be sent immediately from the pharmacy department.

Poison Prevention Packaging Act: Act that requires the use of safety closures on all prescription drugs and most over-the-counter drugs to protect children from accidental poisoning.

powder displacement: The amount of liquid that is displaced by the powder in a powder for reconstitution.

preceptor: Term given to an experienced technician who helps to supervise and mentor a student during clinical experience.

premiums: Monthly fees paid by the patient to the insurance company for coverage of medical expenses.

Prescription Drug Marketing Act: Act that prohibits re-importing drugs into this country except by the manufacturer. It also sets limits for drug samples.

prescription torsion balance: Class A or class III double pan torsion balance calibrated to specific standards acceptable for prescription compounding.

prescription quality weights: Prescription weights that have been checked for accuracy by the Department of Weights and Measures.

prescription weights: A set of finely calibrated metric and apothecary weights approved for use in prescription compounding.

prior authorization: Required by insurance companies when a physician prescribes a drug that is not included in the formulary. The physician must call the insurance company or pharmacy benefit manager to request coverage.

prioritizing phone calls: Answering the phone and transferring the call to the correct person at a time consistent with the work flow.

prioritizing prescriptions: Establishing the order of processing prescriptions based on special needs of patients.

privacy notice: Patients must receive a copy of the organization's privacy policy, and the pharmacy should make an effort to get a signed acknowledgment of the notice from the patient.

prodrugs: Drugs that need to be metabolized to the active form in the body.

professionalism: Term used to describe the conduct of a person who has the knowledge and skills of a profession and incorporates excellent affective behaviors and judgment into their daily work.

professional judgment of a technician: Requires knowledge of the scope and standards of practice for technicians, the state and federal laws governing their practice, and the job description of the practice site to facilitate a competent decision-making process.

prokaryotes: Less-complex cells, including bacteria.

protectant: An agent, such as starch or talc, that is added to ingredients that may form a eutectic mixture if triturated together (prevents two or more chemicals from reacting when mixed).

protected health information (PHI): Any health information that can be used to identify an individual.

protein (amino acids): Parenteral solution required for tissue synthesis and repair.

providers: Individuals or businesses that provide healthcare services to patients (e.g., a physician, laboratory, or pharmacy).

pseudoephedrine dispensing law: Federal law regulating the sale of products containing pseudoephedrine.

PTCB: Pharmacy Technician Certification Board.

PTCE: Pharmacy Technician Certification Exam.

PTEC: Pharmacy Technician Education Council.

purchase order: Document originated by an institution listing the items ordered.

Pure Food and Drug Act: Act passed in 1906 to regulate the quality, strength, and purity of drugs being marketed in the United States.

Pyxis: Automated dispensing machine to provide easy access to patient medications for the nursing staff.

quality assurance: A set formula to analyze and improve pharmacy procedures to provide excellent pharmaceutical care to patients.

rebound congestion: Congestion caused by use of a decongestant for more than 3 days.

recall: Notice that a product must be removed from the shelves due to various problems with the product.

receiving and verifying prescriptions: The technician must check the prescription for completeness of information, legibility, and accuracy.

reconstitution: Purified water or an appropriate liquid is added to a powder to produce a solution or suspension for oral administration.

respondeat superior: When a technician acts as an agent of the pharmacist, the pharmacist is liable for his or her actions.

Reye's syndrome: A serious condition that can occur in children as a result of taking a product containing a salicylate.

rhinitis: An inflammation of the nasal passages.

robot room: A room housing a large automated dispensing system capable of dispensing medications using bar-code technology.

rotating the stock: When stocking merchandise, the newer items should be placed behind the stock already on the shelf to keep expired merchandise to a minimum.

salicylates: Aspirin-containing products or products that contain compounds from the same class as aspirin.

satellite pharmacies: Small pharmacy locations away from the central pharmacy that provide services to a specific area, such as the surgery.

saturated solution: A solution that has the maximum amount of solute that will dissolve in that amount of solvent at room temperature.

scope of practice for pharmacy technicians: List of functions that pharmacy technicians can perform as part of their duties in the pharmacy.

shipper's manifest: Document presented by the person delivering an order describing the number of boxes included in the order.

shotgun preparations: Involves using a combination of drugs in the hope that one or more of them will be effective in treating a condition of unknown cause.

small-volume parenteral (SVP): A single-dose injection containing 100 mL or less of solution for intravenous use (i.e., bypassing the gastrointestinal tract); also called a minibag or piggyback.

solubility: A figure that describes the amount of a solute that will dissolve in a given amount of solvent at a given temperature.

solute: A chemical that is to be dissolved in a liquid.

solvent: A liquid that is used to dissolve a solute.

spacers: Devices that can be attached to an oral inhaler to serve as a holding area for the medication until the patient is ready to inhale.

spatulas: Tools consisting of a wood or plastic handle and stainless steel or plastic blades of various sizes, used for several functions associated with compounding.

spatulate: The process of using a spatula to evenly mix an ointment and eliminate graininess in the final product.

spatulation: The process of mixing an ointment on an ointment slab with a spatula to ensure uniformity of particles.

spirits: Alcoholic or hydroalcoholic solutions of volatile substances, often used for flavoring.

spend-down: The amount of money that a Medicaid recipient is required to pay each month for medications before coverage begins. The figure is based on the income and family circumstances of the recipient.

stability: The amount of time a drug or compound retains its stated potency.

standard of care: The quality of care expected from a professional in the practice of his or her profession.

standards of practice: Quality-assurance guidelines that define the competence required for the performance of pharmacy technician duties.

stat orders: Medication orders written in a hospital setting that should be delivered within 15 minutes.

state boards of pharmacy (BOPs): Groups of pharmacists, usually appointed by the governor of each state, who convene on a regular basis to govern and direct the practice of pharmacy in that state.

stimulant laxative: A laxative that acts by directly stimulating the nerves in the intestine.

stirring rods: Thin glass rods of varying lengths that are used to mix liquids in a beaker to form a homogenous mixture.

stock rotation: Placing items that expire first in front of those with later expiration dates.

subcutaneous (SQ) administration: Injection under the skin.

sublingual tablets: Small, fast-dissolving tablets that are administered under the tongue and absorbed through the oral mucosa.

Supplemental New Drug Application (SNDA): Shortened application used when a manufacturer makes minor changes in an FDA-approved drug.

suppository molds: Aluminum molds of 1- or 2-mL capacity designed to shape a suppository formulation as it cools and hardens. There are also many types of disposable molds for suppositories.

suspension: A liquid in which particles are not dissolved but are dispersed when shaken.

symbiosis: Two organisms living together in a close relationship.

synergism: Relationship in which two organisms work together to produce a desired effect that cannot be produced by either organism alone.

syrup: An oral solution containing a high concentration of sugar.

systemic: A drug intended to be absorbed into the bloodstream and have an action away from the site of administration.

systems approach: Examining the processes and procedures in the pharmacy to determine the cause of medication errors rather than placing blame on an individual.

tare: The process of adding a weighing receptacle to an electronic balance to zero out the weight so that the balance will accurately weigh the chemical.

tech-check-tech: Process in which two certified technicians are allowed to check each other's work without a final check by the pharmacist.

telepharmacy: Use of audio and video links in addition to a computer system so that a pharmacist at a central location can perform the final check and patient counseling for a patient at a remote site whose medication has been prepared by a certified technician.

teratogenic: Capable of causing damage to a developing fetus or the reproductive system.

therapeutic drug class: Drugs are classified according to the use and means of action of the drug.

therapeutic dose range: The dose range in which a drug is effective but not toxic.

therapeutic substitution: Choosing one drug from a given drug class to be dispensed when any drug in that class is prescribed.

third-party billing: Billing process used when the patient's prescriptions are paid for by an insurance company.

tincture: An alcoholic solution of a drug that is much more potent than a fluid extract (do not substitute one for the other); an alcoholic or hydroalcoholic solution containing vegetable materials or chemicals made by a percolation or maceration process.

tineas: Fungal skin infections.

topical agent: An agent intended to be applied to the skin or mucous membrane.

tort: A law concerning personal injury.

total fluid volume: The amount of fluid a patient needs to receive from the TPN to satisfy daily fluid requirements (usually about 2500–3000 mL daily for an average adult).

total parenteral nutrition (TPN): Intravenous therapy designed to provide nutrition for patients who cannot or will not take in adequate nourishment by mouth.

total nutrient admixture (TNA): A three-in-one IV solution that includes a lipid emulsion added to the base components.

TPN compounder: A compounder that can be programmed to simultaneously pump the four basic ingredients of a TPN and dispense the correct amounts of additives into a TPN bag.

trace elements: Small amounts of elements, such as copper, zinc, chromium, manganese, selenium, iron, and iodine, that are commercially available in combinations for addition to TPNs.

transdermal route of administration: Uses a patch formulated to release medication at a predetermined rate to be diffused through the skin.

triage: A process in which the urgency of each situation is determined, and the most urgent problems are resolved first.

trituration: The process of reducing particle size using a mortar and pestle.

tumbling: Mixing powders by placing them in a plastic bag or large jar and rotating it until mixing is completed.

turnover rate: The number of times a given item is dispensed in a given time period.

understanding: Requires that information provided to the patient be presented in lay terms that are clear to the patient so that he or she can assess the benefits and risks.

unit dose packaging machine: A machine capable of packaging medications in individual dose containers with proper labels.

United States Pharmacopeia (USP): The official listing of drugs and the quality standards they must meet to be considered official. The USP also establishes guidelines for the proper preparation of drugs used in the pharmacy.

USP Chapter 797: Guidelines established to provide standards for the areas, personnel, and techniques involved in IV admixture.

vehicle: A liquid (e.g., alcohol, mineral oil, or water) used to dissolve a drug for oral or topical administration.

viscosity: A term indicating the consistency of a substance.

viscous aqueous solutions: Thick solutions that use water as a vehicle and contain high amounts of sugar.

voluntariness: Patients who agree to a course of treatment or drug therapy must do so without the pressure of any coercion.

want book: A book kept in some pharmacies to jot down items that need to be ordered.

weighing boat: Small plastic receptacle used to hold a substance to be weighed.

weighing paper: Coated paper that comes in varying sizes and can be creased to form a pocket to hold the substance being weighed.

wetting agent: A small amount of liquid used to moisten a powder so it can form a smooth mixture.

William Proctor, Jr.: Considered the father of American pharmacy for his lifelong dedication to service in the profession as a retail pharmacist, professor of pharmacy, member of the USP Revision Committee, editor of the American Journal of Pharmacy, and a leader in founding the American Pharmaceutical Association.

W/O emulsion: An emulsion in which the water is the internal phase and the oil is the external phase.

workflow: An established procedure for organizing the daily work in a given practice setting.

zone of turbulence: A disturbance of the airflow pattern created behind an object placed in the laminar airflow hood.

Index

Page numbers in *italic* denote figures; those followed by *t* denote tables.